T0323208

Mental Health Medicines Management for Nurses

3rd Edition

Mental Health Medicines Management for Nurses

Stan Mutsatsa

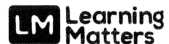

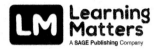

Learning Matters
A SAGE Publishing Company
1 Oliver's Yard
55 City Road
London EC1Y 1SP

SAGE Publications Inc.
2455 Teller Road
Thousand Oaks, California 91320

SAGE Publications India Pvt Ltd
B 1/I 1 Mohan Cooperative Industrial Area
Mathura Road
New Delhi 110 044

SAGE Asia-Pacific Pte Ltd
3 Church Street
#10–04 Samsung Hub
Singapore 049483

Editor: Laura Walmsley
Senior project editor: Chris Marke
Project management: River Editorial
Marketing manager: George Kimble
Cover design: Wendy Scott
Typeset by: C&M Digitals (P) Ltd, Chennai, India
Printed in the UK

Library of Congress Control Number: 2020949654

British Library Cataloguing in Publication Data

A catalogue record for this book is available from the British Library.

ISBN: 978-1-5264-7361-5
ISBN: 978-1-5264-7360-8 (pbk)

At SAGE we take sustainability seriously. Most of our products are printed in the UK using responsibly sourced papers and boards. When we print overseas we ensure sustainable papers are used as measured by the PREPS grading system. We undertake an annual audit to monitor our sustainability.

Contents

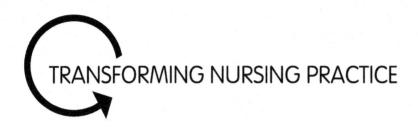

TRANSFORMING NURSING PRACTICE

Transforming Nursing Practice is a series tailor made for pre-registration student nurses. Each book in the series is:

 Affordable

 Full of active learning features

 Mapped to the NMC Standards of proficiency for registered nurses

 Focused on applying theory to practice

Each book addresses a core topic and they have been carefully developed to be simple to use, quick to read and written in clear language.

An invaluable series of books that explicitly relates to the NMC standards. Each book covers a different topic that students need to explore in order to develop into a qualified nurse... I would recommend this series to all Pre-Registered nursing students whatever their field or year of study.

LINDA ROBSON,
Senior Lecturer at Edge Hill University

Many titles in the series are on our recommended reading list and for good reason - the content is up to date and easy to read. These are the books that actually get used beyond training and into your nursing career.

EMMA LYDON,
Adult Student Nursing

ABOUT THE SERIES EDITORS

DR MOOI STANDING is an Independent Nursing Consultant (UK and International) and is responsible for the core knowledge, adult nursing and personal and professional learning skills titles. She is an experienced NMC Quality Assurance Reviewer of educational programmes and Professional Regulator Panellist on the NMC Practice Committee. Mooi is also Board member of Special Olympics Malaysia, enabling people with intellectual disabilities to participate in sports and athletics nationally and internationally.

DR SANDRA WALKER is a Clinical Academic in Mental Health working between Southern Health Trust and the University of Southampton and responsible for the mental health nursing titles. She is a Qualified Mental Health Nurse with a wide range of clinical experience spanning more than 25 years.

BESTSELLING TEXTBOOKS

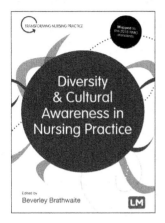

Diversity & Cultural Awareness in Nursing Practice

Edited by Beverley Brathwaite

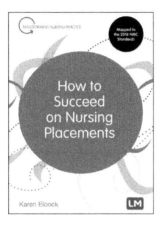

How to Succeed on Nursing Placements

Karen Elcock

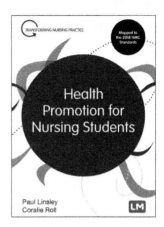

Health Promotion for Nursing Students

Paul Linsley
Coralie Roll

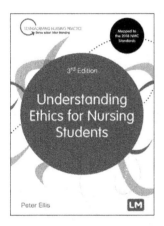

3rd Edition

Understanding Ethics for Nursing Students

Peter Ellis

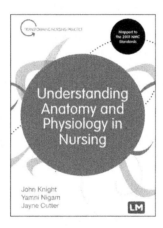

Understanding Anatomy and Physiology in Nursing

John Knight
Yamni Nigam
Jayne Cutter

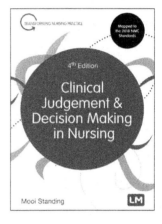

4th Edition

Clinical Judgement & Decision Making in Nursing

Mooi Standing

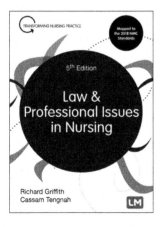

5th Edition

Law & Professional Issues in Nursing

Richard Griffith
Cassam Tengnah

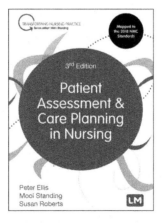

3rd Edition

Patient Assessment & Care Planning in Nursing

Peter Ellis
Mooi Standing
Susan Roberts

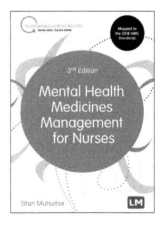

3rd Edition

Mental Health Medicines Management for Nurses

Stan Mutsatsa

You can find a full list of textbooks in the *Transforming Nursing Practice* series at

https://uk.sagepub.com

About the author

Stan Mutsatsa, PhD, RMN, has extensive experience of working in both the clinical and academic settings of mental health. Additionally, he has researched and written extensively on the subject of medicines management. Currently, he is a senior lecturer in mental health nursing at City, University of London.

Acknowledgements

To Simon Thistle for providing artwork under a busy personal schedule.

Lastly, to Joanna, James, Rebecca and Tamira for generally 'putting up with a lot' during the updating of the manuscript.

Introduction

About this book

This book is aimed at supporting pre-registration mental health nursing students to meet the NMC competencies for medicines management. It is structured around the standards of proficiency for registered nurses (NMC, 2018a) to prepare students for a formative and summative assessment for entry into the nursing register. Although the book is primarily aimed at mental health nursing students at the pre-registration level of training, it is important for student nurses of all fields to have an understanding of mental health, and so the book will also serve as a useful reference guide for nursing students of other fields and post-registration nurses, as well as serving as a useful reference for registered nurses throughout their careers. A link between theory and practice is made explicit, and the book is written in a style that is easy to understand, offering academic challenge without diluting academic integrity.

Why is mental health medicines management important for nurses?

Despite the demonstrable importance of psychotropic medication, existing evidence suggests that registered nurses' knowledge and skills in medicines management are deficient. Nurses feel that their practice is hampered by a lack of appropriate educational preparation. In particular, they cite poor knowledge of psychopharmacology as one of the main reasons for a lack of confidence in their role.

Medicines management is a prominent focus of the standards of proficiency for registered nurses (NMC, 2018a). It is a mandatory requirement that all student nurses demonstrate competency in medicines optimisation, administration and calculation, as well as having some knowledge of medicines prescribing prior to registration. This textbook meets the requirements for the application of specific competencies in mental health medicines management. Throughout this third edition, there is an increased emphasis on prescribing to support student nurses' readiness to progress to a prescribing qualification upon registration.

Book structure

The book has 12 chapters. Chapter 1 covers the legal and ethical aspects of medicines management in mental health. Key principles of bioethics, such as consent and autonomy, are described in detail, and legal issues, such as capacity, are also covered in detail. Chapter 2 covers issues relating to the therapeutic alliance, including the health belief model, the self-regulatory model (SRM), the problem of adherence to medication, factors that influence adherence, service barriers to adherence, decision-making capacity, and the use of concordance skills to promote medication adherence.

Chapter 3 provides the necessary baseline knowledge of anatomy and physiology of the brain, as well as forming the basis for an understanding of how psychotropic medications work. Chapter 4 builds on this by looking more closely at the principles of pharmacology and medicine interactions.

Chapter 5 covers the role of the multidisciplinary team (MDT) in medicines management, which includes prescribing, storing and dispensing medicines, as well as administration and record-keeping.

Chapters 6 to 11 cover the management and treatment of various mental health problems: depression, bipolar disorder, psychosis, dementias, anxiety states, and substance use disorders. In these chapters, I cover knowledge of the main clinical features and differential diagnoses of each condition before discussing specific treatment and management options. Each chapter outlines common errors to avoid during treatment and management, as well as summarising how to inform the patient.

Chapter 12 deals with adverse drug reactions (ADRs) and the classification and common side effects of psychotropic medicines, as well as how to manage these with the patient.

Learning features

Activities

Throughout the book, you will find activities that will help you to make sense of – and learn about – the material being presented. All of the activities require you to take a break from reading the text, think through the issues presented, and carry out some independent study, possibly using the internet. Where appropriate, there are outline answers presented at the end of each chapter, which will help you to understand more fully your own reflections and independent study. Remember that academic study will always require independent work; attending lectures will never be enough to be successful on your programme, and these activities will help to deepen your knowledge and understanding of the issues under scrutiny, as well as giving you practice at working on your own.

Case studies and scenarios

Within each chapter, there are case studies that describe real-life situations from the practice environment. The case studies have been included so that you may further understand the material being presented. You may wish to discuss and reflect on the case studies with senior students, as they may have experienced similar situations and could provide valuable insights through their experience.

Scenarios are presented to find a fictitious but realistic perspective on the information being discussed. These have been included so that you may develop the skill of thinking about issues from a number of different viewpoints. For this reason, some of the scenarios require you to put yourself in another person's shoes, considering how and why you would react to a given situation.

There are explanations in the glossary for words in **bold** in the text.

Chapter 1 Legal and ethical aspects of medicines management in mental health

Chapter aims

By the end of this chapter, you should be familiar with:

- accountability as a concept and the four different areas of accountability;
- legislation that impacts on prescribing and medicines management;
- ethical considerations in treatment.

Introduction: a little history

Before 1919, there was no register of nurses, and no national regulations or standards for nurse training. At that time, nurse training was normally for one year, and the general view was that most of what was essential could be learned in that short time; but it became clear that a longer period of training for nurses was necessary to produce a 'professional' nurse.

The Nurses Registration Act 1919 ended many years of conflict within the profession, and set standards for training, examination and registration. This introduced to nursing the concept of legal accountability, which serves to protect the public from malpractice. This chapter will outline the concept of accountability in nursing before discussing specific legislation. It will then discuss the Human Rights Act 1998, the Mental Capacity Act 2005 and the Mental Health Act 1983 before reviewing legislation that deals directly with medicines, such as the Medicines Act 1968, the Misuse of Drugs Act 1971 and the Prescription by Nurses etc. Act 1992. In addition, this chapter will discuss key ethical issues relating to medicines management and prescribing in practice.

Accountability

In common language, accountability may simply mean responsibility to someone or for some activity. In ethics and governance, the term is often used synonymously with concepts such as responsibility, answerability, blameworthiness and liability. However, Swansburg and Swansburg (2002) define accountability as:

> *The fulfilment of a formal obligation to disclose to referent others the purposes, principles, procedure, relationship, results, income, and expenditure for which one has authority.*

(p364)

The Nursing and Midwifery Council (NMC) states that you should 'be accountable for your decisions to delegate tasks and duties to other people' (NMC, 2018b). Although the word 'accountability' is often used interchangeably with 'responsibility', it is important to make a clear distinction. Responsibility means having control or authority over someone or something. You can choose to take responsibility, but you have no power to decide to whom you should be accountable.

Scenario

Tom, a registered nurse who had no prescribing powers, altered a dose on the patient's prescription chart, from 15 mg of diazepam per day to 20 mg per day, without consulting the prescriber. He administered this dose to the patient for a week before it was brought to his manager's attention. Tom defended his action by saying that he knew the patient well and that he was always on a maintenance dose of 20 mg of diazepam. He was adamant that he acted the right way to 'correct' the dose. He was disciplined by his employer and dismissed from his post.

In the above scenario, Tom was responsible for adjusting the patient's dose, and it was his choice to do so. However, he was accountable to his employers for his action, and it was his employers – not him – who decided to terminate his employment.

The purpose of accountability

The nursing profession requires nurses to be accountable for what you do, as it is nurses' obligation to give explanations for their actions and omissions. This is to ensure that the public and patients are not harmed by a nurse's actions and omissions, as well as providing redress to those who have been harmed. Healthcare workers, including nurses, have a moral, professional, ethical and legal obligation to provide care to the highest standard, because patients are entitled to this, irrespective of who is delivering that care. For these reasons, even student nurses are accountable for their actions and omissions.

To achieve this, accountability has the following aims:

- The public must be protected from a nurse's actions and omissions that might cause harm. The nurse can be called to account for their conduct and competence if it is thought that they have fallen below the standards required of a nurse.

- The nurse must be held to account to protect the public and patients by discouraging acts that the professional body (the NMC) considers as misconduct or unlawful. Registered nurses must always act in a manner worthy of a nurse at work, both in public and in private.
- To make the nurse accountable to a range of higher authorities, the law regulates the nurse's behaviour. The regulatory framework makes it clear what standards of conduct and competence a registered nurse should comply with.
- To be accountable, the nurse must: (1) be able to perform the task; (2) accept the responsibility for doing the task; and (3) have the authority to perform the task within the job description, as well as within the policies and protocols of the organisation.

The registered nurse can be called to account and be asked to justify their actions. The public can hear the case, with a view to reassuring patients that the professional body only tolerates the highest standards of nursing. Public scrutiny of a nurse's conduct allows other members of the profession to learn from the mistakes and misconduct of others (Griffith and Tengnah, 2017).

Scenario

A registered nurse was struck off the professional register in 2010 after he was found sleeping on duty and had failed to administer medication to patients in a nursing home. He initially denied the charges, but later admitted to the offence after other employees had testified that he had been caught sleeping on three separate occasions within two months. The committee found him unworthy of being a registered nurse.

Because the registered nurse has a formal obligation to answer for their actions to several higher authorities, they must justify their actions to these authorities, and if they fail to do so sanctions can be applied against them. For example, during training, a university or an NHS trust can take disciplinary action against a nurse or student nurse, which in extreme cases can result in dismissal for the individual. In this regard, the nurse is accountable to:

- the patient;
- the professional body;
- society;
- the employer.

Accountability to the patient

Registered nurses are accountable to the patient who is under their care, and for this reason civil law allows the patient to seek redress if they believe they have suffered harm due to the nurse's actions. Over the years, the NHS has been paying out increasingly large sums of money – over £0.5 billion per year – because of the clinical negligence of staff. A fundamental ethic of healthcare is that you should do your patients no harm. Where harm occurs because of a nurse's negligence, patients can seek compensation from the nurse and the nurse's employer through the courts. The nurse–patient relationship gives rise to a duty of care.

Quite often nurses have argued that they are accountable to themselves for their practice. Although it is accepted that a nurse who harms a patient through their acts will feel remorse, if the definition of accountability is considered, we see that nurses cannot impose sanctions on themselves.

Accountability to the professional body

Registered nurses are accountable to their professional body in accordance with the Nurses, Midwives and Health Visitors Act 1997. This legislation's aim is to protect the public by establishing standards for education, training and conduct. The basis of the NMC's role is to place those who intend to practise on a nursing register. A detailed description of the role of the NMC is beyond the scope of this book, so you are advised to consult a more appropriate textbook in this regard or visit the NMC's website (**www.nmc.org.uk**).

Accountability to society

Registered nurses are subject to the laws of the country they work in, like everyone else. If a nurse is accused of committing a crime at work or outside of work, the country in which they reside may call them to account under its laws. This can have a bearing on the nurse's ability to practise, as the following scenario demonstrates.

Scenario

Bridget was a registered nurse working in a prison, but she was later arrested and convicted of supplying class A drugs to a prison inmate. She was sentenced to three years in prison and was subsequently removed from the professional register.

Accountability to the employer

A registered nurse is accountable to their employing organisation through the terms and conditions of their employment contract. An employer is vicariously liable for the actions of its employees. For example, if a nurse commits a civil wrong, the employer is responsible for the nurse's action. The following scenario gives an example of what this means in practice.

> ## Scenario
>
> Hamid is a patient on phenobarbitone who was found unconscious after a nurse, Shelley, gave him three times the prescribed dose. Hamid had to be admitted to a hospital intensive care ward and fully recovered four days later. The mistake occurred because Shelley did not follow the correct procedures for the administration of medicines. Although Hamid survived, his family persuaded him to take legal action through the courts, and he won a substantial settlement from the hospital. In turn, Shelley was disciplined and was sent for retraining in medicines management.

In the scenario above, we see that Hamid came to some harm because of Shelley's carelessness. However, it was the hospital, not the nurse, that was sued and paid compensation to the patient. The hospital is vicariously liable. 'Vicarious liability' is a legal term that holds one person liable for the actions of another when engaging in some form of joint or collective venture. Both the hospital and the nurse are engaged in a collective venture, but the hospital has vicarious liability. As the number of nurses who prescribe increases, the concept of accountability assumes greater importance, as we will discuss later.

Human Rights Act 1998

Rights can be defined as claims or entitlements that deserve respect. After the Second World War, nations around the world were determined to take steps to guarantee the protection of human rights in national and international law. The first concrete manifestation of this was the American Declaration of the Rights and Duties of Man in 1948. This was followed by the Universal Declaration of Human Rights drawn up by the UN in the same year. These documents concentrate on protecting civil and political rights, such as freedom of expression, freedom of religion and freedom of association.

In the UK, human rights are enshrined in the Human Rights Act 1998, which has its basis in the European Convention on Human Rights (ECHR). All public authorities have a legal duty to act compatibly with the ECHR (and hence the Human Rights Act 1998). The NHS is a public authority and therefore must adhere to the Human Rights Act 1998. Domestic courts are obliged to interpret all laws consistently with the Act. In mental health, courts and mental health tribunals have an obligation to interpret the Mental Health Act 1983 (amended 2007) consistently with the Human Rights Act 1998. The Human Rights Act 1998 thus has the effect of bringing human rights to the centre of both the legal and health systems. The ECHR is divided into 'Articles', which set out the rights that are protected by the Convention. For medicines management and prescribing in mental health, only Articles 2, 3 and 8 are relevant, so it is these that we will discuss next.

Article 2

This Article states:

1. *Everyone's right to life shall be protected by law. No one shall be deprived of his life intentionally save in the execution of a sentence of a court following his conviction of a crime for which this penalty is provided by law.*

2. *Deprivation of life shall not be regarded as inflicted in contravention of this article when it results from the use of force which is no more than absolutely necessary:*

   (a) *in defence of any person from unlawful violence;*

   (b) *to effect a lawful arrest or to prevent the escape of a person lawfully detained;*

   (c) *in action lawfully taken for the purpose of quelling a riot or insurrection.*

The Article imposes on the state the obligation to protect the lives of its citizens, and this responsibility extends to the healthcare system. Before you go any further, complete Activity 1.1.

Activity 1.1   Reflection

You are working on a ward where a patient, detained under section 3 of the Mental Health Act 1983, attacked a fellow patient, causing serious harm. The aggressor was physically restrained and placed in seclusion to allow time for him to 'cool down'. He was then given an injection of 10 mg of olanzapine and a concomitant (augmenting) dose of 2 mg of lorazepam. Two hours after the administration of the injection, the patient fell asleep (at 1900 hours). Although the hospital policy stipulates that a patient who is administered an intramuscular (IM) olanzapine injection must have their vital signs monitored regularly for the first 24 hours, this was not complied with for fear of waking the patient. There were also insufficient staff on duty to cope with any potential acts of violence during the night.

Five hours later, a member of staff found that the patient could not be roused, and immediately sent him to the local general hospital where he was taken to the intensive care unit. After a period in hospital, he fully recovered, but he sued the hospital for breaching his rights under the Human Rights Act 1998.

- Is the hospital in breach of Article 2 of the Human Rights Act 1998?

An outline answer is provided at the end of the chapter.

The most obvious example of the application of Article 2 is in cases where a member of staff deliberately kills a patient, as in the Harold Shipman cases (see the useful websites section at the end of the chapter), but Article 2 extends beyond that, as exemplified by a test case (*Stewart v United Kingdom* [1984]). Moreover, it is not necessary for the victim to die to be in breach of Article 2. It is enough to put the person at 'material risk', as the scenario above demonstrates. Clearly, it was the responsibility of the nursing staff to observe the patient's vital signs regularly after administering an IM injection of olanzapine and lorazepam, but this was not done. As such, the staff placed the patient at material risk by their act of omission, therefore breaching Article 2.

Article 2 further stipulates that where there is a threat to the life of someone in state custody (in this case, the hospital), there is an increased responsibility to provide care and protection. In the UK, this was brought about by a test case (*Osman v United Kingdom* [2000]). After the death of a family member in custody, the family sued the police for failing to protect the family member adequately even though there were clear warning signs of risk to the individual. The judge in the case commented that where the authorities know of a 'real and immediate threat' to a person's life, there is an obligation to take preventive operational measures to protect that person.

The responsibility to protect life is not an unlimited one. Specifically, there is only a breach of Article 2 where there is demonstration that the authorities knew or ought to have known that the person posed a real risk to life. Where the authorities can demonstrate that they took reasonable steps to protect the person, after being deemed to be at risk of losing life, or where there were no indications that the person was at risk of losing life, the death will not result in a breach of Article 2.

In summary, Article 2 imposes both positive and negative responsibilities. It is possible to breach the negative duty not to deprive an individual of life by using excessive or unnecessary force against the person. Another example of a breach of negative duty is when there are failures within the system that may lead to a failure to provide adequate procedures and trained or qualified staff to ensure safety. The positive duty to protect life arises wherever the authorities know or ought to know of a real and immediate risk to the life of a person or group of people. In Activity 1.1, the patient was administered IM olanzapine and should have had his vital signs monitored, but this was not done. This breached the positive duty to protect life under Article 2.

Article 3

Article 3 of the ECHR is the only absolute right, and it states: 'No one shall be subjected to torture or to inhuman or degrading treatment or punishment'. In the UK, the courts have defined degrading treatment as follows:

> *Where treatment humiliates or debases an individual, showing lack of respect for, or diminishing, his or her human dignity, or arouses feelings of fear, anguish, or inferiority capable of breaking an individual's moral and physical resistance, it may be characterised as degrading and fall within the prohibition of Article 3. The suffering that naturally flows from naturally occurring illness, physical or mental, may be covered by Article 3, where it is, or risks being, exacerbated by treatment, whether flowing from conditions of detention, expulsion, or other measures, for which the authorities can be held responsible.*

Before you go any further, complete Activity 1.2.

Activity 1.2   Reflection

Having read the definition of degrading treatment, can you list situations in mental health nursing that could be described as degrading treatment, therefore breaching Article 3 of the ECHR?

Read on for a discussion of this topic.

Although Article 3 is an absolute right that is stated in very simple terms, the problem is that its interpretation can vary. Whether an action is inhuman or degrading treatment will depend on several factors and the unique circumstances of each case. In mental health practice, Article 3 is most likely to be relevant to complaints arising from the conditions of detention, seclusion, forced medication, control and restraint.

Case study: Mr Herczegfalvy

In *Herczegfalvy v Austria* [1992], Mr Herczegfalvy was a Hungarian citizen living in Austria who had served two prison sentences in succession for assaulting his wife, public officials, and customers of his television repair business. In prison, he carried on assaulting fellow prisoners and prison staff. After an assessment, he was deemed to be suffering from a paranoid psychotic disorder, and not responsible for his actions, and was therefore sent to a psychiatric hospital.

Following an assessment in the psychiatric hospital, he was returned to prison, but he protested his detention by staging a hunger strike. He collapsed four weeks later and needed intensive medical care, so was sent to a general hospital for treatment.

On his return to the psychiatric hospital, he was still on hunger strike but was in an extremely weak state. Therefore, he was force-fed in accordance with Austrian hospital law. He refused all medical treatment and was given IM sedation against his will. At this time, he was attached to a security bed, but he managed to cut through the net and straps. He continued his hunger strike, which caused further deterioration of his physical and mental condition, and he was again transferred to a medical intensive care unit.

He was returned to the psychiatric hospital after two weeks and handcuffed, with a belt placed around his ankles because of the continued risk of aggression. Previous physical resistance to forced administrations of antipsychotics had resulted in injuries to him, including loss of teeth, broken ribs, and bruises. He remained in these restraints for 15 days but continued his hunger strike and was force-fed. Gradually, his physical and mental condition improved, and he stopped the hunger strike after a doctor explained to him how it was endangering his life.

(Continued)

(Continued)

Mr Herczegfalvy subsequently took the Austrian government to the European Court of Human Rights, alleging that violent and excessively prolonged measures were used to treat him, in violation of Article 3 of the ECHR. He also argued that these measures contributed to the worsening of his condition. The judge ruled that the established principles of medicine are admittedly decisive in such cases, but concluded, as a rule, that a measure which is a therapeutic necessity cannot be regarded as inhuman or degrading, and the court must satisfy itself that such medical necessity has been convincingly shown to exist. The court accepted that, according to psychiatric principles accepted at the time, medical necessity justified the treatment at issue, and therefore there had been no violation of Article 3.

The above case study demonstrates that the courts can interpret inhuman or degrading treatment in several ways that are dependent on the unique circumstances of each case. In many ways, the treatment of Mr Herczegfalvy could be regarded as harsh and degrading. However, the sole aim and focus were therapeutic. In other words, the aim was always to try to treat Mr Herczegfalvy in the best possible way, and there was never any intention to ill-treat him. Therefore, the judge ruled that Article 3 was not applicable in his case. This court ruling heavily influences UK and European practice in respect of detention of the mentally ill and the deprivation of liberty of a person with no capacity to make a competent decision.

In psychiatric practice, Article 3 is most likely to be relevant to complaints arising from the conditions of detention, seclusion, control and restraint, as the following case study demonstrates.

Case study: Judith McGlinchey

In *McGlinchey and Others v UK* [2003], Judith McGlinchey died in a hospital in West Yorkshire while in the care of the UK Home Office as a convicted prisoner. She had asthma and a long history of intravenous heroin addiction. Soon after arriving in prison, she developed severe opiate withdrawal symptoms with repeated vomiting, leading to dehydration and weight loss. Despite her physical state, there was a gap in monitoring over the weekend. There was a failure to take more effective steps to transfer her to hospital for specialist assessment when her condition deteriorated significantly. She died in hospital after two weeks on a life-support machine. Because of these deficiencies in Judith's treatment, Article 3 was deemed to have been breached.

In this case, it was found that the inadequacy of medical treatment in prison for Judith McGlinchey was deemed to be inhuman and degrading. The prison was found not to have provided necessary healthcare, and it was therefore in breach of Article 3. Although this happened in a penal environment, the case of Judith McGlinchey equally applies in any situation where people are detained, and this includes psychiatric hospitals.

In summary, the general principles of Article 3 are that authorities have an obligation to provide adequate and necessary medical care. However, a treatment or intervention that convincingly shows to be a therapeutic or medical necessity will usually not be regarded as inhuman or degrading, as in the case of Mr Herczegfalvy, and a delay in providing care may be in breach of Article 3, as in the case of Judith McGlinchey. Further, clinical interventions need to balance the potential effect of the intervention with the severity of the presenting clinical problem. In other words, you should respond proportionately to a clinical scenario to avoid the risk of breaching Article 3.

Article 8

This Article states:

1. *Everyone has the right to respect for his private and family life, his home and his correspondence.*
2. *There shall be no interference by a public authority with the exercise of this right except such as is in accordance with the law and is necessary in a democratic society in the interests of national security, public safety or the economic well-being of the country, for the prevention of disorder or crime, for the protection of health or morals, or for the protection of the rights and freedoms of others.*

The key area of Article 8 is to protect the individual's right to privacy and prevent a public authority from intruding unnecessarily into a person's private life. For example, it is possible to breach Article 8 in some cases where people are subjected to undue surveillance, or the interception of their telephone calls, or the publication of newspaper accounts of their private life. Article 8 also protects the right to family life, which means that decisions regarding custody or adoption must consider the right to family life of all those involved. It also protects the individual's right to physical integrity and the right to respect for their home.

Article 8 has been one of the most dynamically applied provisions of the ECHR. It has an extremely wide application (e.g. the use of medical records in court, the right to practise one's sexuality). Before you go any further, complete Activity 1.3.

Activity 1.3   Evidence-based practice and research

A patient detained under section 3 of the Mental Health Act 1983 complained to the European Court of Human Rights that his human rights under Articles 8 and 3 of the ECHR had been breached because he was made to take antipsychotic medication that had unpleasant side effects which had interfered with his private life.

- Can you explain why both Articles 8 and 3 may be relevant in this case?
- What do you think was the outcome of the case?

Outline answers are provided at the end of the chapter.

Article 8 has been used to assess such common, everyday issues as the provision of personal care by same-gender staff, assistance to move to suitably adapted accommodation, the appropriate use of bedpans, and complex end-of-life decisions. Because of the nature of Article 8, it will continue to be tested in many and varied clinical situations, as well as around research. Now we can turn our attention to the key principles of ethics.

Key ethical theories

It is possible to argue that *ethical* and *moral* considerations influence the way we live and interact with others. In turn, our thinking, attitudes, values and beliefs influence our actions. Therefore, when we care for patients, we do so not only because of our professional and legal duty, but because of our moral and ethical values and beliefs. Therefore, who we are and what values we hold influence our professional judgement and reasoning to a degree.

The NMC demands that some specific ethical principles, such as respect for autonomy, confidentiality, compassion, and individual rights and freedoms, should inform nursing practice. Other principles that inform nursing practice include respect for diversity, cultural differences and different values. In this respect, it is important for nurses to be aware of how their value system can impact on the patients they care for (Wheeler, 2013). Above all, the NMC reminds nurses that caring can at times be a very difficult task which involves making difficult decisions, and this in turn demands that nurses make a continuous assessment of their own moral and ethical standpoints. Wheeler (2013) suggests that nurses owe it to their patients to 'do the right thing', including working with them and being guided by a sound moral, ethical and professional code of conduct. In the process, they should show respect for the patient's moral values and belief system, as these help the patient to achieve their health goals. Nurses and healthcare professionals alike cannot justify placing their own autonomy and beliefs ahead of those of the patient. Moreover, if they disproportionately preoccupy themselves with their own values, this may create the potential for conflict with the patient, as well as devaluing the patient as an individual without a belief system and values of their own. In summary, ethical and moral values form the foundation of our care. The following sections cover basic ethical theories that guide and develop us as professionals.

Utilitarianism

This theory bases itself on making decisions from a 'common sense' standpoint by considering the likely outcome of an action. In utilitarianism, a morally correct decision is the one that is likely to produce a more favourable outcome for the person. In other words, it is the the one that produces the best possible outcome and the greatest pleasure to the patient. A well-known utilitarian was John Stuart Mill (1806–1873), who championed that the most important outcome when choosing between two opposing actions is to choose the one that results in people being happy. This philosophy also champions 'the greatest good for the greatest number'. Furthermore, a utilitarian considers that telling the truth to a patient would be dependent on the consequences of the truth. If the truth results in undue sadness or harm to the patient, then telling the truth cannot be the morally correct thing to do in this aspect. However, there are clearly many situations in medicines management and prescribing where this approach may conflict with established values. For example, the ethics of deontology challenges utilitarianism, and we discuss this next.

Deontology

The basis of deontology is the belief that there are basic rules which we should follow. Irrespective of the consequences, duties and responsibilities should be the overriding issue when deciding on an action. Unlike utilitarians, deontologists emphasise that it is important to tell the truth to a patient because it is the right thing to do, not because it will result in happiness. For deontologists, there are certain acts that are wrong or right in themselves. This is because of the sort of acts they are, not because of the consequences they produce. For example, a nurse can justify maintaining patient confidentiality from a deontological viewpoint. Using this example of confidentiality, a deontologically driven nurse may respect a patient's basic right to autonomy irrespective of the consequences. However, like all theories, there are certain instances where the application of deontology can be problematic in practice. For example, if a patient discloses suicidal intentions to a nurse but stresses that the nurse keeps this confidential, then the application of deontology can pose a dilemma for the nurse. It is also important to note that some aspects of deontology can be diametrically opposed to consequentialism (utilitarianism), though there is an overlap between deontology and virtue ethics.

Virtue ethics

The origins of virtue ethics lie in ancient Greek philosophy. Aristotle, Socrates and Plato advocated virtue ethics and defined those characteristics that make a person a good person. For example, the characteristics of a good nurse or a good doctor include virtues such as kindness, honesty, caring, self-discipline, compassion, courage and loyalty (Nuttall and Rutt-Howard, 2015).

These virtues allow nurses to perform with compassion and understanding in all interactions with patients. Furthermore, it can be difficult to manage medicines or prescribe safely and effectively if the nurse does not have some virtuous characteristics. However, according to some authors, virtuous characteristics solely based on religion invite debate and may need to be evaluated, considering the dynamic nature of societies. For example, some religions may be in favour of heterosexual relationships only, but current societal developments favour and respect diversity (Wheeler, 2013). In summary, the application of any form of ethical approach should consider and reflect on patients' needs more holistically, sensitively, widely and deeply.

Bioethics/principlism

Bioethics – or principlism – was advanced most by Beauchamp and Childress (2001), and this is the mainstay ethical approach in healthcare delivery. The four major parts of principlism are autonomy, beneficence, non-maleficence, and justice and veracity.

Autonomy

Autonomy refers to a person's ability to come to their own decisions without undue external influence. Respect for autonomy is one of the most fundamental moral principles that reigns supreme in healthcare ethics because it has important ramifications for a person's health and well-being (Beauchamp and Walters, 1999). In healthcare, behaviours that are contrary to a patient's right to autonomy are typically paternalistic in nature and generally unwelcome.

For this reason, every nurse must respect the patient's right to self-determination. In other words, the patient has a right to choose between agreeing to take part in or refusing treatment. However, in medicines management and prescribing, the concept of autonomy can be fraught with difficulties because each patient is unique and cultures are diverse. In addition, there is a significant group of people for whom autonomy may be absent, compromised or undeveloped.

Scenario

Mrs P attended an outpatient clinic dressed in the style of her immigrant community. She was accompanied by her husband, who greeted the doctor as they entered the consulting room, while Mrs P glanced modestly downward. Upon consultation, it was apparent that Mrs P was suffering from depression and was suicidal. She was experiencing difficulties in coping with activities of daily living (ADLs). It was evident that Mrs P needed a period of being in hospital. When this was suggested to her, her husband responded by saying that they ('we') did not want to be admitted to hospital; rather, they would prefer to get a prescription and go home. When Mrs P was asked what she herself wanted, she merely pointed in the direction of her husband.

For example, a patient may say to the nurse, 'I know you've explained the advantages and disadvantages of each medication to me, but I still can't make up my mind. Can you choose for me, since you're more knowledgeable about treatments than me?' Is the patient giving away their autonomy? Nuttall and Rutt-Howard (2015) argue that by choosing the best medicine for the patient, the nurse is not acting in a paternalistic manner. Rather, the patient is showing respect and trust for the nurse's knowledge and skill, and is willing to accept their professional judgement in deciding what is the best treatment. It is likely that the patient is aware that they control the right to decide, but they pass this responsibility to the nurse because of the respect they have for the nurse.

It is also argued that in theory, non-violation of a person's rights to autonomy is honourable, but it is often difficult to achieve in practice. Moreover, in many circumstances, healthcare professionals may be best placed to make treatment decisions (Fallowfield et al., 1994). In this context, the skills and knowledge relating to medicines management and prescribing could be the rationale underpinning this school of thought. However, an opposing view is that although the knowledge and skills of the healthcare professional are not in question, the professional is likely to lack the ethical understanding and qualifications to allow them to make decisions for others (Kottow, 2004). Overall, our duty and default position as nurses is to respect a patient's right to self-determination but also acknowledge the complex nature of autonomy. Because of this complexity, it is also important to assess whether the patient is sufficiently autonomous. In other words, we need to assess the patient's capacity to consent, a subject we will focus on in later sections.

Dimond (2014) identifies different forms of consent, stating that 'Consent is the agreement by a mentally competent person, voluntary and without deceit or fraud, to an action which without the consent would be a trespass to the person'.

Obtaining consent is a fundamental consideration for the nurse or the prescriber. For prescribers, not only is it necessary to take a thorough patient history (see Chapter 5), but it may be necessary to examine the patient and order clinical investigations to confirm a diagnosis. To be able to perform all aspects of this process, it is important to gain appropriate consent from the patient. However, consent is only valid if the patient is competent to give it. Therefore, gaining a patient's consent is an important part of nursing and prescribing.

First, for consent to be valid, the patient needs to voluntarily give it. Second, the patient must be mentally competent or have capacity to give consent. This latter point poses special problems in mental health, and later sections will discuss this in more detail. Third, the person obtaining consent must not act in a way that could be understood as being deceitful. If any of these elements are absent, then the person obtaining consent may be vulnerable to accusations of infringing on the patient's rights. A closer look at these three components may rightly make the nurse feel unsure, since each component alone is complex and full of ambiguity, inaccuracy and possible misinterpretation. Therefore, it is good practice for nurses to document the process of obtaining consent, even if this may be laborious. Because of the complex nature of consent, it warrants further discussion.

Implied consent

The best illustration of implied – or non-verbal – consent is when a patient displays behaviours of acceptance. For example, if a patient offers their arm to the nurse during subcutaneous injection administration, it can mean that the patient has given consent for the nurse to administer the injection. This is because the patient is acting cooperatively despite not having verbally consented. In mental health, such a scenario is not uncommon because some symptoms of mental health problems may disrupt effective communication. However, some professional bodies, such as the General Medical Council (GMC), warn against relying on a patient's compliance as a form of consent (GMC, 1998). Just because the patient is cooperating with the injection procedure does not in itself indicate that the patient understands what you propose to do and why. Further, in prescribing practice, the reliance on implied consent has limitations and is unsafe, because during an ideal prescribing process a discussion between the prescriber and the patient normally takes place. However, we may use implied consent in some situations during our practice if the consent is valid. If the nurse is not sure about what to do in a specific situation, they should seek advice from their employer, professional indemnity insurance provider, trade union or the NMC, or even independent legal advice. In many situations, obtaining explicit consent from the patient is preferable to implied consent.

Explicit consent

Explicit consent, also known as express or direct consent, is when a patient gives a healthcare professional specific permission to do something. In other words, the nurse presents the patient with clear choices to agree or decline the planned treatment. This type of consent is common in healthcare. In explicit consent, there is a reliance on patients voicing their consent and responding to questions that the nurse may ask. A categorical 'yes' or 'no' from the patient easily confirms or refutes agreement to the planned treatment. However, the problem with this type of consent is that in cases of misunderstanding as to whether the nurse sought consent or not, in the absence of a witness it would simply be the word of the nurse against that of the patient (Dimond, 2014). Therefore, in practice, it is important for the nurse to apply more vigorous approaches to obtaining consent to protect both themselves and the patient. In this respect, explicit written consent offers protection for both parties.

As the name suggests, explicit written consent is the most transparent form of consent. It is an agreement that the patient gives in writing. Written consent is good evidence that the patient agreed to the treatment by providing a signature (Dimond, 2014). Further, in cases that involve higher-risk treatment, such as electroconvulsive therapy (ECT), it is important to gain written consent from the patient (GMC, 1998). This is so that all parties involved understand what was explained and agreed. Written consent forms should include details of the treatment or procedure, and this information forms the basis of consenting or not consenting to treatment. A good example of written consent is the clinical management plan (CMP) in supplementary prescribing. The

CMP usually details enough information for the patient to agree to it. Although written consent is the ideal in supplementary prescribing, and is easy to arrange, such arrangements can be fraught with difficulties in many independent prescribing situations, mainly due to time constraints. In written consent, the nurse or prescriber should provide the patient with details of any significant risks from the treatment or procedure, in addition to gaining the patient's signature. There is no legal requirement to obtain written consent, but it may be advisable in specific cases (BMA, 2018). Ideally, nurses should seek explicit informed consent, a critically important area in clinical practice that we will discuss next.

Informed consent

Informed consent is a term that has wide usage in healthcare law and ethics. The Royal College of Nursing (RCN) defines informed consent as 'an ongoing agreement by a person to receive treatment, undergo procedure or participate in research, after risks, benefits and alternatives have been adequately explained to them' (RCN, 2011).

Informed consent is a difficult principle that many healthcare professionals have problems in understanding. There is some evidence to suggest that nurses and other healthcare professionals seem to show an inadequate understanding of the term 'informed consent' (Nuttall and Rutt-Howard, 2015). This is mainly due to varying levels of information that nurses should provide patients before and during treatment. Therefore, at times, nurses tend to obtain consent imprecisely, without the patient truly understanding the benefits or risks of treatment. For example, many patients receiving psychotropic medication may be doing so without the knowledge of the risks and benefits of these regimens (Gray et al., 2005). Obviously, this is unsatisfactory practice, and for this reason the following section explores the concept of informed consent in more detail to promote a better understanding.

Informed consent has become central to the way that nurses practise. It assumes respect for the individual's right to make free decisions and it is a duty that originates from the moral principle of respect for persons (Tsai, 2008). Further, standard 4.2 of *The Code* says, 'make sure that you get properly informed consent and document it before carrying out any action' (NMC, 2018b). However, many nurses may fail to recognise situations in which patients' ability to provide informed consent may be compromised. Therefore, it is important to give information to patients in a way that they understand. This allows them to exercise their rights and make informed decisions about the care they receive. Whether in medicines or prescribing, it is necessary to assess how much information is enough. There are some situations where the nature of the information is such that the patient's understanding and capacity for decision-making is overwhelmed. In such cases, it is possible that the patient may lack the necessary capacity for informed decision-making (Bester et al., 2016). To compound matters, it may be difficult in practice to establish whether the patient has correctly understood the information and the implications. The following case study illustrates the problematic nature of informed consent.

Case study: *Montgomery v Lanarkshire Health Board* [2015]

Nadine Montgomery, a woman of small stature (5 feet tall), had diabetes. She gave birth to a larger than average-sized baby. The baby suffered from severe disabilities after birth due to shoulder dystocia. Before giving birth, Mrs Montgomery expressed concern to her doctor about whether she would be able to deliver her baby vaginally. The doctor failed to warn Mrs Montgomery of the possible risk of serious injury from shoulder dystocia. Further, the doctor did not suggest the possibility that Mrs Montgomery could opt to have a caesarean section. Lanarkshire Health Board argued that only in circumstances where there is a risk of grave adverse outcome should there be a duty to warn of such risks. They further argued that because the risk of such an outcome was so low and Mrs Montgomery merely expressed concern, this is not the same as asking a direct question that requires an answer. In their view, no warning was required. The lower courts ruled against Mrs Montgomery's claim and staunchly stuck to the view that the failure to warn of risks and alternative procedures would only be negligent if it was not supported as proper by a responsible body of medical opinion (the **Bolam principle**).

However, Mrs Montgomery won her case on appeal to the UK Supreme Court. The Supreme Court ruled that the question should have been about Mrs Montgomery's likely reaction if informed of the risk of shoulder dystocia. The obvious position was that she would have chosen to give birth by caesarean section: 'The test of materiality is whether, in the circumstances of the particular case, a reasonable person in the patient's position would be likely to attach significance to the risk, or the doctor should reasonably be aware that the particular patient would be likely to attach significance to it.' The court emphasised that 'whether a risk is material cannot be reduced to percentages, and instead is based on a variety of factors such as: (1) nature of the risk; (2) effect on the life of the patient; (3) the importance to the patient of the benefits of the treatment; (4) any possible alternatives; and (5) the risk of those alternatives.'

As can be seen from the above case study, the process of informed consent can be fraught with difficulties. The ruling in this case firmly states that the need for 'informed consent' is now part of UK law (England, Northern Ireland, Scotland and Wales). Nurses and other healthcare professionals are now under a clear duty to take reasonable care to ensure that patients are aware of all significant risks to treatment. Previously, it was enough for healthcare professionals to simply explain treatment in broad terms for consent to be valid. In medicines management and prescribing, it is now essential to adequately inform a patient of the potential risks, interactions, contraindications and side effects of medication. The law may regard failure to provide adequate information as negligence. Therefore, nurses and prescribers may find themselves accounting for their practice in a court of law.

Generally, to impose care or treatment on an individual without respecting their wishes and right to self-determination is not only unethical, but illegal. This is also against *The Code*, which states that you must 'respect, support and document a person's right to accept or refuse care and treatment' (NMC, 2018b). However, an exception to this is if the healthcare professional reasonably considers that the disclosure of a risk would 'be seriously detrimental to the patient's health', or in circumstances of necessity. However, lawmakers warn against abuse of this exception.

In prescribing, a general rule to follow is to explain the options to the patient, setting out the potential benefits, risks, burdens and side effects of each option, including the option to have no treatment. The prescriber may recommend an option that they believe to be best for the patient, but they must not put pressure on the patient to accept their advice. The patient can then weigh up the potential benefits, risks and burdens of the various options, as well as any non-clinical issues that are relevant to them. The patient then decides whether to accept any of the options, and if so which one. However, deciding how much information is enough to tell the patient remains a contentious issue.

Healthcare professionals, including nurses, should make their own professional judgement regarding what information to communicate – and to what level. However, the information should be within the sphere and limit of the patient's understanding. This allows the nurse to argue and defend the judgement by saying that it is truly informed. Furthermore, by respecting the patient's right to autonomy, it allows them the dignity of being in control of their own lives and masters of their own well-being (Hendrick, 2000). In prescribing practice, patient participation is high on the agenda, as different healthcare professional bodies ascribe. Platform 4.2 of the standards of proficiency for registered nurses states, 'at the point of registration, the registered nurse will be able to … work in partnership with people to encourage shared decision making in order to support individuals, their families and carers to manage their own care when appropriate' (NMC, 2018a). As discussed earlier, for consent to be valid, the person giving it must do so voluntarily in an uncoerced and non-threatening manner. Above all, the person must be mentally competent to grant such consent.

Patients may not be sufficiently autonomous to make competent healthcare decisions, and in such cases the nurse is best guided by the Mental Capacity Act 2005. We will now turn our attention to beneficence, another key area of bioethics.

Beneficence

The ethical principle of beneficence is about ensuring that patients benefit from the caring relationship. It is the principle of doing good, and refers to the duty of the nurse to act for the benefit of the patient, which is set out by *The Code* (NMC, 2018b). Beneficence also involves the nurse balancing out benefits against risks and costs, thus ensuring that the patient receives the best care. The effects of beneficence should involve both the physical and psychological benefits of caring. Standards set for professionals by their regulatory bodies, such as the NMC, can be higher than the law requires. Therefore, in cases of negligence, the standard that applies is often that set by the relevant statutory body for its members. However, it is worth noting that the 'best care' may be relative to the overall situation which we may encounter in clinical practice. This is because in healthcare, we work within certain restrictions, such as budgetary constraints, and these can be decisive in our decision-making process.

Non-maleficence

At the heart of the principle of non-maleficence is the notion of not knowingly causing harm to the patient. This principle is expressed in the Hippocratic oath. The duty not to harm patients is separate from the duty to help them. Although codes of conduct for various health professions outline duties not to harm patients, many interventions result in some harm to patients, however temporary. In pharmacological treatments, we can describe many interventions as having 'double effect' (i.e. one good effect – the intended pharmacological effect – and one harmful effect – unintended adverse side effects). We can allow the harmful effect if it is, on balance, less impactful than the good effect. In medicines management and prescribing, it is therefore important to review both the potential positive effects of treatment (e.g. symptom control) and the harmful effects (e.g. adverse side effects).

Justice

The concept of justice is not the law in the narrow sense. Rather, this principle involves ensuring that everyone benefits from treatment, as well as the distribution of access to it. To apply this principle, we need to accept and value differences and diversity in our patients. Patients come from different cultural, racial and religious backgrounds. Therefore, fairness and justice in this respect involves respecting and recognising their differences, not acting in a way that disadvantages the patient. In this regard, we need to consider other people's cultural differences when treating them. Importantly, justice is about advocating on behalf of all patients, whether they come in with a Western philosophical perspective or another philosophical perspective. Justice is not about treating all patients the same because it is not possible to justifiably treat all patients the same, since all patients are different and present with different ailments or complaints. We will now return to the issue of capacity to consent and its legal implications.

Mental capacity and consent

A definition of mental capacity is the ability to use and understand information to decide, as well as communicating any decision made. In medicines management or prescribing, it is important to establish if a person has capacity or not. Certain groups of people, such as those with mental health problems, those that are unconscious and those under the influence of alcohol or drugs, may have limited capacity to consent to treatment. However, determining if an individual has mental capacity can be a contentious issue, as the following case study demonstrates.

Case study: Ms B

Ms B was a 43-year-old who suffered from a completely disabling condition, and she requested that her life-support machine be turned off. She did not want to live on a ventilator and had made a living will. Two psychiatrists at the hospital established that she was not competent to refuse ventilation. But later that year, an independent psychiatric reassessment concluded that she was competent to give consent. Thereafter, the hospital regarded Ms B as competent, but her doctors continued to refuse to withdraw her ventilation.

Ms B sought relief from the High Court to refuse life-prolonging medical treatment, as well as attesting that the hospital had been treating her unlawfully. The High Court judge identified that the central issue was whether Ms B was competent to refuse ventilation. In other words, was Ms B able to understand and maintain the information important to the decision, as well as the likely consequences of having or not having the treatment? Furthermore, was she able to use the information and weigh it in the balance as part of the process of arriving at a decision?

The judge ruled that Ms B was competent to make all relevant decisions about her medical treatment including the decision to seek to withdraw from artificial ventilation. Her mental competence was proportionate to the enormity of the decision she made.

Although the case of Ms B occurred in a physical health setting, the key principles of mental capacity to consent to treatment apply equally to medicines management and prescribing in any setting. If we give treatment to a mentally competent person despite their objection, this can be regarded as a trespass – and even an assault – upon the individual. The Mental Capacity Act 2005 reflects the principles of judgement in Ms B's case, and it came into force in October 2007. In English law, a mentally competent person has a right to refuse treatment, even if medical opinion supports the fact that by refusing treatment the patient will die. Outside of the Mental Health Act 1983, a mentally competent person cannot be forced to accept treatment. This is the principle applied by the judge in Ms B's case. However, this situation changes when an individual is deemed not to have capacity to decide. The provisions for lack of capacity are provided for in the Mental Capacity Act 2005.

Mental Capacity Act 2005

Case study: Alan

Alan was a 68-year-old male patient who suffered from paranoid schizophrenia and was detained in a psychiatric hospital. He developed gangrene in one foot but refused to have the leg amputed to save his life. He believed that God would help him through his illness. However, he agreed with the doctors about the consequences of refusing amputation. Further, he issued a court injunction to stop the hospital from amputating his foot without his consent. He won the case in court because the hospital was unable to establish that he lacked adequate understanding of his problem and the medical treatment proposed. The court believed that he possessed mental capacity as: (a) he was able to understand and retain relevant treatment information; (b) he believed the information; and (c) he had arrived at a clear conclusion, for better or worse.

The Mental Capacity Act 2005 covers all personal decisions on the welfare of people who temporarily or permanently lack mental capacity to decide for themselves. It defines someone as lacking in capacity if 'at the time, he [*sic*] is unable to decide for himself because of an impairment of, or a disturbance in the functioning of, the mind or brain.'

Despite its title, the Mental Capacity Act 2005 applies to anyone who lacks capacity to make decisions, as well as those who wish to plan for others to make decisions on their behalf in the event of losing capacity to make their own decisions in the future. Anyone who delivers care or treatment to a person who lacks capacity aged 16 years and over living in England or Wales should consider the Act. For example, informal carers, health and social care professionals, and the emergency services may rely on the Act.

The term 'decision-maker' is used for those who make decisions on behalf of incapacitated people.

The five principles of the Mental Capacity Act 2005

Section 1 of the Act outlines five principles that intend to protect people who lack capacity to make their own decisions, as well as maximising people's ability to make their own decisions as far as possible. These five principles are as follows:

1. An individual must be assumed to have capacity unless it is determined otherwise.
2. An individual is not to be regarded as unable to decide unless all practicable steps to help the individual to do so have been taken without success.
3. An individual is not to be regarded as unable to decide merely because he or she makes an unwise decision.

4. An act done, or a decision made under the Act, for or on behalf of a person who lacks capacity, must be done in their best interest.

5. Before the act is done, or the decision is made, consideration must be given as to whether the purpose for which the decision or act is needed can be as effectively achieved in a way that is less restrictive of the person's rights and freedom of action.

The Act enshrines in law best practice and common law principles concerning people who lack mental capacity to decide for themselves and those who make decisions on their behalf. It also deals with the assessment of a person's capacity and those who may act on the patient's behalf. The law does this by setting out a clear test to assess whether someone lacks capacity to make a decision at a specific time. You cannot label someone 'incapable' simply because of a medical condition or diagnosis.

In section 2 of the Act, you cannot establish a lack of capacity merely by reference to a person's age, appearance, or any condition or aspect of a person's behaviour that might lead others to make unjustified assumptions about capacity. In other words, a mentally ill adult can refuse treatment if they are mentally competent when they make the decision, as in the case of Alan above. Being mentally ill by itself does not automatically deprive the person of capacity. Section 2 of the Act requires the person making the decision to establish two facts: (1) Is there a specific decision to be made now? (2) Is the person unable to make that decision because of an impairment of – or a disturbance in the functioning of – the mind or brain, whether temporary or permanent? If the decision-maker answers 'no' to one or both questions, then the Act will not apply to the person. In Alan's case, a decision to amputate his leg had to be made, but he understood what his condition was and the likely consequences of refusing treatment. Therefore, the Act did not apply in his case, even though he suffered from paranoid schizophrenia. The judge ruled that Alan was able to decide competently.

Another important consideration relating to consent is that when a patient refuses treatment, we must be sure that they have the capacity to make that decision, and have not been unduly influenced by other persons. The following case study clearly demonstrates this point.

Case study: Ms Re T

Ms Re T, a pregnant woman who was injured in a road traffic accident, needed a life-saving blood transfusion following a caesarean section. Before the operation, she informed the medical staff that she would not accept a blood transfusion and signed a form to that effect. Her mother was a Jehovah's Witness and influenced her into refusing the transfusion. The patient's partner applied to the court for permission for the medical staff to give her the transfusion. The court ruled that the blood could be given. This was because the evidence showed that at the time of deciding, she did not have the necessary capacity to make a valid decision because her mind was unduly influenced by her mother.

What is important here is not that the court consented for a mentally competent adult by proxy, but rather at the time of making the decision Ms Re T was not in a competent state of mind due to her mother's influence. For the best interest of her child and her-self, Ms Re T was given the blood to save her life. This decision may sit uncomfortably with many nurses and healthcare professionals. However, where possible, the competent person's wishes must be respected.

Section 3 of the Act sets out a legal test to determine whether the person is competent of making their own decisions. As previously discussed, just because someone has a mental illness or a disorder in the functioning of the mind does not necessarily mean that they have no capacity to make all of their own decisions. Section 3 of the Act states that an individual has an 'inability to make decisions' if they are unable to:

(a) understand the information relevant to the decision;

(b) retain the information;

(c) use or weigh that information as part of the process of making the decision;

(d) communicate his decision (whether by talking, using sign language or any other means).

The decision-maker must decide what information is relevant and impart with that information in a way that the person can understand.

If the decision-maker is satisfied that the person fulfils all four of the above require-ments (a–d), then that individual must have capacity to make the decision. However, if the decision-maker believes that the person is unable to demonstrate one or more of the four requirements, then the person is deemed to lack capacity to decide. The decision-maker is then able to make decisions on the individual's behalf, acting in the person's 'best interest'.

Section 4 of the Act does not define 'best interest', but sets up a list of factors that the decision-maker must consider. The purpose of the list is to ensure that any decisions made – or actions taken – are in the best interest of the incapacitated person. Aspects to consider are broad, allowing them to be applied to all decisions and actions. When determining what is in the patient's best interest, a quick summary of the code of prac-tice offers guidance for the decision-maker.

Code of practice guidance

Encourage participation. Whenever possible, encourage the person to participate, or enhance their ability to participate, in the decision-making process. Identify all relevant situations and try to find out all the things that the person who has no capacity would have considered if they were making the decision or acting for themselves.

Find out the person's views. Try to find out the views of the person who is lacking capacity, including:

- their past and present desires (these may have been expressed orally, in writing, or through behaviours or habits);
- any credible ideals (e.g. religious, cultural, moral, political) that would have been likely to impact on the decision in question;
- any other aspects the person would likely have considered if they were making the decision or acting for themselves.

Avoid discrimination. Do not make assumptions about the person's best interest simply based on their age, appearance, condition or behaviour.

Assess whether the person might regain capacity. Consider whether the person is likely to regain capacity (e.g. after receiving medical treatment). If so, can the decision wait until then?

If the decision concerns life-sustaining treatment, then it should not be motivated in any way by the wish to bring about the person's death. Further, the decision-maker must not make assumptions about the person's quality of life.

Consult others. If it is practical and appropriate to do so, consult other people for their views about the person's best interest, as well as seeing if they have any information about the person's wishes, feelings, beliefs and values. Specifically, try to consult:

- anyone previously named by the person as someone to be consulted on either the decision in question or on similar issues;
- anyone engaged in caring for the person;
- close relatives, friends or others who may take an interest in the person's welfare;
- any attorney appointed under lasting power of attorney or enduring power of attorney made by the person;
- any deputy appointed by the Court of Protection to make decisions for the person.

For decisions relating to major medical treatment or where the person should live, and where there is no one who fits into any of the above categories, the decision-maker must consult an independent mental capacity advocate (IMCA). When consulting, the decision-maker should remember that the person who is lacking in capacity has a right to keep their affairs private. Therefore, it is inappropriate to share every piece of information with everyone.

Avoid restricting the person's rights. The person making the decision should see if there are other alternatives that may be less restrictive of the person's rights.

To determine a person's best interest, the decision-maker should take all of the above into account. There are no statutory forms for either the best interest checklist or the capacity test. Nevertheless, the advice to the decision-maker is to document their decision-making process, as this will provide weight for their actions and help protect them from liability. In addition to the best interest decision-making checklist, an important area to cover is the Mental Capacity Act 2005 checklist from Barber et al. (2016), which I will turn to next.

Case study: Mental Capacity Act 2005 checklist

Has the decision-maker:

- applied the five principles?
- established that the person's age is 16 years or over?
- established that there is a specific decision to be made?
- established that the person is lacking capacity because of an impairment of – or a disturbance in the functioning of – the brain or mind?
- ensured that the person is lacking capacity in relation to a specific matter at a specific time?
- ensured that the decision is not based on assumptions about the person's age, appearance, behaviour, etc.?
- established that the person is unable to make their own decisions because they have not been able to respond positively to one or more of the of the following questions?

  o Do they understand the relevant information?
  o Can they retain it?
  o Can they weigh up the information?
  o Can they communicate a decision?

- taken all practicable steps to help the person make their own decision?
- ensured that this is a genuine lack of capacity, not merely an unwise decision?
- applied the best interest checklist?
- considered whether there might be a less restrictive option?
- ensured that the care or treatment is a mere restriction of movements rather than a deprivation of liberty?

Before reading any further, complete Activity 1.4.

Activity 1.4   Critical thinking

May is a 25-year-old chemistry graduate who has had numerous admissions to hospital, usually on a section order of the Mental Health Act 2005. She suffers from schizophrenia, and on her last discharge from hospital the consultant psychiatrist prescribed a depot injection instead of the usual tablets. The doctor wanted May to break the cycle of hospital admissions by ensuring compliance with medication. May was unhappy about taking a depot injection and argued that she suffers worse side effects on a depot than she does while taking oral medication. The consultant psychiatrist refused May's request, arguing that she has made similar promises in the past without honouring them. In his view, she lacked capacity.

- Does May lack capacity?
- What other factors might be leading May to refuse medication?

Outline answers are provided at the end of the chapter.

Section 5 of the Act allows decision-makers to carry out actions in relation to care or treatment if they follow the requirements of the Act. However, there are restrictions, which in effect means that certain actions are not permitted under Section 5. Going beyond these restrictions would amount to unlawful practice. Section 5 of the Act allows persons to make decisions and carry out acts for or on behalf of the incapacitated person, provided that:

- before carrying out the act, the decision-maker takes reasonable steps to determine whether the person lacks capacity specifically to the matter;
- when carrying out the act, the decision-maker believes the person lacks capacity specifically to the matter;
- the act is in the person's best interest (determined in accordance with section 4 of the Act).

If these criteria are met, the decision-maker should be protected from liability, if they do not exceed the limitation detailed below and do not act negligently.

Limitation section 5

Section 6 of the Act sets out several conditions that must be met to ensure that section 5 of the Act is lawful. If the decision-maker follows the procedure explained above and does not exceed the limitation detailed below, their acts of care or treatment will fall within the scope of section 5 of the Act.

Section 6 of the Act defines restraint as 'the use or threat of force where a person who lacks capacity resists, and any restriction of liberty or movement whether the person resists'. If restraint is needed to prevent harm to others, then the decision-maker needs to establish if the Mental Health Act 2005 or the common law would provide more appropriate means of meeting the person's needs or safeguarding others.

Restraint can be used provided the following criteria are met:

- the decision-maker believes that the restraint is necessary to prevent harm to the person and the act is a proportionate response to the likelihood of the person suffering harm and the seriousness of that harm.

While restraint is permitted in certain circumstances, it will only be permitted where it amounts to a restriction of the person's movements, rather than a deprivation of the individual's liberty. This leaves the decision-maker with a complex question to answer: What amounts to deprivation of liberty? Subsequent sections partially address this question through case law examples.

Another limitation of section 5 of the Act is that it prevents decision-makers from carrying out acts if they conflict with:

- a person's advance refusal of treatment;
- the authority of an attorney appointed by the person;
- the authority of a deputy appointed by the Court of Protection.

The deprivation of liberty safeguards

The deprivation of liberty safeguards (DoLS) are an amendment to the Mental Capacity Act 2005, introduced in 2009. The DoLS were put in place to protect any deprivation of liberty of an adult who may lack capacity to decide. The aim of the DoLS is to ensure that the Act complies with the provisions of Article 5 of the ECHR. The following case study serves to highlight the importance and complex issues relating to the concept of deprivation of liberty.

Case study: *G v E v A Local Authority v F* [2010]

E, aged 19, had a physical health problem, a learning disability, and language skills comparable to those of an 18–25-month-old child. He was removed from the care of his long-term carer by the local authority to residential care. While in residential care, he showed some behavioural challenges, and these appeared to worsen over time. The judge determined that the local authority care arrangement deprived E of his liberty. He based his conclusions on having noted that the residential place had complete control over his care and movements. These included complete control over assessment, treatment, contacts and where he resides. The judge was also influenced by the high level of confinement of E to a residential institution. He could have visits, but these were under escort, and he had no private space or possessions. His social contacts were very limited. More importantly, he was administered psychotropic medication, which he had no control over, to manage his behaviour.

There is no single classification of what deprivation of liberty is, or what is a restriction of movement. It is essential to recognise that giving care and treatment that amount to restriction of a person's movement does not necessarily breach Article 5 of the ECHR. Depriving a person of their liberty, as in E's case, on the other hand, is unlawful unless it meets the conditions of Article 5. But the problem is that the ECHR does not define 'deprivation of liberty', and Article 5 does not provide examples of what constitutes deprivation of liberty. It is possible to argue that in E's case, he was being restricted, not deprived of his liberty. However, the degree and intensity of the restrictions imposed were enough to sway the judge's opinion and rendered these restrictions a deprivation of liberty. It is important that any decision to provide care and treatment to people should make the distinction between the two. Nurses need to make the decision to determine what restrictions are being placed on the individual and then decide if these amount to a deprivation of liberty. If a person is deprived of their liberty, or at risk of it, then the deprivation must be compliant with Article 5 of the ECHR for it to be lawful.

Several cases have been before the courts regarding the issue of the difference between restriction of movement and deprivation of liberty. These cases have set standards and provide decision-makers with some direction on how to differentiate between the two in clinical practice. Potentially, actions such as the use of force, restraint (physical or through medication), seclusion, 'timeout', overly intrusive observation, use of electronic devices, locked doors/wards, and freedom to interact with others outside the institution may – in certain situations – amount to a deprivation of liberty. However, each situation is likely to have its own unique set of circumstances, and consideration of these is important.

The assessment procedure for DoLS

Where an adult who lacks capacity is deprived – or at risk of being deprived – of their liberty within a residential care or hospital setting, the managing authority should initiate the DoLS procedure by making an application that is in the prescribed form. The form's content varies depending upon whether the request is within England or Wales.

After making the application, the 'supervisory body' should consider the request and commission the six assessments. If the assessment meets the criteria, the supervisory body will authorise a deprivation of liberty.

Once an application has been made, there is an expectation that certain people should be informed of the request. If the supervisory body considers the request appropriate, and has all the relevant information, it should commission assessors to perform the six assessments (age, no refusals, mental capacity, eligibility, best interest, authorisation). The assessors have 21 days in which to complete the assessment for a standard authorisation of deprivation of liberty. If the equivalent of these assessments has not been carried out within the last 12 months, new assessments will be required.

Scenario

Mr Jones is 73 years old, lives in the community on his own, and has no known living relatives. When he was 66 years old, he made an advance decision regarding how his affairs should be managed should he lose capacity. He is showing early signs of Alzheimer's disease.

(Continued)

(Continued)

A care worker visits daily to ensure that his needs are attended to. Recently, the care worker has noticed deterioration in Mr Jones' level of coping with ADLs, and a care conference has been arranged to make an application to the court to appoint a person to make decisions on his behalf and look after his welfare.

The Mental Capacity Act 2005 allows a person to appoint an attorney to act on their behalf if they should lose capacity in the future, as in the case of Mr Jones above. In addition, it provides for a system of court-appointed deputies to make decisions on welfare, healthcare and financial matters, as authorised by the Court of Protection, but the appointee will not be able to refuse consent to life-sustaining treatment on behalf of the patient.

In addition to the above, the Act provides for an IMCA, who is appointed to support a person who lacks capacity but has no one, such as family or friends, to speak for them. Mr Jones is likely to need an IMCA. The IMCA will only involve themselves where decisions are being made about serious medical treatment provided by the NHS or about a change in the person's accommodation, where it is provided by the local authority. The IMCA makes representations about the person's wishes, feelings, beliefs and values at the same time as bringing to the attention of the decision-maker all of the factors that are relevant to the decision. The IMCA can challenge the decision-maker on behalf of the person lacking capacity, if necessary.

Ethical conflicts

There is little doubt that the principle of justice comes into conflict with other ethical considerations in mental health practice. In particular, the principle of autonomy, which focuses on the needs and rights of the individual, gives rise to ethical dilemmas more in mental health than in other fields of nursing. This may be because of the highly patient-oriented approach that is more common in the mental health field (Berghmans et al., 2004; Szasz, 2009). The patient-oriented approach stresses the importance of taking the values and preferences of the individual into account in treatment decisions. For example, Pound et al. (2005) conducted the qualitative equivalent of a meta-analysis of issues surrounding the way in which patients are non-adherent to medication as prescribed. They identified that the concept of 'resistance' to taking medication was linked to the patient's sense of self or autonomy. Continued taking of psychotropic medication may undermine the feeling of autonomy, and therefore may result in less than optimal adherence, despite the obvious benefit that the patient may derive from taking such medicines, and

Chapter 2 dicusses this theme in greater detail. Clearly, this situation generates conflict in the nurse. On the one hand, the nurse needs to respect patient autonomy and the patient's right to make decisions; on the other, the nurse's duty is also to promote good mental health through adherence to treatment. In addition to ethical considerations in mental health, you need to be aware of the legislation that specifically governs the use of medicines.

Mental Health Act 1983 (amended 2007)

We have seen that a mentally competent adult must consent to treatment before we give it. However, there is a legal exception to this rule under the the Mental Health Act 1983 (as amended by the Mental Health Act 2007). The Mental Health Act 1983 provides a far-reaching legal framework for the detention of people in hospital who are suffering from a 'mental disorder' for treatment and care. The aim of the Act is to protect the rights of people in England and Wales who have a mental disorder. The following section briefly examines some of the political drivers that led to amendment of the Mental Health Act 1983, as well as the key concerns that the amendments were trying to resolve.

One of the key principles underpinning the Mental Health Act 1983 is *parens patriae*. This is when the state assumes both the right and the responsibility to treat people who are unwell when it is necessary. In other words, the state acts as the parents of its citizens, and must do so to protect those citizens who are mentally ill and need treatment. The state can override the right to freedom of a mentally ill person both to protect the person from themselves and others from any harmful actions of the mentally ill person. In addition to the *parens patriae* principle, the murder of Jonathan Zito in England by Christopher Clunis accelerated the 2007 amendments. Christopher Clunis was a patient suffering from paranoid schizophrenia who had stopped taking his medication while under the care of community mental health services. The second event was the murder of Lin and Megan Russell in 1996 by Michael Stone, a man who suffered from 'personality disorder'. Stone had been refused admission to hospital just days before he committed the murders, the reason given being that he suffered from an 'untreatable disorder'. Because of these events, it became necessary to amend the Mental Health Act 1983.

There is a procedure to follow to protect patients from inappropriate detention or treatment without consent. In summary, the legislation ensures that people with serious mental disorders which threaten their health and safety, or the safety of the public, can be treated, if necessary, without their consent. This is to prevent them from harming themselves or others. In medicines management and prescribing, we mainly concern ourselves with sections 2, 3 and 37.

Section 2

Case study: Yosuf

Yosuf is a 36-year-old man with no history of mental health problems. After the death of his mother nine months ago, he became withdrawn. His appetite and sleep pattern deteriorated. He denied experiencing any mental health problems but admitted to hearing the voice of his mother at night. He was recently rushed to hospital after being found unconscious due to taking a mixture of alcohol and sleeping tablets. After he regained consciousness in hospital, he asked to be discharged but was referred to the duty psychiatrist. The duty psychiatrist thought Yosuf was suffering from a mental disorder and was a risk to himself. Yosuf was not in agreement with the doctor's assessment and insisted on being discharged. The doctor recommended that Yosuf be admitted to a psychiatric unit for assessment under section 2 of the Mental Health Act.

Section 2 of the Mental Health Act allows compulsory admission for assessment, or for assessment followed by treatment. An approved mental health professional (AMHP) or the nearest relative can make an application within 14 days of the last doctor seeing the patient, such as in the case of Yosuf above. Two medical recommendations must support the application and they must have seen the patient within five days of each other. One of the medical recommendations should be from a suitably qualified and experienced doctor (often referred to as the responsible clinician) who is approved under section 12 of the Mental Health Act. In practice, the approved doctor is normally a psychiatrist or a senior registrar with special experience in the diagnosis and treatment of mental disorder. Wherever possible, a doctor who has previous knowledge of the patient should provide the other recommendation. In practice, the second doctor is usually the patient's own GP. If their GP is not available, then a doctor from an independently approved section 12 list can complete the second recommendation.

Both medical recommendations must agree that the detention is in the best interest of the patient and is for the patient's own safety, or that of others. In the above case study, Yosuf was at risk of harming himself and therefore neded to be detained for his own personal safety. The medical reports should also state that the patient is suffering from a mental disorder of a nature or degree that warrants detention for assessment, or assessment followed by treatment. The patient must be admitted to hospital within 14 days of the last medical examination. The detention can last up to 28 days and the patient can appeal to the Mental Health Review Tribunal (MHRT) within 14 days of admission. Under section 2, the patient cannot refuse treatment, but some treatments cannot be given without the patient's consent unless certain criteria are met, such as ECT.

In most cases, the responsible clinician can discharge the patient from section 2. The reasons for discharge can be that the patient has been assessed as not needing further detention, or because they are willing stay in hospital informally or can return to the community with support. In this case, the responsible clinician can rescind section 2. The other basis for discharging a patient from section 2 is if the responsible clinician concludes that the patient no longer needs treatment. In addition, the hospital managers or an MHRT can discharge the patient if they feel that the criteria for detention are no longer met.

Section 3

Scenario

Jane has a history of depression, suicide attempts and alcohol abuse. She has had numerous previous admissions to hospital, usually after taking a drug overdose. She was admitted informally to a ward but she wanted to discharge herself within hours of admission. Because Jane presented a high risk to herself, her consultant psychiatrist recommended that she be detained in hospital under section 3 of the Mental Health Act.

Section 3 is like section 2, differing only in the period of detention. Unless it is not practicable to do so, or if consultation would result in 'unreasonable delay', the AMHP must consult the nearest relative before detaining someone under section 3. In cases where the AMHP is unable to consult with the nearest relative, the reasons for this should be justified and documented. If the nearest relative objects, detention under section 3 cannot go ahead unless legal action is taken to remove the title of nearest relative (and the rights that accompany the title) from the person who is objecting. However, there is a subtle difference between agreeing and objecting to the application. In some cases, relatives may not precisely agree with the decision, but are not objecting, and so the application can proceed. The AMHP needs two medical recommendations to be able to make an application. One of the medical recommendations should be from a suitably qualified and experienced psychiatrist (often the responsible clinician) who is approved under section 12 of the Mental Health Act. The other medical recommendation should be, as far as possible, from the patient's GP. If their GP is not available, then a doctor from an independently approved section 12 list can complete the second recommendation. The grounds for detaining a patient under section 3 are:

- the patient suffers or is suffering from a mental disorder in accordance with the definition of mental disorder in the 2007 amended Mental Health Act;
- it is necessary for the health or safety of the patient or for the protection of other persons, and such treatment cannot be provided unless they are detained under this section.

In the case of Jane above, she has a history of suicide attempts, and for her own protection it is necessary to detain her under section 3. Section 3 can last up to six months, and the patient has no right to refuse treatment under section 3. If they do refuse treatment, they can be treated against their will for the first three months, but after this time a second opinion appointed doctor (SOAD) must see the patient. The SOAD will carry out an assessment to determine if the patient needs treatment. In other words, after three months, the patient can only compulsorily receive treatment with SOAD approval. The patient has the right to appeal to the MHRT within the first six months after section 3 initiation, and then once a year afterwards. There is an automatic referral to the MHRT if the patient does not appeal. As soon as the patient no longer meets the criteria for detention, section 3 can be rescinded.

If there is a need to renew section 3, the responsible clinician must apply for a renewal, which a second professional must support. The second professional must:

- come from a different professional discipline than the responsible clinician;
- be involved with the care of the patient;
- be able to reach independent decisions;
- have enough expertise and experience to make a judgement about whether the patient meets the criteria to continue detention.

There may be instances where the responsible clinician disagrees with the view of the second professional, and in such cases the section 3 renewal of detention cannot go ahead. In very exceptional circumstances, where there is a difference of opinion between the professionals, they should bring this to the attention of the hospital managers, who will consider and approve the renewal of the detention.

Section 37

Section 37 of the Mental Health Act 1983 (amended 2007) is similar in its application to section 3 but refers specifically to offenders seen before the courts. Appeal against this section can only occur in the second six months of treatment. However, the courts can apply section 41 of the Mental Health Act to restrict the discharge of people committed to hospital under section 37. If there is an application of a restriction under section 41, it is not possible to discharge, grant leave or transfer the patient without Home Office consent.

Community treatment orders

The hospital can discharge a person after detention under section 3 or section 37 using a community treatment order (CTO). The responsible clinician can decide to place someone on to a CTO with a supporting recommendation from an AMHP. Normally, conditions accompany a CTO, and these might include staying at a particular address, attending for treatment at a particular time or place, or taking medication. Failure to comply with these conditions, or a significant deterioration in mental health, may result in the individual being recalled back to hospital. On recall to hospital, which can last for up to 72 hours, an assessment is made. After the assessment, the individual can return to the community, be admitted to hospital as a voluntary patient, be discharged from the CTO, or revoke the CTO. Revocation of a CTO means that the person will be readmitted to hospital and the section under which they were initially detained will come back into force. Because principles of compulsory treatment evoke moral and ethical debates, we will briefly turn to these next.

Ethical considerations of compulsory treatment

Case study: Trish

Trish, a 30-year-old woman who works as teacher, recently approached her doctor after feeling stressed at work. There had been disagreements at work that verged on conflict, particularly with her line manager. She felt belittled by her manager and some of her co-workers. She wanted something to help her sleep for a few nights. On further investigation, Trish showed all the signs and symptoms of major depression and she expressed suicidal ideation. Her doctor suggested a referral to a psychiatrist, but Trish declined, saying that she wanted medication and believed this was the key to resolving the problems she was experiencing at work. Because the doctor deemed Trish a risk to herself, he recommended admission to hospital under the Mental Health Act 1983.

Apart from legal considerations, the use of compulsory treatment for people suffering from mental illness has ethical ramifications. To understand the origins of compulsory treatment, as well as the moral and ethical issues surrounding it, we need to briefly review earlier work by some anti-psychiatrists, most notably Thomas Szasz, and we will turn to this later.

In the above case study, if you consider Trish's feeling of humiliation and her depressed mood, it is possible to conclude that Trish is suffering from major depression as a result of the situation at work. However, some authorities have suggested that depression is not a psychiatric illness, but simply a variation in normal mood. This originates from the view that some events are so horrific that depression seems a reasonable response, and the concept of 'depressive realism' applies (Alloy and Abramson, 1988). Thus, people with depression appraise their situation more realistically. It has been argued that 'depression has a keener eye for the truth' (Freud, 1957) and that 'depressives' thoughts are painfully truthful whereas non-depressives' thoughts are unrealistically positive' (Alloy and Abramson, 1988). If we accept the concept of depressive realism, is it then ethically correct to administer pharmacological treatment, and perhaps to do so coercively?

In *Coercion as Cure*, Thomas Szasz provides an extensive history of the use of coercion throughout psychiatry, including the early use of various mechanical restraints such as the 'tranquillising chair', moral treatment, the 'resting cure', insulin shock therapy, ECT, lobotomy, and, of course, medication (Szasz, 2009). He argues that each one of these breakthrough 'discoveries' in psychiatric medicine is simply a reworking of old ideas, and that they all share the common thread of coercion, thus depriving people of their liberty. He further argues that the 'liberation' of patients from mental hospitals by virtue of medicines such as chlorpromazine in the 1950s amounted to no more than drugged coercion, with patients still under CTOs in the community. He rejects the use of medicines and coercion in psychiatry altogether and calls for an abolition of psychiatric coercion as a 'crime against humanity'.

Szasz also makes the point that in assessing any therapeutic intervention outcome, what we should consider is not its effectiveness, but whether it was brought about consensually or coercively. To an extent, Szasz's views inform the absolutist civil liberties approach, which is that psychiatric hospitalisation of a person against their will is a dangerous assault on individual freedom. In other words, in the above case study, if Trish has not given consent, her hospitalisation is totally unacceptable and a breach of her human rights – her right to liberty is supreme.

Another current – and perhaps more influential – civil liberties position is to accept compulsory treatment under certain circumstances but only when exercising extreme caution. Medical necessity is regarded as insufficient reason to justify the use of coercive powers. Only in circumstances where a person is at physical risk of harming themselves or others can treatment coercion be applied.

A third view is informed by medicine, which regrets the necessity for involuntary hospitalisation but regards it as an essential last resort, enabling the care and treatment of a small proportion of patients whose severe mental illnesses substantially interfere with their capacity to accept such treatment voluntarily, and this is the view that Trish's doctor took in the above case study.

As you can imagine, these opposing views evoke lively and polarising debates, and this is best exemplified by Trish in the above case study. The fact that the doctor and Trish took differing views that are equally valid is a case in point. Nurses may be caught up in the moral dilemma of patients' needs versus patients' rights, but what is important here is to be aware that we are dealing primarily with questions of values, not facts. One person may have a different perception from that of other members of the multidisciplinary team (MDT) regarding a situation, thus making it very difficult to arrive at common ground with colleagues. Clearly, there is a need to be aware of the ethical dilemmas that may confront nurses from time to time during the treatment of patients. Nurses should let legislation assist them in making decisions, and the Medicines Act 1968, discussed below, is an important element in medicines management.

Medicines Act 1968

This important Act, with which nurses must comply, deals with the prescribing, supply, storage and administration of medicines, and defines three categories of medicines:

- prescription-only medicines (POMs), which are available only from a pharmacist if prescribed by an appropriate practitioner;
- pharmacy (P) medicines, which are available only from a pharmacist but may be obtained without a prescription;
- general sales list (GSL) medicines, which may be bought from any shop without a prescription.

Under the Act, possession of POMs such as antibiotics, with or without a prescription, is not a specified offence. Possession of POMs without a prescription is only an offence if the drug is also controlled under the Misuse of Drugs Act 1971.

Misuse of Drugs Act 1971

The main purpose of this Act is to prevent the non-medical use of certain medicines or drugs. It achieves this by imposing a complete ban on the possession, supply, manufacture, import and export of controlled drugs, except as allowed by regulations or licence from the Secretary of State. In addition to banning the possession of illegal drugs, the Act prohibits their import, export, production and supply. It also makes it illegal to incite another person to do any of the above. It is also an offence to knowingly use or allow usage of premises for drug misuse. Under the Act, cannabis plant cultivation, possession of opium pipes, and possession of hypodermic syringes for illegal drug injection are all banned. Initially, the Act divides drugs into three classes, A, B and C:

- *Class A* includes heroin, cocaine, crack, LSD, ecstasy, 'magic mushrooms', morphine and amphetamines for injection. The penalty for possession of these drugs can be an unlimited fine and/or up to seven years in prison. The penalty for dealing can be an unlimited fine and/or up to life in prison.
- *Class B* includes cannabis, dihydrocodeine, methylphenidate (Ritalin), pholcodine and amphetamines. The penalty for possession of these drugs can be an unlimited fine and/or up to five years in prison. The penalty for dealing can be an unlimited fine and/or up to 14 years in prison.
- *Class C* includes **anabolic steroids**, benzodiazepines, gammahydroxybutyrate (GHB) and ketamine. The penalty for possession of these drugs can be an unlimited fine and/or up to two years in prison. The penalty for dealing can be an unlimited fine and/or up to 14 years in prison.

Because most controlled drugs have medical uses or are of scientific interest, the Act allows the government to authorise possession, supply, production, and import or export of drugs to meet medical or scientific needs. These exemptions are expressed in the form of 'regulations' made under the Act. Controlled drugs are classified as follows:

- *Schedule 1* drugs are the most stringently controlled. They are not authorised for medical use, and can only be supplied, possessed or administered in exceptional circumstances under a special Home Office licence, usually only for research purposes. Examples include cannabis, coca leaf, ecstasy, LSD, raw opium, and psilocin.
- *Schedules 2 and 3* drugs are available for medical use and can be prescribed by doctors. It is illegal to be in possession of these drugs without a doctor's prescription. Schedule 2 drugs include amphetamines, cocaine, dihydrocodeine, dipipanone (Diconal), heroin, methadone, morphine, opium in medicinal form, pethidine, and methylphenidate (Ritalin), and they are subject to strict record-keeping and storage in pharmacies. Schedule 3 drugs include barbiturates, flunitrazepam (Rohypnol), and temazepam tranquillisers, and are subject to restrictions on prescription writing.
- *Schedule 4* is divided into two parts. Part 1 comprises most minor tranquillisers (other than Rohypnol and temazepam) and eight other substances. It is now illegal to be in possession of these minor tranquillisers without a prescription. Part 2 comprises anabolic steroids, which can be legally possessed in medicinal form without a prescription, but they are illegal to supply to other people.
- *Schedule 5* drugs are considered to pose minimal risk of abuse. Some of these are diluted, small-dose, non-injectable preparations that pharmacists can sell over the counter without a prescription, and all may be possessed by anyone. But once bought, they cannot be legally supplied to another person. Among these are some well-known cough medicines, anti-diarrhoea agents and mild painkillers.

An understanding of the Misuse of Drugs Act 1971 is important in the administration of medicines, as well as in prescribing.

Medicinal Products: Prescription by Nurses etc. Act 1992

Non-medical prescribing relates to prescribing by professional groups, other than doctors or dentists, who have been granted prescribing rights. These professionals include nurses, pharmacists, optometrists, midwives and health visitors. In 1992, the Medicinal Products: Prescription by Nurses etc. Act was passed, leading to amendments of the Medicines Act 1968 and the NHS Act 1977. The Act came about as a result of the changes in healthcare and the realisation that there are significant potential benefits to nurses having prescribing rights. These rights now extend to community nurses. There are two types of prescribers: independent prescribers, who would be responsible for the assessment of patients with undiagnosed conditions and for making decisions about the clinical management of these patients, and supplementary prescribers, who would be responsible for the continuing care of patients who have been clinically assessed by an independent prescriber.

Chapter summary

Nurses play an extremely critical role in people's lives, particularly at times when they are most vulnerable. The decisions they make can have a long-term impact on people's physical and mental health. For this reason, it is only proper that nurses should be accountable for their actions and omissions. There is a plethora of legislation that regulates the way nurses practice, such as those based on the ECHR, which states that every human being is entitled to life, that no one should be subjected to degrading and inhuman treatment, and that everyone has a right to privacy. The Mental Capacity Act 2005 gives recognition to the view that everyone should be regarded as mentally capable of deciding for themselves unless proven otherwise. Furthermore, if someone lacks capacity, a procedure for appointing someone to act on behalf of the individual ought to be followed. This Act is closely linked to sections of the Mental Health Act 1983 (amended 2007), which states that treatment can be given to people against their will should criteria be satisfied.

Regarding legislation that deals with the supply and administering of medicines, the Medicines Act 1968 classifies medicines depending on whether a person requires a prescription or not to obtain them. It is not an offence under this Act to be in possession of POMs. However, it is an offence to be in possession of controlled drugs without a prescription under the Misuse of Drugs Act 1971.

Activities: brief outline answers

Activity 1.1 Reflection (page 9)

The answer is 'yes'. To breach Article 2, death does not necessarily need to occur. The hospital policy, as well as good practice, states that vital signs should be recorded regularly if someone is administered intramuscular or intravenous antipsychotic medication. This was not done, therefore putting the patient at material risk. This alone is enough to breach Article 2 of the Human Rights Act 1998.

Activity 1.3 Evidence-based practice and research (page 14)

Article 8 has been breached because the patient had no choice of medication. Article 3 has been breached because of the imposition of antipsychotic drugs resulting in unpleasant side effects.

The outcome was that the case was dismissed, because even if the medical treatment in question and the applicant's lack of choice of therapist had breached Article 8(1), this could be justified under Article 8(2) because of the need to maintain public order and to protect the applicant's own health. As for the patient suffering unpleasant side effects, the patient is not protected under Article 3 because the purpose of giving antipsychotics to the patient was not to inflict side effects, but to treat a psychiatric condition that the patient suffered from.

Activity 1.4 Critical thinking (page 28)

It is unlikely that May lacks capacity. She appears to understand that she needs medication, but it does appear that she is not involved in the decision-making process, and it is therefore not surprising that May finds ways of avoiding medication. The issue of side effects, as well as how to manage them, may be impacting on her willingness to take medication.

Further reading

Griffith, R. and Tengnah, C. (2017) *Law and Professional Issues in Nursing*, 4th edition. Exeter: Learning Matters.

This is a very useful book that covers most aspects of nursing practice law.

Szasz, T. (2009) *Coercion as Cure: A Critical History of Psychiatry*. Piscataway, NJ: Transaction Publishers.

This is an interesting book that looks at ethics from an anti-psychiatry perspective.

Useful websites

www.legislation.gov.uk/ukpga/2007/12/contents

This is the government publication of the entire Mental Health Act 1983 (amended 2007).

www.the-shipman-inquiry.org.uk

Harold Shipman was a GP who murdered his patients, and this inquiry into his conduct sets out recommendations.

Chapter 2 The therapeutic alliance and the promotion of adherence to psychotropic medication

Chapter aims

By the end of this chapter, you should be able to:

* understand adherence and the factors that mediate the concept;
* understand health beliefs and illness perception concepts, as well as their impact on health-seeking behaviours;
* understand the therapeutic alliance and strategies for improving adherence.

Introduction

The treatment of psychological problems goes as far back as the fifth century BC when mental disorders, particularly psychotic disorders, were considered supernatural in origin. Less enlightened treatment of people with mental disorders was prevalent, with those people often labelled as witches and assumed to be inhabited by demons. This view was prevalent during both ancient Greek and Roman times, but early writings in the fourth century BC suggest that even then, the role of biology in mental disorders was recognised, particularly by Hippocrates. The ancient Greek physician considered mental disorders as diseases to be understood in terms of disturbed physiology, rather than reflections of the displeasure of the gods or evidence of demonic possession. However, religious leaders and others who were powerful at the time continued to use forms of exorcism to treat mental disorders, and these methods were often barbaric. It was not until the medieval age that care for the mentally ill significantly changed.

In medieval Europe, from the thirteenth century on, psychiatric hospitals were built to house patients with mental disorders, but they were used only as custodial institutions and did not provide any type of treatment. In complete contrast to the prevailing Christian approach, which relied on demonological explanations for mental illness, the medieval Muslim approach was based mostly on clinical observations. Records also show that from as early as the eighth century BC, Muslims were among the first to provide psychotherapy and moral treatment for those who were mentally ill. Other forms of treatment included baths, medication, music therapy and occupational therapy. In the Western world, it was not until the early 1950s that there was a dramatic change in the treatment and care of people with mental disorders, particularly those with psychosis. This was mainly due to the discovery of antipsychotic medication.

The introduction of psychiatric medications altered the relationship between mental health professionals and their patients. This shift was interpreted as a lack of concern for patients, which in part gave birth to an 'anti-psychiatry' movement in the late twentieth century. This was also due to the much-publicised view that mental illness was a myth and psychiatry was a form of social control. The movement demanded that institutionalised psychiatric care be abolished. Although the popularity of the anti-psychiatry movement has declined, it had the positive outcome of helping mental health professionals become more sensitive to the needs of those with mental health problems.

Now we turn to the role of the nurse in the care of people with mental illness.

The history of the mental health nurse

While the formal recognition of psychiatry occurred early in the nineteenth century with the development of the modern cognitive sciences, psychiatric nursing as a profession was not recognised until the latter part of the century. As with psychiatry in general, mental health nursing suffered from many misinformed theories of cognition and mental illness, leading to practices that would now be deemed counterproductive or even harmful. Subsequent advances in cognition and psychology produced a more balanced approach that combined medical procedures, medicines and cognitive therapy to improve the mental health of the individual. Mental health nursing had difficulties with the shifting environment of the mental health profession, often being caught between competing viewpoints, and this has been reflected in the debate regarding the 'medical model' and the 'psychosocial model' of care.

Where available, care has tended to become more intimate and holistic, taking various approaches and applying them to the complete person, where applicable. This has brought the concepts of medication adherence and the **therapeutic alliance** into being.

This chapter will initially explore the concept of medication adherence before dealing with issues relating to forming an effective therapeutic alliance. The importance of a therapeutic alliance in promoting treatment and recovery will be covered before dealing with strategies for improving patient adherence to medication. The final sections will cover what the patient needs to know, as well as common errors that occur during the formation of a therapeutic alliance.

Medication adherence

The terminology used when discussing medication-taking behaviours is rather complex; according to National Institute for Health and Care Excellence (NICE) guidelines cited by Horne et al. (2005), there are at least three common definitions in use: compliance, adherence and concordance.

- *Compliance.* The extent to which the patient's behaviour matches the prescriber's recommendations.
- *Adherence.* The extent to which the patient's behaviour matches agreed recommendations from the prescriber. Adherence emphasises the need for agreement, and that the patient is free to decide to adhere to the doctor's recommendation or not. In contemporary literature, there is a preference for the term 'adherence' over 'compliance', because we consider adherence to be non-judgemental, whereas 'compliance' carries negative connotations and suggests blame for the patient (Julius et al., 2009).
- *Concordance.* This is a recent term whose meaning has changed. It was initially applied to the consultation process in which the doctor and the patient agree therapeutic decisions that incorporate their respective views, but it now includes patient support in medicine-taking and prescribing communication.

Concordance reflects normative values, but it does not necessarily address medicine-taking behaviour and may not lead to an improvement in adherence. The National Co-ordinating Centre for NHS Service Delivery and Organisation (NCCSDO) recommends using the term 'adherence' to describe patients' medicine-taking behaviour (Horne et al., 2005).

Medication adherence defined

Early conceptions of medication adherence originate from an authoritarian traditional medical model that equated adherence with compliance. A more recent conceptualisation involves medication adherence as a **collaborative process** that includes the patient as an active participant in their own treatment (Inder et al., 2019). This concept of adherence places the therapeutic alliance at the heart of the process, as well as using the relationship between the nurse and the patient as the vehicle for exchanging information and opening a discussion that aims to reach **concordance** about treatment.

From a practical aspect, adherence involves several behaviours that include accessing treatment, obtaining medication, understanding and following instructions about taking medication, and remembering to take medication. When the patient intentionally decides not to adhere to treatment, this non-adherence is voluntary, and it is involuntary where the lack of adherence is unintentional. An example of involuntary non-adherence is when a patient forgets to take their medication.

Nurses may observe that some patients modify, rather than completely accept or abandon, treatment. This behaviour is called *partial adherence*. For example, a patient may only take part of their full dose or may stop and restart treatment sporadically for varying intervals.

Another form of non-adherence is *over-adherence* through possible abuse of prescription medication. An example of this is where there is a requirement for a patient to take, say, one tablet, but instead they take three. This is particularly common in people who are prescribed anti-anxiety or pain relief medicines. A further form of adherence behaviour is *selective adherence*. This is when a patient may choose to be fully adherent to one type of medicine and non-adherent to another. A good example of selective adherence is a person who suffers from depression and diabetes who is fully adherent to medicines for diabetes but is not adherent to antidepressants. We can see from these examples that adherence is a dynamic and changing process that varies in several ways. It is a profound problem, but we should not conceptualise this as the patient's problem. Rather, it reflects a limitation in the delivery of healthcare, often due to a failure to fully agree on the prescription in the first place or to identify and provide the support that patients need later on. Therefore, as a nurse or prescriber, it is important to discuss adherence with the patient repeatedly throughout the treatment process. However, to determine the extent of adherence is a difficult task that will be discussed in a later section. Despite the challenge posed by the measurement of adherence, its importance in the treatment and recovery of people with mental health problems is clear, and it is this that we will discuss next.

The importance of medication adherence

There is enough research evidence to suggest that medication plays a crucial role in determining the outcome and recovery of people suffering from all types of illnesses, and this is also true for those suffering from mental health problems. As such, treatment with **psychotropic medication** plays a pivotal role despite advances in other forms of treatment. There is also evidence to suggest that non-adherence to medication is a widespread problem in all types of illness, including mental illness (Haynes et al., 2008). Relapse of illness due to non-adherence has many personal, social and economic consequences, particularly for those suffering from mental health problems.

Relapse causes patients to suffer distressing symptoms that can lead to hospitalisation. In turn, hospitalisation usually results in disruption to the patient's life, and this can lead to a family losing income, particularly if the patient is the breadwinner. In this regard, unsuccessful management of medication adherence has links with poor clinical response and may be the most common cause of illness relapse. Thus, many people who may benefit from medications do not, and this undermines much of the investment and research in healthcare (Nieuwlaat et al., 2014). In addition, non-adherence to medication has a high economic cost (Cutler et al., 2018). According to NICE (2009a), the NHS in England spent £10.6 billion on drugs, around three-quarters of which was in primary care. The estimate is that between one-half and one-third of all medicines prescribed for long-term conditions, including mental health problems, are not taken as recommended (Horne et al., 2005), and this can lead to patient relapse and hospitalisation.

In people with schizophrenia, the approximate annual total cost of patient hospitalisation due to non-adherence is at least £5,000 per patient per year (Knapp et al., 2004). Evidence also suggests that the intermittent pattern of medication-taking associated with non-adherence increases the incidence of **tardive dyskinesia** (see Chapter 8). Further, prolonged untreated psychosis may diminish the effectiveness of medication treatment, and some researchers have noted that non-adherence to medication has a link with longer hospitalisations and an increase in suicidal behaviour (Qurashi et al., 2006), and this is also true for those in primary care (Saini et al., 2018). These findings are also compatible with a relatively recent study which found that partial adherence and non-adherence to antipsychotics were associated with up to 12-fold risks of completed suicide (Forsman et al., 2019).

From a social perspective, relapse caused by non-adherence in people with psychosis may be more problematic than relapse that occurs while a patient is taking medication, being more severe and disruptive (Torrey, 1994). NICE guidelines assert that 'improving medicines taking may have a far greater impact on clinical outcomes than an improvement in treatments' (NICE, 2009a). Despite the importance of medication adherence, medicine-taking is controversial because it often indicates a fundamental mismatch between the service providers' therapeutic advice and patients' actual illness behaviour (Horne et al., 2005). Further, it has so far not been possible to introduce an accurate way of measuring adherence. We now look at possible solutions to this problem.

The measurement of adherence

It is now known that adherence to medication is not 'all or nothing', and may be partial, irregular or selective. This poses a challenge to nurses who need to estimate adherence accurately, but currently there is no universally agreed method of doing adherence. Current methods of assessing the concept include:

- patient self-reports;
- reports by family members or significant others;
- biological tests;
- pill counts;
- pharmacy refill records;
- electronic methods.

All of these methods have limitations. For example, it has been suggested that self-reporting by patients is potentially unreliable as patients may overestimate or over-report their treatment adherence. In the case of using blood plasma levels of the medicine as a measure of adherence, this method could potentially overestimate adherence to long **half-life** medicines, such as antipsychotics or fluoxetine. Also, the assessment of some medicines with great inter-individual variations of serum levels, such as antidepressants, would be confusing. Although electronic medication packs may provide more reliable information about adherence, associated costs tend to be prohibitive for use in clinical practice. Information from pill count assessments may be unreliable as patients may not necessarily be ingesting the pills after removing them from their packaging.

Clearly, the estimation of adherence is difficult, and an individual's health belief system shapes the concept of adherence. Before proceeding, you may wish to work on Activity 2.1.

Activity 2.1 Reflection

In a group or on your own, discuss and list reasons why a patient may decide to be partially adherent to medication.

An outline answer is provided at the end of the chapter.

Health beliefs and health-seeking behaviour

We can define health-seeking behaviour as any action that an individual who is perceived to have a health problem undertakes for the purpose of finding an appropriate remedy. The behaviour starts with a decision-making process that depends on an individual's family, community values and expectations. A person's characteristics and the behaviour of the healthcare provider also determine health-seeking behaviour. These factors interact to produce a final choice of a health-seeking option that may typically involve recognition of symptoms and the perceived nature of the illness, followed by appropriate care and monitoring.

Several theories that seek to explain health-seeking behaviour are in existence. The most common are the biomedical and health belief models.

The biomedical model

Early biomedical theories were formulated in terms of the institutionally defined roles of 'authority' and 'supplicant' (the patient). In this approach, the doctor prescribes and the patient complies with the medication regimen. This autocratic outlook views non-adherence as a failing of the patient through lack of knowledge, motivation and will. Vestiges of this approach are occasionally witnessed, particularly when people use expressions such as 'the patient failed the treatment', but usually there is little research evidence to support these biases because – as seen later – no specific patient characteristic consistently relates to non-adherence behaviour.

Despite obvious flaws in the biomedical model, it has several aspects that may be useful. First, it makes a critical contribution to the concept of adherence by specifying several factors that impact on medication adherence. Among these is the prescribed treatment regimen as the criterion against which we evaluate adherence behaviour. The biomedical model also focuses on medication side effects as undesirable outcomes that affect medication adherence and efficacy. This model has shown endurance in the face of other models that potentially have more explanatory value. One such model is the health belief model.

The health belief model

The health belief model was first developed in the 1950s by social psychologists Godfrey Hochbaum, Irwin Rosenstock and Stephen Kegels, working in the United States Public Health Service. It was developed in response to the failure of a free tuberculosis health screening programme, and since then the health belief model has been adapted to explore a variety of long- and short-term health behaviours, including sexual risk behaviours and the transmission of HIV/AIDS. It attempts to explain and predict health behaviours of people by focusing on the attitudes and beliefs of individuals. It considers five main areas that are likely to influence health-seeking behaviour. Put simply, from the patient's viewpoint, these are as follows:

- *Perceived susceptibility*: Am I going to get the disease?
- *Perceived seriousness*: How bad would it be?
- *Perceived benefits and barriers*: How easy would it be to get something done about it? What is it going to cost me?
- *Self-efficacy*: Am I able to make any changes?
- *Cues to action*: OK, now I am going to do something about it!

Perceived susceptibility

For a given condition, a patient will have a perception of how susceptible they are to develop the illness. They may base this perception on experience: they might have a parent or sibling with the disease, and therefore convince themselves that they too will get it. Conversely, they may feel that they are somehow not vulnerable to certain diseases. For example, you may have come across a smoker who refuses to give up smoking because the person knows a lifelong smoker who has never had any health problems. Another important factor that shapes the perception of susceptibility is awareness of illness, and this is particularly relevant in people with psychosis. When someone believes they are not suffering from an illness, the person is unlikely to feel susceptible to the illness despite the presence of symptoms and may offer an alternative explanation for these symptoms.

Perceived seriousness

Patients differ in how serious they consider different conditions to be, and this interacts with their perception of susceptibility. For instance, a patient may be at low risk of developing bowel cancer, but since the person perceives it as a very serious condition they may feel the motivation to see the doctor about persistent loose stools. Another patient may consider a headache a triviality and feel that seeing the doctor will be a waste of the doctor's time, and therefore possibly fail to have a serious condition diagnosed.

Perception of seriousness can affect not only if a patient presents to a healthcare service, but also where they present. If a patient feels that coughing up green phlegm is serious, they may consult their doctor; but if the patient considers it trivial, they may take the problem to a pharmacist. This last point is important because it also interacts with cultural factors. Before proceeding further, complete Activity 2.2.

Activity 2.2   Critical thinking

Julio is a 33-year-old man who has a long history of reluctance to seek help from psychiatric services even though he suffers from an unspecified psychotic illness. Although Julio acknowledges that he becomes unwell, he believes that this is due to a jealous relative who cast an evil spell on him when he was a child in South America. He has on several occasions travelled to South America to see a traditional healer who 'exorcised' the evil spirit.

• Is Julio's view of his condition invalid?

An outline answer is provided at the end of the chapter.

Perceived benefits and barriers

Quite often patients face different options in choosing how to deal with their health concerns. They will often weigh up the potential benefits and drawbacks to each course of action and consider any perceived potential barriers to health-seeking activity. How patients decide which route to take, as well as the importance they attach to individual benefits, disadvantages and barriers, may differ markedly from person to person. These perceived benefits and barriers generally interact with the concept of self-efficacy.

Self-efficacy

Self-efficacy describes how people view their own ability to carry out a particular action. We define self-efficacy as people's beliefs about their capabilities to exercise control over events that affect their lives, as well as their beliefs in their capabilities to mobilise the motivation, cognitive resources, and courses of action needed to exercise control over task demands (Bandura, 1977). Therefore, self-efficacy attributions are concerned not with the skills one has, but with the judgements of what one can do with whatever skills one possesses. This includes a patient's perception of how likely they are to change behaviours. For example, a patient may realise that if he stops taking medication for his heart condition, he may well relapse and die from heart disease. Although he has spoken with his GP on several occasions and has been assisted to continue taking medication, he thinks that he will never be able to continue taking medication for the rest of his life, so does not think it worth the bother of seeking help to continue taking medication. A perception of low self-efficacy is the barrier to taking action in this case.

Cues to action

Even when a patient develops a perception about their health, there is usually a trigger to turn this into action. From a communication viewpoint, the nurse or prescriber will want to uncover what triggered a patient to seek healthcare. The possible triggers may be quite varied (e.g. the media, a relative, an overheard conversation, a reminder letter). Such a prompt may increase a patient's perception of their susceptibility to a disease or of its seriousness. It may remind them of the increased benefits of seeking healthcare. The prompt may increase the patient's motivation to change or convince them that they may in fact be able to make any required changes themselves. Like all theoretical models, the health belief model has some limitations. For this reason, it has been modified over time through the influence of modifiers such as culture, society and the media, as well as demographic factors. Other health-seeking models based on illness perception have been formulated.

The self-regulatory model

The basis of illness perception models in mental health is the self-regulatory model (SRM) (Leventhal and Ian, 2012). In turn, the SRM is built on at least four components:

- People are active problem-solvers and they strive to make sense of their world as they search for suitable, effective ways of controlling and adapting to their world.
- Multilevel information processing, which includes both emotional and intellectual levels, drives people's conceptualisations of health threats.
- There is simultaneous generation of emotional reactions and intellectual notions of a disease and its treatment.
- Contextual factors, including cultural, environmental and social relationships and personality dispositions, influence the way that individuals understand health threats and how they manage them.

Because of its reliability and **validity** in exploring important patient beliefs across a range of physical illnesses, the SRM currently enjoys wide usage, and it allows us to make advances in understanding self-management of and recovery from illnesses. Much of the work carried out in mental illness is consistent with this model.

As previously mentioned, Leventhal and Ian (2012) first conceptualised the SRM in the late 1970s when they examined how fear messages in relatively acute situations might lead people to take health-promoting actions, such as wearing seat belts or giving up smoking. They found that people need different types of information to influence attitudes and actions to a perceived threat to health and well-being.

The SRM proposes that during illness, two parallel processes are in operation: first, the intellectual or objective interpretation of the threat to health; and second, the emotional or subjective reaction to the threat to health. These parallel processes of intellect and emotion are interactive. For example, adherence to medication in mental health includes intellectual processing of information to understand the complex relationship between medication adherence and the diminishing of symptoms. However, socioculturally related emotional values about illness and medication-taking experiences may be more important than intellectual processes. In such situations, people may choose not to take medication because they feel a social obligation not do so. Before proceeding further, undertake Activity 2.3.

Activity 2.3 Reflection

Alone or in a group, think of a situation where a person recognises that they are ill but decides not to seek treatment. It may be that you have been in this position yourself.

• What factors might be influencing the person not to seek treatment?

An outline answer is provided at the end of the chapter.

The key beliefs identified in the SRM refer to a specific illness episode rather than intellectual beliefs about a potential illness. In applying the SRM to physical illness, it is possible to identify five specific components as key to guiding an individual reaction to a threat to health. The original four components are:

• the perceived identity of the illness (including a label and signs/symptoms);
• the perceived consequences (physical, social and behavioural);
• the causes of the illness;
• the timeline or sense of how long the illness will last.

A fifth belief about the potential for control or cure of the illness has also been added to the model.

Although originally developed around physical illness, the SRM is also applicable to mental health situations. A good example is that of hypochondriasis. This condition begins when an individual believes they have an illness in response to a perception of bodily sensations. The individual's viewpoint is that they have a serious illness, but medical investigations do not confirm this view, and the medical practitioner's view is that the patient is experiencing anxiety. Repeated reassurance does not work in the long term because it fails to provide the individual with an alternative coherent argument that explains why they experience the bodily sensations. Until this is provided, re-experiencing the bodily sensations will trigger the old belief in the illness and the accompanying concern.

There is considerable support for the model. For example, how an individual summarises and labels these experiences may have an important impact on their responses, and this is linked to a perception of quality of life. Mechanic et al. (1994) found that people who attributed their mental illness to a physical, medical or biological problem, as opposed to psychological problems, scored higher on a perceived quality of life measure, as well as reporting less personal stigma and greater self-esteem. Also, the dimension of the likely consequences of having a health problem on their daily lives has an association with variations in coping levels, depression and medication adherence. This leads to our understanding of how some patients with certain types of illness might cope during illness episodes.

Patients suffering from schizophrenia, for example, can identify strategies they use to cope with their symptoms. Their beliefs about the likely consequences of symptoms appear to influence this relationship. For example, Kinney (1999) showed that patients who perceived their symptoms as more taxing and burdensome were more likely to report difficulties in coping.

Overall, evidence suggests that the SRM is a potentially useful way to understand health-seeking behaviour, although this approach may require modifications before it can be usefully employed in people suffering from psychosis. For example, Kinderman and Bentall (1997) reported that patients experiencing psychosis did not identify their experiences as separate 'illnesses' and did not have 'illness beliefs', which makes it difficult to apply the model without modifications. Those patients who are in remission conceptualise their experiences as separate from their normal behaviour and use a conceptual framework that differs significantly from conventional health belief models.

Finally, it is important to recognise that the illness models in use, which help to increase our understanding of people's responses to mental health problems, are theoretical. They are tools to help nurses in potentially important areas of intervention. These conceptualisations have limitations and cannot replace an individual's perception of illness, which provides a far more complex and useful guide to understanding their illness and what it means for them. If we integrate health-seeking behaviour theories into our understanding of adherence to psychotropic medicines, it is possible to divide factors that pertain to adherence into three broad areas: those that relate to the patient, the illness and the treatment.

Factors influencing adherence

If we integrate the role of health belief and illness perception models, we can see that adherence is a complex behavioural process strongly influenced by the environments in which people live and work, the healthcare provider's culture, and the healthcare system's way of delivering care. Health belief and illness perception models are associated with people's knowledge and beliefs about their illness, their motivation to manage it, their confidence in their ability to engage in illness management behaviours, their expectations regarding the outcome of treatment, and the consequences of poor adherence.

It is important to recognise that a person may have multiple risk factors for medication non-adherence. Also, the factors that influence a person's medication-taking behaviour may change over time. Because of the dynamic nature of these factors, nurses need to assess a person's adherence throughout the course of treatment. Furthermore, because there is usually no single reason for non-adherence, there can be no 'one-size-fits-all' approach to improving adherence. Before we discuss strategies for enhancing medication adherence, we need to discuss factors that have been identified to predict adherence.

Illness-related factors

In mental health, there is consistent evidence supporting the link between medication adherence and severity of illness, called 'condition-related factors' in Figure 2.1. For example, in those suffering from psychotic illness, the severity of symptoms such as

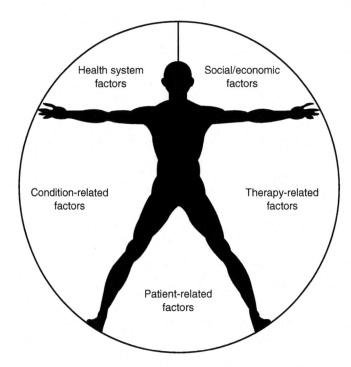

Figure 2.1   The factors associated with adherence to medication (adapted from WHO, 2003, p27)

paranoia, hostility and delusional beliefs has been linked to poor adherence to medication. One of the earliest studies to identify this link was by Van Putten et al. (1976), who identified the severity of grandiose delusions as particularly predictive of poor adherence. Additionally, people with more severe negative symptoms, such as motivational impairment, are likely to be non-adherent to medication according to some studies (Subotnik et al., 2014).

A relatively recent prospective longitudinal study examined the relationship between adherence and symptoms in a group of patients suffering from schizophrenia. The investigators found that those who were non-adherent with medication had worse positive symptoms (Subotnik et al., 2014). Thus, across a wide range of mental illnesses, the severity of illness has an association with poor medication adherence. Before proceeding further, complete Activity 2.4.

Activity 2.4 Critical thinking

Chris is a 41-year-old man who believes he has telepathic powers and does not like watching television because he can hear his name being discussed on the TV. From time to time, he says he hears 'the voice of God' telling him to leave his flat and sleep on the streets. He does not believe that he suffers from a mental illness, and therefore he is reluctant to take medication.

- Can you suggest factors that may lead someone to think they have no mental health problems despite evidence to the contrary?

An outline answer is provided at the end of the chapter.

Awareness of illness (insight) and adherence

The relationship between awareness of illness and adherence has been studied in a wide variety of settings, such as at hospital admission, on discharge, post-discharge and in outpatient clinics. In people with psychosis, awareness of illness or **insight** consistently predicts adherence behaviour (Garcia et al., 2016; Sendt et al., 2015). This is further buttressed by a relatively recent study that combined samples from the Clinical Antipsychotics Trials of Intervention Effectiveness (CATIE) and the European First Episode Schizophrenia Trial (EUFEST). The study found that poor adherence to psychotropic medication has an association with impaired insight (Czobor et al., 2015).

Adverse side effects and adherence

Many medicines for the treatment of mental health problems, though effective at controlling symptoms, have adverse side effects, making many patients reluctant to take them. The problem of non-adherence due to adverse side effects is probably more acute in people suffering from psychosis. Older or conventional antipsychotic medicines such as chlorpromazine, haloperidol and zuclopenthixol (Clopixol) tend to cause a wide variety of adverse side effects. In a systematic review of 13 observational studies of people taking antipsychotics, the investigators found that adverse side effects were modestly and inconsistently associated with adherence with medication (Sendt et al., 2015). In people suffering from depression, antidepressant side effects such as sedation, sexual dysfunction and dry mouth can influence whether people take medicines or not (Hung, 2014). Moreover, people on antidepressants tend to discontinue taking them within the first 12 weeks of treatment. In some situations, patients may not be willing to take medication because of their pre-existing attitudes towards it.

Attitudes towards medication and adherence

Case study: Mark

Mark is a 23-year-old university student who was admitted to a ward because he believed he could not cope with his coursework. He became increasingly isolated at university and expressed suicidal ideas. He was prescribed antidepressants by his doctor, but he refused to take them for fear of becoming dependent on medication. He was, however, prepared to see a psychologist to talk about his problems.

The case of Mark illustrates a common attitude towards medication. He is reluctant to take prescribed medication, but nevertheless acknowledges that he needs treatment. For this reason, he is prepared to see a psychologist. Whether or not someone takes medication depends very much on their attitude towards it.

A patient's attitude towards treatment is an important factor in medication adherence, and several factors influence attitudes (see the earlier sections on health beliefs and health-seeking behaviour). There is abundant evidence to support a relationship between adherence and attitudes towards medication. In the area of psychosis, one of the earliest studies to find such a relationship was by Van Putten et al. (1976), who examined the reactions of 29 patients who habitually refused medication and 30 patients who readily took medication. They found that those patients who refused medication experienced an **ego-syntonic** grandiose psychosis after they discontinued medication. In contrast, those who consistently complied with medication developed **decompensation**, characterised by effects such as depression and anxiety. This finding has been confirmed by at least 20 studies that examined a link between adherence and attitudes towards medication. Further, a systematic review and meta-analysis of 14 studies that examined attitudes and adherence found that a positive attitude towards medication had an association with a better adherence to antipsychotic medication (Richardson et al., 2013). Other studies have found a role for the therapeutic alliance in medication adherence.

The therapeutic alliance and adherence

There is a general acceptance that the quality of communication between the mental health nurse and the patient contributes to the welfare of patients in every aspect. Patients regard nurses and doctors as respectable and trustworthy sources of health information, and this suggests that the health advice nurses and doctors give may have a greater impact than that from other sources. Also, the attitude of the nurse or prescriber can influence patients with mental health problems, and this can affect whether they take medication or not. Furthermore, a beneficial therapeutic alliance between patients and staff is one of many effective strategies for improving treatment retention, adherence and subsequent outcomes. Proactive patients, autonomous individuals who feel respected as a treatment partner and who express confidence in their healthcare environment, tend to fare better than patients who lack a voice in their own treatment course (Zeber et al., 2008).

With regard to improving adherence to medication, there is indirect evidence suggesting that a positive relationship with the nurse or prescriber is essential (Chakrabarti, 2018). A patient's perception of the nurse or prescriber's interest in them, as well as how they explain the reasons for taking medication and its side effects, all seem crucial in creating a positive therapeutic relationship. A strong therapeutic relationship based on trust, clear information and reinforcement via educational programmes using patients' coffee groups showed improvement in adherence with medication, according to findings by Dorevitch et al. (1993). Another study exploring patients' attitudes to a collaborative care model, as well as how individuals with bipolar disorder perceive treatment adherence, supports this finding. These individuals perceived the ideal collaborative model as one in which the patient has specific responsibilities, such as coming to appointments and sharing information, and in which the provider likewise has specific responsibilities, such as keeping abreast of current 'state-of-the-art' prescribing practices and being a good listener. Treatment adherence was identified as a self-managed responsibility within the larger context of the collaborative model. The study places emphasis on the interactional component within the patient–health provider relationship, particularly with respect to times when the individual may be more symptomatic and more impaired (Sajatovic et al., 2005). In patients with schizophrenia, a study found that a better therapeutic relationship is associated with better medication adherence (Tessier et al., 2017). In summary, the therapeutic alliance between the practitioner and the patient is a necessary factor in medication adherence, and later sections will continue this discussion. An equally important factor in medication adherence is the role of socio-economic factors. There is also enough evidence to suggest that socio-environmental factors influence medication adherence.

Socio-environmental factors

The more support people get from family and friends or significant others, the better the outcome in any health intervention. The evidence shows that patients living with family members are likely to be more adherent to medication, and this is particularly true for those suffering from psychotic illnesses. As early as 1984, Caton and colleagues noted that involving families in planning the discharge of patients from hospital can improve adherence and treatment outcomes (Caton et al., 1984). Several studies support this finding, including one by Olfson et al. (2000), who found that patients with families who refuse involvement in their care are at high risk of non-adherence to antipsychotics. Further, a relatively recent systematic review and meta-analysis of 13 observational studies found that social support in younger patients has an association with good adherence with antipsychotic medication (Sendt et al., 2015). In other long-term conditions such as HIV, good social support has a direct link with better adherence to antiretroviral medication (Cox, 2002). Similarly, the emotional environment of the patient's family appears to play a role in medication adherence (Scott et al., 2012; Wang et al., 2017b).

In schizophrenia and related disorders, high levels of critical comments by significant others have an association with early relapse. In a study of patients with bipolar disorder, low levels of medication adherence were seen in patients who perceive high levels of criticism and who have a family member with poor knowledge and understanding (Scott et al., 2012). In a later study, the rehospitalisation rate of patients with high expressed emotion (HEE) caregivers was higher than in those with low expressed emotion (LEE) caregivers (Wang et al., 2017b). These findings support earlier findings about the important role that **expressed emotion** plays in medication adherence (Sellwood et al., 2003). More importantly, there is some evidence supporting the use of family intervention techniques to improve adherence with medication and reduce relapse in those suffering from schizophrenia (Pharoah et al., 2010; Zhao et al., 2015). In summary, there is abundant evidence suggesting that negative socio-environmental factors impact negatively on medication adherence. Similarly, the use of **psychoactive** substances, such as cannabis, is known to retard recovery because it makes a patient's non-adherence to medication worse. Before the role of psychoactive substances is discussed, complete Activity 2.5.

Activity 2.5   Critical thinking

Jane is a 35-year-old single woman who lives with her two young children on the sixth floor of a high-rise building owned by the council. She has suffered from depression since her first child was born and she is prescribed antidepressants. As she cannot often go out in the evenings, her social life is restricted, and there are no family members living nearby. She accepts that the medication helps, but she finds it difficult to be fully adherent to her treatment.

- What factors impede Jane from being fully adherent to her medication?

An outline answer is provided at the end of the chapter.

Substance misuse and adherence to medication

Most mental health nurses or prescribers will have come across some patients suffering from a mental health problem who also use illicit drugs or alcohol. These patients are commonly referred to as suffering from a **dual diagnosis** or **co-morbid substance misuse**. Previous research has consistently established that patients with a dual diagnosis are less likely to adhere to medication (Jonsdottir et al., 2013; Kashner et al., 1991). A relatively early study by Kashner et al. (1991) discovered that patients who abuse substances are 13 times more likely to be non-adherent to medication than those who do not. More recently, a systematic review of 13 observational studies concluded that lower rates of substance abuse have an association with better adherence with antipsychotic medication in people with schizophrenia (Sendt et al., 2015). Overall, there is accumulating evidence supporting the negative role that psychoactive substances play in medication adherence.

However, even if there is an improvement in factors pertaining to adherence, there are a variety of reasons why some patients are unlikely to experience the full benefit of medication because of its limited efficacy.

Benefits and limitations of medication

Despite the effectiveness of medication in assisting people with mental health problems, there may occasionally be patients who fail to respond to these medicines. This is because, despite evidence of efficacy, most patients show an **idiosyncratic response** to psychotropic medication. In other words, while a medication might be effective in one individual, the same medicine and dosage could be totally ineffective in a second person or cause severe adverse effects in a third person. Considering this situation, when is non-adherence to medication a problem? As early as 1997, Weiden et al. (1997) suggested that non-adherence to medication is a problem only in situations where treatment is effective. Therefore, a necessary step towards understanding non-adherence behaviour is first to understand medication effectiveness.

For example, if we consider the efficacy of antipsychotic medicines, we may find that most patients continue to have symptoms despite being on medication, and many others will relapse even if they are taking medication. In addition, it is well known that some psychotropic medication causes adverse side effects such as Parkinsonism, akathisia and dystonia (see Chapter 7). Patients experiencing these side effects are less likely to be adherent with medication, which in turn compromises outcomes. The newer generation of antipsychotic medicines, such as olanzapine, have much lower neurological side effects profiles, but they can cause other problems such as weight gain and sexual dysfunction. With respect to antidepressants, the older or classical antidepressants, such as the **tricyclics**, have adverse side effects such as **sedation** and **cardiotoxicity**, and can induce movement disorders. The newer antidepressants, such as the selective serotonin reuptake inhibitors (SSRIs), can cause sleep disturbance and sexual dysfunction. The problem of poor effectiveness of medication also occurs for those taking antidepressants and anti-anxiety medication. Therefore, even if patients are adherent to medication, some are disappointed by its lack of efficacy, so it may not be fair to call someone non-adherent when they are only gaining a modest benefit from medication. In cases where patients find medication helpful, nurses and prescribers need strategies for improving adherence. To enable the nurse to work effectively with patients, nurses and prescribers need to develop a therapeutic alliance with patients.

The therapeutic alliance

In the classical medical relationship, the person receiving the help is the patient and the person making the decisions is the doctor. There is the expectation that the patient complies with the doctor's orders as a passive recipient of help. Further, the doctor decides who is sick by providing them with a sick certificate. In turn, there is the expectation that the sick person adopts a sick role. Unfortunately, this paternalistic approach is fraught with problems. Also, the growth of consumerism means that patients are increasingly taking an active part in their treatment. More importantly, there is research evidence suggesting that people who play an active role in their treatment are more likely to recover a lot quicker than those who play a passive role (Zeber et al., 2008). As a mental health nurse, the need to establish a therapeutic relationship or alliance is a basic tenet of your practice. It is an essential tool that facilitates effective care. So, what is a therapeutic alliance?

The therapeutic alliance has been discussed in the psychotherapy literature for nearly a century, and historically it was the first concept to be developed to capture the special role of the patient–psychotherapist relationship. The therapeutic alliance is described as a patient's capacity to collaborate productively with the nurse or the prescriber because there is the perception that they are helping professionals with good intentions. In other words, the goals of treatment, as well as the tasks needed to accomplish those goals, generally involve an agreement between the nurse and the prescriber. Furthermore, there should be a sense of a personal bond between the nurse or the prescriber and the patient. In 1912, Sigmund Freud outlined the first references to the therapeutic alliance by highlighting its importance as a vehicle for success in psychoanalysis (Levy, 1982). In this regard, one of the most consistent findings emerging from psychotherapy research is that the quality of the therapeutic alliance is a robust predictor of outcomes across a range of different treatments. Conversely, a weak or ruptured alliance correlates with treatment drop-out. In some instances, it is possible to assume that the quality of the therapeutic alliance is more important than the type of psychotherapy in predicting positive therapeutic outcomes (Safran et al., 2011).

In a landmark **empirical study**, the therapeutic alliance was found to have the same effect on outcomes, regardless of whether the treatment was psychotherapy or **pharmacotherapy**. In another study, Krupnick et al. (1996) examined 225 individuals with depression having outpatient treatment and either interpersonal psychotherapy, cognitive behavioural therapy (CBT), medication with clinical management, or a placebo with clinical management. The study found that the quality of the therapeutic alliance accounted for most of the variance in treatment outcomes, regardless of the kind of therapy. These findings are now supported by a relatively recent systematic review of 17 studies that examined the relationship between the effects of the clinician–patient alliance and communication on treatment adherence. The systematic review revealed that there is a consistent association between a good therapeutic relationship with treatment adherence of all types (Thompson and McCabe, 2012). As a result, there is the suggestion that a good therapeutic alliance is a prerequisite for all therapies.

Regarding medication adherence, there is evidence to suggest that a relatively strong therapeutic alliance during the opening phase of treatment may be the best predictor of a good outcome. Another important study that underscored the role of the therapeutic alliance found that patients with schizophrenia who are adherent to prescribed medications are more likely to be satisfied with their doctor, to feel that their doctor understands them, and to feel that their treating doctor has their best interest at heart (Marder et al., 1983).

Developing a therapeutic alliance

Mental health nurses can help to foster a positive alliance with the patient by identifying both with patient treatment goals and with those healthy aspects of the patient's self that are striving to reach these goals. A patient will then experience their nurse as a collaborator who is working with them rather than against them. Developing a good alliance with patients requires the nurse not only to be positive and empathetic, but also to work within a collaborative framework – a partnership in which the patient sees themselves as a respected participant.

Gabbard (2005) provides a good example of how to foster a therapeutic relationship, and notes that the 'therapeutic alliance may be the most essential element of adherence'. Therefore, the nurse should collaborate with the patient to identify mutually agreed treatment goals and strategies, including medications, and view the patient as a key stakeholder in the treatment planning process. Sharing decision-making between the patient and the nurse to determine the most appropriate treatment approach should be the focus of adherence. The nurse listens to the patient with empathy to build a strong relationship with them. This involves identifying patient concerns regarding medications and addressing any barriers to adherence that the nurse may identify to establish a strong nurse–patient therapeutic alliance. At the same time, the nurse needs to be aware of their own feelings that may arise in dealing with the non-adherent patient. Patients and nurses do not always agree on the causes of non-adherence. By discussing patients' perceptions regarding medications, the nurse can address the patient's concerns without assuming that they already know the barriers which may be contributing to adherence problems.

In people with schizophrenia, establishing rapport with the patient can be challenging. However, a therapeutic alliance with a patient increases the likelihood of the patient staying in therapy, adhering to prescribed medications and achieving a better outcome. In his discussion of the therapeutic alliance, Gabbard (2005) notes that mental health professionals ought to be innovative and find some common ground with patients, such as music, films, holiday places and sports. This allows the patient and nurse to share common interests and provides an opportunity for the therapeutic relationship to grow. If the patient expresses delusions, the nurse should neither challenge nor confirm these, but should view them as metaphors that can provide insights into the patient's inner conflicts.

The nurse can further help to foster the alliance by focusing on a patient's strengths, and accepting without judgement bizarre behaviour, feelings and thoughts that others do not understand. As the alliance develops, the nurse can work with the patient to identify specific relapse triggers to assist the patient in relapse prevention.

As noted above, engaging patients with schizophrenia in a therapeutic alliance can be difficult. The process can take up to six months, and it is important to remain optimistic, even if the patient is not engaging in the collaborative therapeutic relationship after several months. Frank and Gunderson (1990) assert that if there is no formation of an alliance after six months, then there is a need to re-evaluate the therapy.

In establishing a therapeutic alliance with individuals with depression, the nurse should simply listen and empathise with the patient's point of view while attempting to gain a better comprehension of the patient's understanding of the illness. It is important to empathise with the painfulness of the depression and to enlist the patient's help in a collaborative search for the underlying causes. It is also important to avoid making 'cheerleading' comments such as 'You have so much to live for'. These comments are often understood to be a lack of empathy, and can lead to the patient feeling worse and not understood. Also, it is important to avoid interpreting a patient's behaviour or mood. Typically, the nurse should avoid making statements such as 'You are not really depressed – you're angry', as the patient may understand this as a lack of empathy by the nurse. In addition to developing a sound therapeutic alliance with the patient, the nurse should aim to understand strategies in common use to improve adherence.

Strategies for improving adherence to medication

Medicine-taking is a complex human behaviour, and patients evaluate medicines – and the risks and benefits of medicines – using the resources available to them. As has been said previously, there is growing acceptance that non-adherence to medication is a significant problem that affects recovery and outcomes in people with mental health problems. Despite this, there is insufficient evidence for the use of interventions that target the specific factors causing non-adherence. This is due in part to the complex multifactorial nature of the concept of adherence, and the measurement of adherence is problematic. However, interventions such as psychotherapy have had some measure of success in alleviating poor medication adherence.

The nurse can use several intervention strategies, such as alliance-building, motivational interviewing, psychoeducation, psychotherapy and/or CBT. NICE guidelines (NICE, 2009a) suggest the observation of some general principles in improving adherence, and these are as follows.

Concept summary: key principles on adherence (NICE, 2009a)

- Healthcare professionals should work in such a way as to involve individual patients in decisions about their medicines at the level they wish.
- Establish the most effective way of communicating with each patient.
- Offer all patients the opportunity to be involved in making decisions about prescribed medicines. Establish what level of involvement in decision-making the patient would like.
- Be aware that increasing patient involvement may mean that the patient decides not to take or to stop taking a medicine. If in the healthcare professional's view this could have an adverse effect, then the information provided to the patient on risks and benefits, as well as the patient's decision, should be recorded.
- Accept that the patient has the right to decide not to take a medicine, even if the nurse does not agree with the decision, as long as the patient has the capacity to make an informed decision and has been provided with the information needed to make such a decision.
- Be aware that patients' concerns about medicines, and whether they believe they need them, affect how and whether they take their prescribed medicines.
- Offer patients information that is relevant to their condition, potential treatments and personal circumstances. The information should be easy to understand and free from jargon.
- Recognise that non-adherence is common and that most patients are non-adherent sometimes. The nurse should routinely assess adherence in a non-judgemental way in all prescribing, dispensing and reviewing of medicines.
- Be aware that although patients can improve adherence, there is no specific intervention which is suitable for all patients. Tailor any intervention to increase adherence to the specific difficulties with adherence that the patient is experiencing.
- Review patient knowledge, understanding and concerns about medicines, and the patient's view of their need for medicine, at intervals with the agreement of the patient, because these may change over time. Offer repeat information and review to patients, especially when treating long-term conditions with multiple medicines.

Psychotherapy

Psychological counselling may produce an emotional improvement that can increase the desire and ability of some patients to improve self-care. This is particularly so for those who are depressed, and there is some evidence to support the use of psychotherapy to improve medication adherence. It is assumed that by coming to understand their treatment rights and responsibilities, patients can break the cycle. Improvements in feelings of self-worth and independence may then produce positive behavioural outcomes, which may include improvement in adherence to medication. Thus, addressing depression using psychotherapy appears to be a logical approach for some non-adherent patients.

Psychoeducation

Psychoeducation is a specific form of education that aims to help people with mental health problems to access the facts about a broad range of mental illnesses in a clear and concise manner. It is also a way of accessing and learning strategies to deal with mental illness and its effects. It remains a consistently popular tool for families and carers to use to make sense of what is happening to a person who is experiencing a mental health problem, as well as helping them to care for that person. With regard to improving medication adherence, psychoeducation has been the mainstay intervention, although evidence is modest. A systematic review of 13 studies evaluated psychoeducational interventions for patients' families, and patients' responses showed that an increase in knowledge about depression and its treatment had an association with better prognosis in depression, as well as with the reduction of the psychosocial burden for the family (Tursi et al., 2013). This finding is supported by recent systematic reviews of 16 studies that evaluated the role of psychoeducation in adherence with medication in people with bipolar disorder. The study found that psychoeducation appears to be effective in preventing relapse in bipolar disorder (Bond and Anderson, 2015). Other studies that have directly examined the relationship between adherence and psychoeducation support its effectiveness (Chen et al., 2019; Rahmani et al., 2016).

Many of these psychoeducation strategies involve individual or group counselling sessions and/or use of written and audiovisual materials on diagnoses, medications and side effects. For maximum benefit, we can use psychoeducation in conjunction with other therapies.

CBT

CBT is a form of psychotherapy that emphasises the importance of finding new ways of thinking and behaving to deal with current problems. It conceptualises adherence as a coping behaviour that has its basis in the individual's perception of their illness and their beliefs about medications. Hence, interventions that have their basis in CBT seek to assist the patient in questioning their automatic thoughts regarding medication. The emphasis on CBT is to help the patient mentally link medication adherence to symptom reduction and personal health. The nurse should follow a programme manual and have several individual sessions with patients.

However, there is only modest evidence to support the use of CBT in improving adherence in people with mental health problems. A Cochrane systematic review of 182 randomised controlled trials found that only five studies reported improvements in both adherence and clinical outcomes, and no common intervention characteristics were apparent. Even the most effective interventions did not lead to large improvements in adherence or clinical outcomes. The authors concluded that across the body of evidence, effects were inconsistent from study to study (Nieuwlaat et al., 2014).

Other behavioural approaches to improve adherence include conditioning, rewards, cues, reminders and skills training. These interventions seek to promote, modify and reinforce behaviours related to adherence in patients, including those with psychotic disorders. More recently, motivational interviewing principles have been added to CBT approaches to enhance adherence.

Communication style: motivational interviewing

Motivational interviewing is a directive, client-centred counselling style for stimulating behaviour change in people by helping them to explore and resolve **ambivalence**. In practice, this means that the content of the session centres on the individual's viewpoint (i.e. it is person-centred). In addition, the therapist uses the spirit of motivational interviewing to guide the discussion in the direction of behaviour change (directive) through the resolution of ambivalence. Therefore, the focus on the resolution of ambivalence is central and the therapist is deliberately directive in following this objective. Motivational interviewing has many applications in the health field, including the treatment of addictions. Before we go further, we need to discuss the concept of motivation within the context of motivational interviewing.

Case study: Jane

Jane is a 24-year-old female who has been admitted to hospital and has a diagnosis of paranoid schizophrenia. She was brought in involuntarily by the police for displaying violent behaviour, and she said that ward staff, the police and her mum were conspiring to poison her. She believes that she does not suffer from any mental illness and refused all food and medication. She has had two previous admissions to hospital since the age of 20. She has a history of medication non-adherence and each of these admissions to hospital were under the Mental Health Act 1983 (amended 2007).

Motivation

It is easy to confuse lack of motivation with lack of activity, but the two are different. For example, a person may have an inner desire (motivation) to take medication but fail to achieve this (lack of activity) for a variety of reasons. Equally, a person may take medication due to external factors without having the motivation to do so. Therefore, when these external factors disappear, the person may stop taking medication again. To put this differently, you can change a person's behaviour by applying external punitive action if they do not take their medication. The person is likely to take their medication but is also likely to stop once the punitive action stops. In the above case study, Jane most likely took her medication while in hospital because of external factors but stopped taking her medication when she was discharged from hospital. A more lasting approach is to motivate the individual so that they decide for themselves to want to take their medication. This desire or intrinsic motivation to take their medication will still be present despite barriers or pressure from other people to stop taking their medication. The nurse should apply these principles to support and encourage the patient through the process of behaviour change, and this requires specific skills. One of the most important skills is to gain a patient's confidence and to work collaboratively with them.

Collaboration

A collaborative approach is at the heart of motivational interviewing, and is one that emphasises working together with patients as equal partners in a relationship that is supportive and conducive of change. In the above case study, it is important that Jane sees herself as an equal partner in the treatment process where her views are valued. In this regard, the relationship should not be – or be perceived as – coercive. During the collaborative process, the nurse's own awareness of their own motives, values and views is vital in ensuring that they do not impose these on others. Another useful and necessary skill of motivational interviewing is evocation.

Evocation

Evocation is about the nurse's own skills to listen to, understand and remind the patient of their own reasons for change. Although the nurse may have their own views on why the patient should take medication, the emphasis here is on exploring the patient's own knowledge, efforts and motivation. This involves eliciting information from the individual rather than imparting knowledge, insight or reality. In this case, it is important to explore and elicit information from Jane as to the reasons why she does not want to take medication. Useful approaches might include **Socratic questioning** – exploring ambivalence without judgement by presenting both sides of the decisional balance – and avoiding giving an unsolicited opinion. The nurse should notice, reflect and ask questions to elaborate on *change talk*. It is important to ask the patient questions from a perspective of curiosity rather than from a position of assumption, as making assumptions might run the risk of giving the impression that the nurse is advancing a viewpoint or interrogating the patient. In addition to evocation, the nurse should support and emphasise autonomy in the patient.

Autonomy and support

A key element of motivational interviewing is that the responsibility for change lies with the patient. It is important that the nurse always respects the patient's free will and autonomy. Your main aim is to understand the patient's arguments for change and then support them. In addition to autonomy and support, the provision of direction plays an important role in motivational interviewing.

Direction

The nurse should honour all of the above principles and approaches while still moving in the direction of change to deliver a directed intervention without confrontation, education or authority. This should occur through careful listening, summarising, affirming and reflecting on just the right information in the person's own words that emphasises their own intent, reason or need for change, as well as their hope and optimism in achieving this. Part of providing direction should initially involve assessing readiness to change.

Assessing readiness to change

Several factors influence the behaviour of an individual during the change process: desire, ability, reason, need and commitment. The acronym 'DARNC' is generally applied:

- *D*esire for change
- *A*bility to change
- *R*eason for change
- *N*eed for change
- *C*ommitment to change

The nurse should assess these aspects of motivation when talking to the patient. The assessment should also include how the patient is feeling and thinking about changing their current behaviour. For some people, this may involve a lengthy discussion. For others who are ready to act, the assessment may only be brief before planning action. We will look at these aspects of motivation in turn.

Desire for change

This relates to how much the patient wants to change. It is what the patient wants to do, regardless of logic, need or reason. For example, if Jane has no desire to change (i.e. to take medication), she may continue not to take medication, whether medication is available or not. This is because Jane may not have that deep-down desire to change her current behaviour. This is important because desire guides change. In addition to having the desire for change, the patient must have the ability to change behaviour.

Ability to change

Jane may already be thinking about change, but it is still important to assess the patient's ability to change and their beliefs about this ability. This is because although most people can change their behaviour, they may face real or imaginary obstacles that may undermine their efforts to change. In people with mental health problems, real obstacles may include cognitive deficits such as poor memory, which may prevent them from effecting behaviour change. In some cases, the use of substances such as cannabis and alcohol can have a negative impact on memory and thinking, creating an obstacle for change. In other instances, psychotropic medication can induce side effects such as drowsiness, restlessness, constipation, and many more that may interfere with the ability to effect change. Another area of real obstacles is the patient's social circumstances. It is important to assess the patient's social circumstances as some patients may experience peer or family pressure to continue with their current behaviour. For example, it is possible that Jane may face pressure from her friends not to take medication. In addition to real obstacles, patients may also face belief obstacles in their quest for change.

Belief obstacles are those beliefs that undermine a plan for change. For example, Jane might believe that she cannot continue to take medication because she may not have enough willpower to continue to do so. Belief obstacles become firmer when previous experiences seem to support that viewpoint. In Jane's case, the belief obstacle may be firmer due to her previous attempts to continue taking medication that ended in failure. To help patients overcome this, the nurse needs to acknowledge their previous attempts to change behaviour and reframe this as being partially successful. This helps to minimise the failure beliefs that the patient might have, as well as strengthening beliefs about their ability. It is important to also assess why the patient wants to change behaviour, to gain a more rounded view.

Reason for change

Consider a situation where a patient such as Jane acknowledges that she needs to take medication because it helps to keep her well. Jane may feel that there is a need to keep taking medication. However, she also feels that she does not have a good reason for taking medication as she believes that there are many other things which contribute to keeping her well, and taking medication will not make any difference. Besides, Jane feels that she is able to relax and socialise better without medication. Further, the reason for change interacts with the need for change.

Need for change

In some cases, a patient may not express a desire to be adherent to medication but can clearly identify problems with non-adherent behaviour. For example, Jane's non-adherence to medication led to frequent relapses and admissions to hospital. This does not mean that Jane is ready to act or will change. Therefore, Jane may have a *desire* for non-adherence, but she has a *need* to adhere to medication (change behaviour) because of frequent relapses and hospitalisation. Frequent relapses and hospitalisation are potentially a *need* to change, and the patient acknowledges the advantages and disadvantages of behaviour change. The patient may be *ambivalent* to change or *contemplate* change because of their *desire* for non-adherence. The patient may react by denying the need to change behaviour and become *pre-contemplative* (see the later section on the transtheoretical model of change). Therefore, you need to distinguish between *need* and *desire* to change.

Commitment to change

This is when patients want to put in the necessary effort to change and sustain these changes. In general, the factors that influence commitment are the desire, ability, reason and need for change ('DARN').

Therapeutic skills required for motivational interviewing

There are four major skills of intervention to remember (using the acronym 'OARS') when using motivational interviewing:

- Ask *O*pen-ended questions.
- *A*ffirm patients' self-efficacy.
- *R*eflect on patients' thoughts via active listening.
- *S*ummarise patients' narratives to help resolve ambivalence and promote change.

Let us now look at these in turn.

Open-ended questions

From the outset, the patient should do most of the talking during therapy as this allows the nurse to shape the patient's speech, such as by eliciting change talk. Ask a mixture of open-ended and closed questions. Closed questions are those that a person can answer with a short, simple phrase, a word, or a 'yes' or 'no'. For example, 'How old are you?' and 'Where are you going?' are closed questions. Closed questions tend to give you facts; they are easy and quick to answer, and you can keep control of the conversation.

In contrast, open-ended questions encourage the patient to explain or expand upon their answer. Open-ended questions tend to start with 'what', 'why' or 'how' (e.g. 'What did you do on Christmas Day?' 'How did you manage to do all of that work in an hour?'). You frame open-ended questions in such a way as to encourage further discussion. Open-ended questions have the following characteristics: they ask the patient to think and reflect, they will give the opinions and feelings of the patient, and they will hand control of the conversation over to the patient. In this respect, they encourage the patient to 'open up'. The nurse should avoid asking more than three questions in a row – intersperse questions with affirmations, reflections and summaries (see the following sections).

Affirmations

At its most basic, an affirmation refers to positive mental attitude and self-efficacy. Affirmations can include the positive statements a patient makes about changing behaviour. The nurse needs to recognise these as encouraging without being excessive in the acknowledgement of them. Sometimes it can be worth checking back on how the comments feel to the individual.

Reflective listening

This is a communication approach that involves two key stages. The first stage is to try to understand the patient's point of view. The second important stage is to offer the point of view back to the patient to confirm that the nurse has understood it correctly. In other words, the nurse should attempt to 'reconstruct' what the patient is thinking and feeling, and then communicate this understanding back to the patient. To be effective in reflective listening, it is important to step back from the words used and think about alternative meanings for what has been said. In reflective listening, the nurse checks if the guessed meaning is correct before moving forward. Another skill requirement in motivational interviewing is summarising, and we will turn to this next.

Summarising

The main purpose of summarising is to link information together, to recap and to reinforce important change talk from the patient. In summaries, the nurse can collect information together and then conclude with an open encouragement to the patient. Summaries can link different information, such as the two sides of ambivalence, which you can link with 'and' or 'at the same time' that emphasise the ambivalence, rather than using 'but' or 'yet', which can be more confusing. For example, you may say, 'So, on the one hand, you have concerns about how much medications help you to keep well; and, on the other, you have worries about side effects?'

Express empathy

Empathy is the experience of understanding another person's condition from their point of view. When you express empathy, you place yourself in your patient's position and imagine – to the best of your ability – what they are feeling. There is evidence suggesting that empathy increases helping behaviours (prosocial). In this respect, accurate empathy or 'acceptance' is the process of seeking to understand and accept the patient's feelings and their point of view through skilful reflective listening. You do not need to agree with the patient; it is possible for the nurse to have a different view from the patient and still express that view if the patient asks. However, the nurse should be able to respect the fact that the patient asked while at the same time having respect for the patient's own different stance. This approach is likely to help the nurse build collaboration while promoting a sense of autonomy in the patient.

Develop discrepancy

The aim of developing discrepancy is to draw the patient's attention to the difference between where they are now and where they ideally want to be in terms of change. For example, if the patient's life goal is to be able to find employment, then there is a potential disparity between non-adherent behaviour and this goal. The nurse may develop discrepancy by prompting the patient to consider the cost of their current behaviour (e.g. their strained relationship with their family) and the benefit of change (e.g. an improved relationship with their family), relating these to the chance of achieving their life goal of finding employment. The greater the importance the patient attaches to a life goal (e.g. getting a job) and the greater the discrepancy between this goal and their current behaviour (e.g. non-adherence), the more likely it is that the patient will move towards change. There is a need for caution here to ensure that the goals are the patient's, not the nurse's. Every patient has different life experiences and skills. In comparison to others, some patients may need to make more changes to reach the same goal.

Avoid argument

It is not acceptable to try to force or argue for a behaviour change in the patient, because in doing so they are more likely to argue for things to remain as they are. The nurse may offer new information and a new perspective to the patient, but this should be done with the patient's agreement that they can take it or leave it. In addition to avoiding argument, rolling with resistance is critical.

Roll with resistance

If the nurse meets with resistance, they should not see this as a negative development on the part of the patient. Rather, it is a sign that the conversation with the patient is perhaps proceeding far too quickly. Instead of fighting this resistance, which may develop into an argument, one way of overcoming it is to respond differently by reframing the resistance and actively involving the patient in problem-solving, which respects the patient's autonomy. That way, the patient can perceive themselves as having the answers to their problems, and the nurse can focus on asking questions rather than answering them. An approach that focuses on answering a patient's questions may encourage the patient to find fault with these answers. For example, if the nurse faces a question such as 'What do you think I should do about taking medication then?' an inappropriate response might be, 'Well, I think if you continue to take medication, it always helps to suppress the symptoms that you experience.' The patient might find fault in this and may respond, 'Yes, but taking medication is very unnatural.' Instead, the nurse should elicit reasons why the patient wants to stop taking medication. Alternatively, the nurse can give a response that emphasises the patient's own ability to answer the question. For example, you could say, 'I think that you know more about your situation than I do, and you're good at coming up with ideas as to what to do.' Or, 'I am just wondering what ideas you have?' This type of response promotes self-efficacy and encourages change talk in the patient.

Support self-efficacy

Self-efficacy describes the belief that an individual has in their ability to change or overcome difficulties. The nurse's belief in the patient's ability to change behaviour should enhance their self-efficacy. The nurse can demonstrate this by emphasising any success the patient might have had in overcoming obstacles. Without this belief, the patient is unlikely to change behaviour, as any change needs to come from the individual rather than from external others. The patient is likely to change behaviour if they are getting support from carers.

Collaboratively address risk factors for non-adherence

Earlier, we identified the risk factors associated with non-adherence (see page 54), and it is important to be aware of – and to identify – these potential barriers early in the treatment process. Unfortunately, one of the main disadvantages of current intervention strategies for improving adherence is that they are not designed to target specific risk factors; therefore, further research is necessary in this area. However, the goal of recognising risk factors for medication non-adherence is to identify individuals at high risk of non-adherence and allocate time to spend with them to address medication issues.

During the first interview, the nurse can explore the patient's expectations to help them accept treatment that is in some way consistent with their expectations. Initiate a discussion of adherence by asking the patient directly, 'Is there anything that may be preventing you from taking your medication?' At all times, the nurse should avoid taking an authoritarian approach, as this may backfire, leading to the patient being non-adherent. The nurse should provide education for the patient on the reasons for recommending types of medicines and discuss potential side effects, but the nurse should always ask if the patient is happy to be given unsolicited advice, as some patients may object. This type of approach is likely to have a positive impact on the therapeutic alliance and minimises resistance. Patients and mental health professionals sometimes differ in their opinions regarding the value of various medication selection factors. Therefore, there is a need to promote an open discussion about medication and the decision-making process to increase the likelihood that the patient will adhere to prescribed medications. More importantly, it is essential to assess the patient's level of motivation to change their behaviour.

Incorporating the transtheoretical model in improving adherence

To be able to assess the likelihood of a patient's adherence to medication and adopt a treatment recommendation, it is critical to assess the patient's motivation. The nurse can begin by discussing psychoeducational information about medications without assessing the patient's motivation to take medication. Unfortunately, most patients do not come forward and say, 'I want to change my behaviour.' In particular, the unmotivated patient is less likely to initiate and maintain recommended treatment. Behaviour change requires motivation, and it is therefore important for the nurse to understand the theory underpinning the motivation to change behaviour. One model with wide usage to motivate people to adhere to medication is the stages of change, or the transtheoretical model, formulated by Prochaska (Prochaska and Diclemente, 1984). In health psychology, the transtheoretical model assesses an individual's readiness to act on new, healthier behaviour. It provides processes taken over a period to guide the individual through the stages of change to action and maintenance (see Figure 2.2).

Patients in the *pre-contemplation stage* may not believe that medication adherence is important and may not have any desire to change. Those patients in the *contemplation stage* are thinking of changing but are not yet fully dedicated to changing. These patients are more aware that non-adherence can be problematic to their health. Patients in the *preparation stage* are intending to adhere to their medication regularly but may have several barriers preventing them from doing so. Patients who are *taking action* are actively working to take their medications regularly, while patients in the *maintenance stage* are doing so on a consistent basis.

In deciding to change a current behaviour, patients must balance the pros and cons of the change (decisional balance) according to their lifestyles and health beliefs. As patients move from unawareness of any problem, through contemplating a change, to carrying out the action, the pros increase and the cons decrease. Once the patient accomplishes the change, self-efficacy – the confidence to overcome difficulties and maintain the new behaviour pattern – is important (Julius et al., 2009).

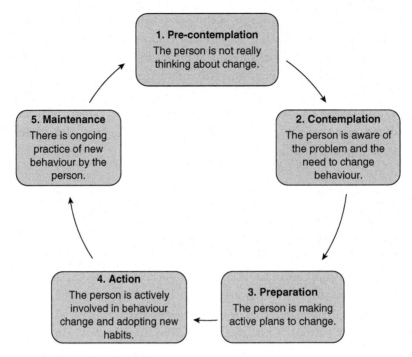

Figure 2.2   Stages of change model

There is a need to reinforce any progress and encourage the patient during the entire process of change. In the early stages, emotional and cognitive factors are important to raise consciousness and increase motivation to take the first step. In the later stages, there is more emphasis on commitment, action and avoiding relapse, and defining goals and teaching medication administration skills and relapse prevention strategies become more important. The nurse should gear motivation and supplying information specifically to the patient's stage of readiness to change. However, it is important not to pressure the patient as this may lead to resistance.

In assessing motivation and readiness to change, start by agreeing on an agenda with the patient to address medication adherence and related issues, including the following, suggested by Borrelli et al. (2007):

- 'I'd like to take some time to discuss your medication.'
- 'How many times this past week did you take your medication?'
- 'How does taking your medication fit into your daily routine?'
- 'On a scale of 1 to 10, how motivated are you to take your medication?'
- 'What do you think it would take to make you a 10 on this scale as opposed to where you are now?'
- 'What do you feel is preventing you from taking your medications as prescribed?'
- 'What are the positive/negative aspects of taking your medications?'
- 'How would taking your medications regularly change your life?'
- 'How would taking your medications regularly help you?'

Table 2.1 Integrating the transtheoretical model and basic intervention strategies to improve medication adherence

Stage of change	Process in operation/ explanation	Patient characteristics	Possible intervention
Stage 1: Pre-contemplation	1. Consciousness raising 2. Social liberation	1. Rebellion 2. Resignation 3. Rationalisation 4. Reluctance	1. Provide choices 2. Build hope 3. Encourage reflection 4. Give information 5. Reinforce progress
Stage 2: Contemplation	1. Consciousness raising 2. Social liberation 3. Emotional arousal 4. Self-evaluation 5. Commitment	1. Open to information 2. Ambivalence	1. Provide information 2. Help to weigh pros and cons 3. Increase self-efficacy 4. Reinforce progress
Stage 3: Preparation	1. Social liberation 2. Emotional arousal 3. Self-evaluation	1. Determination	1. Help set goals 2. Provide strategies for change 3. Reinforce progress
Stage 4: Action	1. Social liberation 2. Commitment 3. Reward 4. Environmental control 5. Helping relationships	1. Actively changing 2. Self-evaluation	1. Teach skills and self-management 2. Guide attribution process 3. Reinforce progress
Stage 5: Maintenance	1. Commitment 2. Reward 3. Countering 4. Environmental control 5. Helping relationships	1. At risk/relapse 2. Self-evaluation	1. Teach relapse prevention strategies 2. Encourage continuation 3. Reinforce progress

Encourage the patient to discuss the positive and negative aspects of taking medication as prescribed. It is important that you prompt the patient to verbalise their own intent to change to increase the likelihood that they adopt the behaviours necessary for change. Use reflective listening skills, and after the patient has verbalised their thoughts summarise the pros of taking the prescribed medications in their own words. The nurse should help the patient make associations between the benefits of taking medication and symptom reduction (Julius et al., 2009). Finally, when the patient makes steps towards behaviour change, the nurse should give positive feedback to reinforce these behaviours.

Carer involvement

As discussed previously, families can have an impact on patients' adherence to prescribed medications. Family members with negative attitudes regarding medications and other misconceptions about the nature of their loved one's mental illness can be a barrier to adherence to prescribed medications (Julius et al., 2009). Evidence shows that there is an improvement in adherence and reductions in relapse in patients whose family members have an active engagement with the patient's treatment and receive some level of intervention from mental health professionals. With the permission of the patient, it is important to involve family members in treatment planning and addressing potential concerns about recommended treatment. The nurse should also involve them in the provision of educational information, diagnosis and treatment. It is also important to identify and discuss the family's ability and willingness to support the patient and encourage adherence to recommended treatments. The nurse should provide emotional support to families to enable them to cope with the mental illness of their loved one. For example, the nurse might encourage family members to participate in local support groups, such as those sponsored by voluntary organisations (Julius et al., 2009).

Chapter summary

Current methods of treating and aiding recovery in people with mental health problems place special emphasis on establishing a shared decision-making approach where patients take an active part in their treatment, and this necessitates building a therapeutic alliance.

Despite potential benefits derived from taking medication, people with mental health problems sometimes do not take medication, and this can have enormous personal, social and economic consequences on their lives. The reasons for poor adherence are many but include adverse side effects, attitudes to treatment, and severity of illness. Because of the importance of medication adherence, several strategies have been devised to improve it. One of the more popular strategies is a combination of CBT and psychoeducation. In all of these interventions, the application of motivational interviewing principles to aid communication is important. Patient involvement and establishing a good therapeutic alliance are central to the recovery model of care.

Activities: brief outline answers

Activity 2.1 Reflection (page 48)

Some reasons why patients are partially adherent include that they may not consider themselves to be ill, a lack of family support, adverse side effects, or they believe that their illness can be treated by other means instead of medication. A poor relationship with the mental health professional can impact on adherence.

Activity 2.2 Critical thinking (page 50)

Julio's view of his illness is valid if we consider his cultural background. People's health belief systems are in part shaped by their culture. More importantly, Julio accepts that he is unwell, but it is his explanation of his circumstances that is culturally based. For this reason, he seeks a culturally appropriate remedy because it makes sense to him. This is in line with the self-regulatory and health belief models.

Activity 2.3 Reflection (page 52)

There are many barriers to seeking help. The most common tend to be lack of understanding regarding the illness, financial constraints, language, cultural differences between the patient and the provider in the interpretation of symptoms, and inappropriate services that do not reflect the needs of the people they serve.

Activity 2.4 Critical thinking (page 55)

Some of the factors that may lead someone to think they have no mental health problems despite evidence to the contrary include severity of the illness, social isolation and cultural beliefs.

Activity 2.5 Critical thinking (page 58)

Reasons that may impede Jane from benefiting fully from medication include environmental factors – she lives on the sixth floor of a high-rise flat, which is hardly ideal for someone with two young children. Also, it appears that she has little support from family and friends, and this contributes towards poor adherence.

Further reading

Amador, X.F. and David, A. (2004) *Insight and Psychosis: Awareness of Illness in Schizophrenia and Related Disorders.* Oxford: Oxford University Press.

This is a valuable book that details awareness of illness and how it is a barrier to seeking health.

Blackwell, B. (1998) From compliance to alliance: a quarter century of research. In B. Blackwell (ed.), *Treatment Compliance and the Therapeutic Alliance.* Amsterdam: Harwood Academic, pp1–15.

This is a very useful book that comprehensively covers factors that affect medication adherence in serious mental illness. This chapter on treatment compliance in schizophrenia explains adherence from a public health viewpoint.

Leahy, R. (2006) *Roadblocks in Cognitive-Behavioral Therapy: Transforming Challenges into Opportunities for Change.* London: Guilford Press.

This book addresses difficult questions – or 'roadblocks' – in CBT. It explores how and why they arise and suggests effective, practical solutions. Topics include overcoming obstacles in the treatment of specific disorders.

Miller, W.R. and Rollick, S. (2012) *Motivational Interviewing: Preparing People to Change,* 3rd edition. London: Guilford Press.

This is a very useful book that deals with motivational interviewing.

Useful websites

www.babcp.com

The British Association for Behavioural and Cognitive Psychotherapies (BABCP) is the leading organisation for the theory, practice and development of CBT in the UK. It has over 8,000 members, including nurses, trainees, counsellors, psychologists and psychiatrists.

Chapter 3 — Essential anatomy and physiology of the brain related to psychopharmacology

---

Chapter aims

By the end of this chapter, you should be familiar with:

- the anatomy and physiology of the brain regions relevant to psychopharmacology;
- the role of ion channels and classical neurotransmission;
- neural connectivity and the importance of synapses.

Introduction

The human brain is the result of at least four billion years of evolution and is the most complex object known; it is an electrical and chemical powerhouse that sends messages where needed in a perfectly targeted way. The brain is soft and grey, and weighs about 1.5 kg. It is not only where we experience and manipulate the world, but it is also responsible for the control of our breathing, body temperature, blood pressure and hormones. Unlike the heart or lungs, the brain has no moving parts; and unlike the kidney, liver or spleen, it does not make anything. Unlike the skin or bones, the brain serves no *obvious* purpose, yet we know it is responsible for thoughts, emotions and free will. In short, the simple view of the brain as the most fundamental of all organs may seem rather obvious, but how did we come to such a conclusion? To answer this question, we need to go back into the past and find out what people before us believed about the brain.

In ancient Egypt, the brain was regarded to be a form of 'cranial stuffing' that served no useful purpose. The heart was instead thought of as the seat of intelligence. This belief is best exemplified by the way that ancient Egyptians prepared bodies for mummification, by taking great care in the preparation of organs such as the heart, lungs, liver and stomach, while the brain was simply scooped from the skull. As much as we now know that the brain is the seat of intelligence, colloquial expressions such as 'learning something by heart' or 'suffering from heartache' remain in common use to this day.

Around 450 BC, the Greek physician Alcmaeon was among the first to recognise the brain's importance, but his view was not universally accepted. One hundred years later, Aristotle reasserted the importance of the heart and suggested that the brain was little more than a cooling system for the heart.

From the first century BC, the prevailing view was that of Galen, a Greek doctor who suggested that the heart controlled the four humours: blood, phlegm, yellow bile and black bile. This theory was untrue, of course, but Galen did manage to recognise the link between the brain and memory, as well as emotions and the processing of senses. It was not until the 1800s that progress regarding brain physiology was made.

Thomas Willis (1621–1675), an English neurologist, is largely credited with advancing knowledge about the brain, being the first person to examine the brain with real scientific rigour. After years of research, he published his groundbreaking *Cerebri Anatome*, providing the first complete description of the brain's regions. He correctly linked memory and higher function with the cerebral hemispheres, as well as laying down the basis of brain science terminology. Another breakthrough by Willis was to correctly propose that the liquid-filled spaces deep inside the brain, the ventricles, served no significant purpose, whereas before many believed that the ventricles were the centre of high brain function. Several other scientists contributed to our knowledge of the brain, including Emanuel Swedenborg (1688–1772), Franz Joseph Gall (1758–1828), Pierre Paul Broca (1824–1880) and Carl Wernicke (1848–1905). Most importantly, Santiago Ramón y Cajal (1852–1934) published a textbook regarded by many as one of the greatest scientific texts: *Manual of Normal Histology and Micrographic Technique*. He was the first to suggest that the brain and the nervous system consist of discrete cells called neurons. He described the nervous system and the brain with unparalleled clarity, and for his work he received the Nobel Prize in Physiology or Medicine in 1906. These breakthroughs inspired many surgical techniques and drug discoveries that remedy brain dysfunctions. But the greatest advance of all was observing the activity of the living brain using brain scanning.

Brain scanning

Our knowledge of the brain has been greatly enhanced by scanning techniques. The first major attempt at scanning the human brain was by Hans Berger in 1924. He used an electroencephalogram (EEG) to measure human brainwaves, and this laid the groundwork for future research into computerised axial tomography (CAT/CT) and positron emission tomography (PET). CAT scans use powerful computers to convert two-dimensional X-ray pictures into three-dimensional images for further study. PET scans use a radioactive 'tracer' substance that is injected directly into the human body. This substance gradually accumulates inside the major organs while at the same time emitting positron radiation, which is detected by a sensor. A more recent and non-invasive technique is functional magnetic resonance imaging (fMRI). This technique uses a magnet weighing several tons. It relies on the metal-charged ions in our body, including iron. The magnetic properties of the metal charges change in the presence of oxygen. A change in oxygen concentration reflects brain activity and a powerful computer processes this information to construct a two- or three-dimensional image of brain activity. This technique allows us to observe the global behaviour of the brain during different types of activities, such as mental arithmetic, reading a book or watching a movie.

In summary, it has taken us centuries to understand even the basic functions of the human brain. Although there is still much that we do not know about the brain, we now have a good knowledge of the basic anatomy and physiology of each region of the brain.

Brain regions

In neuroscience, the brain is considered to have at least six main regions: the cerebral hemispheres, the diencephalon (thalamus and hypothalamus), the midbrain, the cerebellum, the pons, and the medulla oblongata. Each brain region has a complex internal structure.

The brainstem

This is the stalk-like part of the brain connecting to the spinal cord and the forebrain, and it is made up of the pons, the medulla oblongata and the midbrain (see Figure 3.1). The brainstem functions as an important relay station for every electrical impulse that passes between the brain and the spinal cord to allow the body to function normally.

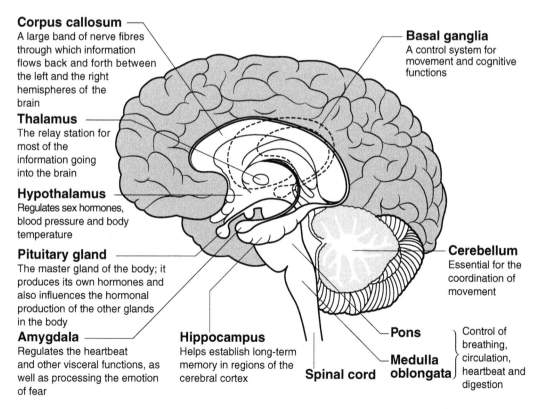

Figure 3.1   A cross-section of the brain showing the major regions and their functions

The medulla oblongata controls the unconscious or autonomic parts of bodily function, such as blood pressure, heart rate and muscle tone. It also plays a part in regulating other reflexive functions, such as sneezing, coughing and vomiting.

The pons is situated between the midbrain and the medulla oblongata. The pons' function is to relay signals from the cortex to assist in the control of movement, and it is also involved in the control of sleep and arousal. The pons also plays an important part in fine-tuning motor messages as they travel from the motor area of the cerebral cortex down to the cerebellum. The midbrain is positioned between the hindbrain and the forebrain. It forms part of the brainstem and connects the brainstem to the forebrain, and it is mainly responsible for controlling sensory processes. Before you read further, undertake Activity 3.1.

Activity 3.1   Critical thinking

If a person is pronounced to be 'clinically dead', what part of the brain plays an important part in coming to this conclusion, and why?

An outline answer is provided at the end of the chapter.

The cerebellum

The cerebellum, or 'little brain', is found behind the brainstem, to which it connects. It is split into two hemispheres and it has a convoluted surface that makes it look somewhat like a giant walnut (see Figure 3.1). It is one of the earliest brain regions to evolve and the human version is comparatively like that of other mammals. The cerebellum fine-tunes and smooths out movements, especially those necessary for quick changes in direction. For example, when a person reaches out to catch a moving object, the cerebellum is involved in the timing of movement.

As the motor systems of mammals became more sophisticated, there was a need to coordinate increasingly accurate movements, such as those of the eyes, hands and fingers, and this has resulted in the evolution and enlargement of the cerebellum. This is evident in its structure, in which the central part is the oldest and most primitive and the outer part is concerned with functions unique to humans. It has strong connections with the motor parts of the cortex. The cerebellum has two lobes, but – unlike the motor cortex – it controls movements on the same side of the body as itself. When the cerebellum goes wrong, it results in awkward, jerky movements and an impairment of coordination called *ataxia*. Professional boxers are particularly susceptible to slight cerebellum damage, which can result in 'punch-drunk syndrome'. The most common cause of temporary ataxia is consuming alcohol. Now we need to turn our attention to another part of the brain called the diencephalon.

The diencephalon

The diencephalon, or 'interbrain', is part of the forebrain that is located between the cerebral hemispheres and above the midbrain. This region of the brain includes the thalamus, the hypothalamus, the epithalamus, the prethalamus or subthalamus, the pineal gland, the pituitary gland, and other structures (see Figure 3.1).

The egg-shaped thalamus that is above the hypothalamus consists of two oval-shaped lobes that lie side by side, one in each hemisphere. It is essential for gating and processing sensory information entering the brain. The only exception to this is that it does not process information from the nose. The thalamus processes information and decides whether it needs to be sent to the cortex for conscious consideration. Also, information from the cerebellum and other areas that are involved in movement is sent to the thalamus for processing. Just below the thalamus is the hypothalamus, which controls a multitude of functions.

The hypothalamus is about the size of a pearl or grape, but despite its small size it is the control centre for many autonomic functions, and it connects to almost every other part of the brain. It is the control centre for many autonomic functions of the central and peripheral nervous systems. The hypothalamus influences various emotional responses through its influence on the pituitary gland, the skeletal muscular system and the autonomic nervous system. The hypothalamus directs a multitude of important functions in the body. It is essential to motivation, including seeking out pleasurable rewards. Its connection with structures of the endocrine and nervous systems allows it to play a vital role in maintaining **homeostasis**. Blood vessel connections between the hypothalamus and the pituitary gland allow hypothalamic hormones to control pituitary hormone secretion (see Table 3.1). Some of the physiological processes that the hypothalamus regulates include blood pressure, body temperature, cardiovascular system functions, fluid balance and electrolyte balance.

Table 3.1 Hormones produced by the hypothalamus and their function

Hormone	Function
Anti-diuretic hormones	Regulate water levels and influence blood volume and blood pressure.
Corticotropin-releasing hormone (CRH)	Central role is the regulation of stress. It causes release of adrenocorticotropic hormone (ACTH) from the pituitary gland. CRH also acts on many other areas within the brain, where it suppresses appetite, increases anxiety, and improves memory and selective attention. CRH is also produced throughout pregnancy in increasing amounts by the foetus and the placenta, with the effects of increasing cortisol. Ultimately, it is the high levels of CRH, along with other hormones, that are thought to start labour.
Oxytocin	Influences sexual and social behaviour. Its release during labour is triggered by the widening of the cervix and the vagina.
Gonadotropin-releasing hormone	Produced and released into tiny blood vessels in the pituitary gland, where it stimulates the production of follicle-stimulating hormone (FSH) and luteinising hormone (LH), or lutropin.
Somatostatin	Somatostatin from the hypothalamus inhibits the pituitary gland's secretion of growth hormone (GH) and thyroid-stimulating hormone (TSH).
GH-releasing hormone	Stimulates the pituitary gland to produce and release GH into the bloodstream. This then acts on virtually every tissue of the body to control several physical functions and processes.
Thyrotropin-releasing hormone (TRH)	Stimulates the pituitary gland to release TSH, which regulates metabolism, growth, heart rate and body temperature.

The limbic system

In addition to the structures that make up the diencephalon, there are further major brain structures buried deep beneath the folds of the cortical hemispheres: the basal ganglia, the amygdala and the hippocampus (see Figure 3.1), as well as the cingulate gyrus, the fornix, the thalamus, the olfactory cortex, the spinal cord and the cerebrum. These structures and others form the limbic system.

The limbic system, which includes portions of all the lobes of the cerebral hemispheres, is a complex set of three C-shaped structures containing both grey and white matter. It is buried under the cortex and can be located on top of the brainstem. It is one of the more primitive parts of the brain. Limbic system structures are parts of the brain that are most closely associated with emotional expression and motivations, particularly those that connect to our survival. Such emotions include fear and anger, as well as emotions related to sexual behaviour. The system influences both the peripheral nervous system and the endocrine system. Damage to or stimulation of sites within this system may profoundly affect emotional expression, either by causing excessive reactions to situations or greatly reducing emotional response. Clinical conditions involving the limbic system include epilepsy, congenital syndromes, dementias and various psychiatric disorders, as will be seen in later chapters. Here, we describe key structures that are important to mental health pathology and treatment.

Basal ganglia

Connected to the cortex and the thalamus are swollen structures called the basal ganglia (see Figure 3.1). The basal ganglia consist of substructures, including the caudate nuclei, the putamen, the nucleus accumbens, the olfactory tubercle, the globus pallidus, the ventral pallidum, the substantia nigra and the subthalamic nucleus. In general, the basal ganglia structures receive most of their input from the cortex and are responsible for the coordination of fine movement. Parkinson's disease provides an excellent example of what happens when there is damage to the basal ganglia through the progressive destruction of dopamine neurons. This destruction leads to a decrease in the activity of other structures within the basal ganglia. A related movement disorder, tardive dyskinesia, may result from long-term use of antipsychotic medication (see Chapter 11).

Nucleus accumbens

A part of the basal ganglia that deserves special consideration is the nucleus accumbens. It is a paired structure (one in each hemisphere) located near the amygdala and is part of a group of structures that form the dopamine pathway originating from the brainstem (upper pons), terminating in the frontal cortex. The nucleus accumbens itself is separated into two anatomical components: the shell and the core. These two connecting areas have overlapping connections but make different contributions to its function. The most widely accepted role of the nucleus accumbens is in the 'reward circuit' of the brain. When we do anything that we consider rewarding (e.g. eat food, have sex, take drugs), dopamine neurons (along with other types of neurons) in the ventral tegmental area (VTA) of the brain are activated, increasing dopamine levels in the nucleus accumbens (see Chapter 10). However, this theory is under challenge as new insights seem to suggest that dopamine levels also increase when we experience unpleasant events (Volman et al., 2013).

Amygdala

The term 'amygdala' comes from the Greek word for 'almond' and is a reference to its size and shape. The amygdala is found below the hypothalamus, deep in the temporal lobe (see Figure 3.1). Despite its relatively small size, the amygdala plays an important part in generating emotional responses, such as fear, anger and desire, and it is responsible for the way we relate to the world and those around us. The amygdala is also responsible for determining what memories to store and where to store them in the brain. The decision of what memory to store is believed to be based on how big an emotional response an event invokes in us. Scientific studies of the amygdala have led to the discovery of neurons that are responsible for fear conditioning – an associative learning process where we learn through repeated experiences to fear something (see Chapter 10). Our experiences can cause brain circuits to change and form new memories. For example, when we hear an unpleasant sound, the amygdala heightens our perception of the sound. We then consider this heightened perception as distressing and we form memories associating the sound with unpleasantness. If the noise surprises us, we have an automatic fight or flight response. This response involves the activation of the sympathetic division of the peripheral nervous system. In turn, the activation of the nerves of the sympathetic division results in an accelerated heart rate, dilated pupils, an increase in metabolic rate, and an increase in blood flow to the muscles. The amygdala coordinates this activity and allows us to respond appropriately to danger.

Hippocampus

Close to the amygdala is the hippocampus (see Figure 3.1), which takes its name from its seahorse-like shape. It is a paired structure, with one hippocampus located in each hemisphere. It is particularly important in creating new memories and connecting emotions and senses, such as smell and sound, to memories. It acts as a memory indexer by sending memories out to the relevant part of the cerebral hemisphere for long-term storage and retrieving them when necessary. It is also here that experiences turn into neural pathways that are then stored for future reference. People who experience damage to this structure have difficulty in storing new information, and Alzheimer's disease is a prime example.

Alzheimer's disease severely affects the hippocampus first, before other parts of the cortex, so memory is usually the first thing to falter (i.e. the ability to make new memories). The hippocampus also seems to be involved in severe mental illnesses such as schizophrenia and some severe depressions, where it appears to shrink. Accumulating evidence also suggests that the hippocampus undergoes significant alteration because of stress or post-traumatic stress disorder (PTSD). Before you proceed further, consider Activity 3.2.

Activity 3.2   Critical thinking

The hypothalamus is part of a collection of brain tissues called the diencephalon, and it is connected to every part of the brain. What may cause hypothalamic dysfunction?

An outline answer is provided at the end of the chapter.

The cerebral cortex

The crowning achievement of brain evolution in many respects must be the cerebral cortex (see Figure 3.2). This is a rippling outer layer that gives the human brain most of its unique powers. The cortex grew a lot during a relatively short evolutionary period, and to accommodate its growth it became increasingly folded. It is estimated that the human cortex has an area of about 1.5 m² and is 4 mm thick. The grey surface of the cortex is due to a vast network of specialised neurons, six layers of which travel down towards the underlying white matter. In the white matter region, the same neurons form a vast number of connections with other neurons. This vast matrix allows for swift intercommunication, facilitating our powers of thought.

The cortex is not a homogeneous region as it is divided into many areas (Gibb, 2012). First, it is divided into two hemispheres (left and right), which are themselves divided by deep grooves into four major areas called 'lobes': the frontal, parietal, occipital and temporal lobes (see Figure 3.2).

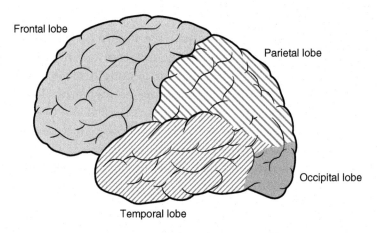

Figure 3.2   The four lobes of the cerebral cortex

The frontal lobe lies directly beneath the forehead and is involved in what are collectively termed 'higher functions'. These higher functions include attention, planning, language and movement. It is like a master control unit that helps to integrate information and govern what the rest of the brain does. Behind the frontal lobe and at the top of the head is the parietal lobe, which processes sensory information, allowing us to perceive the world and our place within it. At the back, the occipital lobe deals primarily with vision, and it is here that signals from the eyes become transformed into useful visual representations. Finally, the temporal lobes are located on each side of the brain, and they mainly process sound and language. Because they connect to the hippocampus, they are also concerned with memory formation and retrieval.

The corpus callosum

A bundle of tissue called the corpus callosum holds the brain's hemispheres together. The corpus callosum is the largest bundle of nerve fibres in the brain and it is also the main channel through which information flows from one side of the brain to the other. If there is damage to the corpus callosum, this can give rise to illnesses such as epilepsy. Now turn your attention to Activity 3.3.

Activity 3.3   Research

The cerebral cortex is a highly evolved part of the brain. Name the subregions of the cerebral cortex and their functions.

An outline answer is provided at the end of the chapter.

Table 3.2   A summary of the parts of the brain and their functions

Part	Function
Frontal lobe	Memory, consciousness, motor activities, judgements, controls emotional response and language.
Parietal lobe	Visual attention, touch perception, goal-directed voluntary movements, manipulation of objects, integration of different senses.
Occipital lobe	Vision.
Temporal lobes	Hearing ability, memory, visual perceptions, object categorisation.
Midbrain	Connects the brainstem to the forebrain, controls sensory processes.
Pons	Relays signals from the cortex, involved in sleep arousal.
Thalamus	Processes sensory information entering the brain.
Hypothalamus	Connected to every part of the brain, important in motivation and seeking reward.
Cerebellum	Controls movement.

The neural network

The nervous system consists of the brain, the autonomous nervous system (ANS) and the central nervous system (CNS). It is made up of specialised cells that communicate with each other and with other cells in the body. These specialised cells are called neurons, or nerve cells in common parlance, and the human brain consists of approximately 200 billion of them.

There are three main classes of neurons: sensory neurons, motor neurons and interneurons. Each neuron links with thousands of other neurons through small spaces called synapses. The brain has trillions of these specialised connections. Sensory or afferent neurons carry messages to the central nervous system from sensory receptors in the the skin, eyes, nose, and so on, as well as some organs, muscles and joints. The brain and at times the spinal cord interpret these messages and send appropriate responses through motor or efferent neurons, which cause sensory organs (muscles, glands, etc.) to respond. For example, a sensory neuron from the ear will detect a loud bang and send messages to the brain. The brain will interpret the message, and in turn send information to the motor neurons of the neck muscles and eyes to act. Interneurons are located within the CNS and work to bridge communication between the sensory and motor neurons.

When neurons malfunction, this can result in behavioural symptoms (Stahl, 2013). We can correct the malfunction of neurons through medicines that work on these neurons to relieve behavioural symptoms. The following section will describe the function of a normal neuron as a first step for understanding mental health disorders, and – as you will see in later chapters – this helps us to understand how psychotropic medicines work.

The structure of the neuron

Many textbooks portray the neuron with a generic structure, but the reality is that many neurons have unique structures. They vary so much in shape that it is not possible to describe a 'typical' one, but they have three major features in common. All neurons have a cell body called the *soma*, which contains a *nucleus* and an extension called the *axon*. The soma receives information from other cells and the axon transmits electrical impulses to other cells. It also determines the overall shape and behaviour of the neuron by producing protein in accordance with instructions that the **deoxyribonucleic acid (DNA)** issues. The third major feature of neurons is one or more tree-like branching extensions called *dendrites*, which make connections with other neurons (see Figure 3.3).

When activated, neurons transmit a wave of electrochemical charge called an *impulse.* The starting point of an impulse can be a sensory organ, such as the skin, an eye or an ear, as mentioned in earlier sections, or it can be at a dendrite that has received a message from another neuron.

The dendrites collect information and send it to the neuron's control centre, which is the *cell body* (see Figure 3.3). The cell body pools together the data from each branch of the dendrite to create an overall signal. The signal then passes to an area called the *axon hillock* (see Figure 3.3), which serves as an electrical integrator. Here, the axon hillock decides whether to fire an electrical impulse in response to incoming electrical information or not. If the overall charge from the dendrites reaches a threshold, the neuron fires a signal. The axon propagates chemical signals within the internal cell matrix, but it also propagates these electrical signals travelling along the membrane to the presynaptic zone.

The firing of an electrical impulse down an axon is less straightforward than the flow of electrons down a copper wire (Gibb, 2012). However, just as in copper wire, which is often insulated with plastic, many axons are insulated with a fatty substance called the *myelin sheath*, which reduces the risk of short circuits caused by nearby axons. The **myelin** sheath also helps to speed up electrical impulses, which jump from one node of Ranvier to the next (see Figure 3.3), a process called *saltory conduction.*

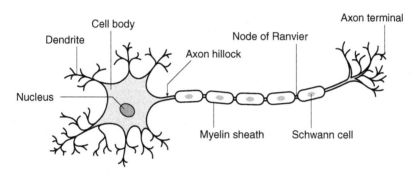

Figure 3.3   The structure of a neuron, showing dendrites, the cell body axon and the myelin sheath

When the electrical impulse reaches the end of the neuron, it causes the activation of the *synaptic vesicles,* which contain chemical substances called *neurotransmitters.* These neurotransmitters amplify or modulate electrical signals being passed to the neighbouring neuron. We will look at neurotransmission in more detail in later sections.

In the human brain, each neuron makes thousands of synapses with other neurons to create an estimated 1 trillion chemically neurotransmitting synapses. Synaptic communication between all of these neurons is chemical (via neurotransmitters), not electrical. Finally, neurotransmission continues in the postsynaptic neuron either by converting the chemical information back into an electrical impulse or remaining unchanged. Later sections describe the action of neurotransmitters in more detail. Meanwhile, turn your attention to Activity 3.4 to test your understanding.

Activity 3.4   Evidence-based practice and research

Search the internet and find out what illnesses are associated with a dysfunction of the following regions of the brain:

- cerebral cortex;
- amygdala;
- hippocampus;
- pons;
- substantia nigra.

Outline answers are provided at the end of the chapter.

Neural development

As previously discussed, it is not possible to overstate the importance of understanding how the brain develops. It is another necessary step towards understanding how psychotropic medicines work. This section will discuss the basic concepts of neural development. Initially, the section will focus on describing the anatomical basis of neurotransmission, before discussing how neurons migrate, form synapses and demonstrate plasticity.

Time course of neural development

The understanding of human neural development is changing at an extremely fast pace thanks largely to stem cell research and advances in forms of brain imaging techniques. The process of neural development starts when the egg fuses with the sperm and a process of cell division (mitosis) commences.

Cells differentiate into immature neurons, and those that are selected migrate to different parts of the brain and differentiate into different (specialised) types of neurons. The formation of new neurons, or *neurogenesis,* continues throughout adult life in some parts of the brain, particularly in the hippocampus. The hippocampus is an area that appears to be particularly sensitive to the effects of stress, ageing and disease. Learning, psychotherapy, exercise and even certain types of psychotropic medicines can stimulate neurogenesis of the hippocampus. Neurogenesis may also occur in other brain areas, including the substantia nigra, the striatum, the amygdala and the neocortex, and several new potential sites of neurogenesis have been described in recent years. We also know that a neuron may fail to develop during childhood, either because of a developmental disease or a lack of appropriate neural or environmental stimulation (Stahl, 2013). Part of neural development takes the form of neural migration.

Neural migration

As much as it is surprising that the production of neurons occurs in the mature adult brain, it is also surprising that periodically, under specific conditions, neurons can kill themselves. We call this form of cell suicide *apoptosis*, and up to 90 **per cent** of the neurons that the brain makes during foetal development commit apoptosis. The reason for apoptosis is that there is an excess of neurons during the prenatal stage of neural development and only a few neurons will be selected for migration. Some of these neurons are healthy and others are defective. In normal brain development, only healthy neurons migrate and the defective neurons commit apoptosis. However, if there is a neurodevelopmental disorder, some defective neurons may migrate, and this will cause neurological or psychiatric disorders in later life.

Scenario

A 46-year-old mother with a son suffering from schizophrenia informed a nurse that while she was seven months pregnant with her son, she contracted a viral infection that lasted three weeks.

Trauma or infection to the mother during pregnancy can have profound effects on the neural development of the unborn child. There is a robust link between viral infection during the third trimester of pregnancy and schizophrenia (Blomstrom et al., 2015; Khandaker et al., 2013). It is possible that via the immune system, microbial agents interfere somewhat with the process of neural selection, whereby defective neurons are selected for migration.

As has been previously discussed, in addition to selecting the correct neurons for migration, the neurons must migrate to the right parts of the brain. Incorrect migration of neurons can dispose an individual to a neurodevelopmental disorder such as epilepsy, schizophrenia or attention deficit hyperactivity disorder (ADHD). We will now turn our attention to another process that involves the formation of the synapse: synaptogenesis.

Synaptogenesis

Once neurons settle down in their respective areas, they specialise and form synapses (see Figure 3.4). A synapse is the space between two dendritic neurons. It is a structure that permits a neuron to pass an electrical or chemical signal to another cell.

During normal development, neurons from different parts of the brain are appropriately directed to their target dendrites to form correct synapses with other neurons.

Therefore, synaptogenesis is the formation of synapses between neurons in the nervous system. Although it occurs throughout a healthy person's lifespan, an explosion of synaptic formation occurs during early brain development, known as *exuberant synaptogenesis*. In abnormal neural development, the wrong dendrites will form synapses with the wrong neurons, resulting in incorrect wiring. In later life, this could lead to abnormal information transfer, which affects neural communication and the ability of neurons to function normally under certain conditions. We now turn our attention to the concept of neural plasticity.

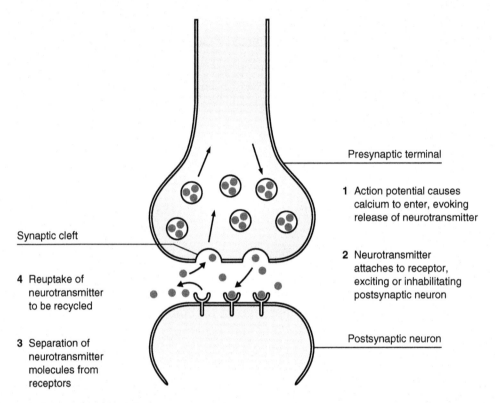

Figure 3.4 A synapse with neurotransmitters

Neural plasticity

The synapses can form on any part of the neuron and not just on the dendrites. Synapses that form on any part of the neuron other than the dendrites are called *asymmetrical*. Once a synapse forms, it remains a dynamic area of intense molecular activity, and in many ways a synapse is under constant revision if it is functional, with molecular maintenance and alterations constantly taking place to respond to changing conditions. For example, the surface area of the pre- and postsynaptic membrane can increase to accommodate numbers and types of receptors that facilitate communication. An increase in neurotransmission may lead to an increase in the number of postsynaptic receptors, or in some cases whole axons can develop. Also, if the brain stays active, this preserves neurons, and new ones can even form, but if it is not active the neural connection becomes weak and may be 'pruned off'.

As life proceeds, some neural connections get stronger and some get weaker, and the brain can even form new ones. This is how practising a new activity makes us better. In other words, our experiences of repeating interaction with the outside world transform into a strengthened neural interaction or connection between the relevant neurons inside our brain. For example, after one lesson of learning how to administer medicines, little will probably happen in our brain to keep that knowledge intact. However, as we continue to stimulate the neural pathway responsible for learning how to administer medicines, our neurons will eventually reach a critical threshold and the neurons will physically change. The synaptic connections between the neurons become firmer and new synaptic connections can form.

In summary, the dendritic tree of a neuron not only sprouts new branches; it grows and establishes a multitude of new synaptic connections throughout its life, and can also remove, alter, trim or destroy such connections when necessary.

Now that you have read about the mechanism of neural plasticity, undertake Activity 3.5 to test your understanding.

Activity 3.5   Critical thinking

In a group or as an individual, find out the typical age of onset for psychosis.

- How does this period of onset relate to neural pruning?

An outline answer is provided at the end of the chapter.

Chemical neurotransmission

We can define neurotransmission as the passing of signals from nerve cell to nerve cell through chemicals. Chemical neurotransmission constitutes the cornerstone of neuroscientific principles, and the concept has been in existence in various forms since early Greek civilisation. However, it was not until 1877 that the German physiologist Emil du Bois-Reymond (1818–1896) suggested that there might be substances in the body, electrical in nature, responsible for neurotransmission (Lopez-Munoz and Alamo, 2009). We now call these substances *neurotransmitters*. In 1904, the neurotransmission phenomenon was postulated by Thomas Renton Elliott (1877–1961) and his mentor John Newport Langley (1852–1925).

Neurotransmitters are chemicals that the body uses to transmit messages from one neuron to the next across synapses. They are relatively low molecular weight amines that originate from dietary amino acids. We find neurotransmitters at the axon terminal end of neurons, where they stimulate the muscle fibres or other neurotransmitters. To classify these chemicals as neurotransmitters, they must meet the following criteria:

- they must be present within a neuron;
- they must be released in response to neuron stimulation;
- they must have a postsynaptic receptor present.

Neurotransmitters can be excitatory or inhibitory. *Excitatory neurotransmitters* are the nervous system's 'on switches', increasing the likelihood of sending a signal that excites a neuron. They are like the accelerator of a car: when we press it, it makes the car move or move faster. In other words, excitatory transmitters act as the body's natural stimulants, generally serving to promote wakefulness, energy and activity. An example of an excitatory neurotransmitter is glutamate or adrenaline (see Table 3.3).

Table 3.3   Classical neurotransmitters and their postsynaptic effects

Neurotransmitter	Location	Function postsynaptic effect
Acetylcholine	Can be found in the parasympathetic nervous system, spinal cord and cortex.	Excitatory
GABA	Most of the brain and spinal cord.	Inhibitory
Glutamate	Brain and spinal cord.	Excitatory
Dopamine	Limbic system and basal ganglia.	Excitatory/inhibitory
Serotonin	Brainstem and most of the brain.	Excitatory/inhibitory
Adrenaline	Brain neurons and adrenal cortex.	Excitatory
Noradrenaline	Spinal cord and limbic system, targeted organ of the sympathetic nervous system.	Excitatory

Inhibitory neurotransmitters are the nervous system's 'off switches'. They decrease the likelihood of sending an excitatory signal. They are like the brakes of a car: when we press them, they slow the car down or stop it moving. In other words, inhibitory neurotransmitters act as the body's natural tranquillisers, generally serving to induce sleep, promote calmness and decrease aggression. The main inhibitory neurotransmitter is gamma-aminobutyric acid (GABA) (see Table 3.3).

It has been proposed that there may be several hundred to several thousand neurotransmitters in the body, but only half a dozen or so are pharmacologically relevant, and these are acetylcholine, serotonin, noradrenaline, adrenaline, dopamine, glutamate and GABA. These neurotransmitters are sometimes referred to as the classical neurotransmitters. In the long term, we may discover many more neurotransmitters, and many more will become pharmacologically important as we discover new medicines.

Classical neurotransmitters

As previously discussed, neurotransmitters mediate neuron-to-neuron communication in the nervous system. Although these neurotransmitters show great diversity in many of their properties, they are all stored in small pockets called *synaptic vesicles* in the axon terminals. During neurotransmission, the synaptic vesicles fuse with the cell membrane and release their contents (neurotransmitters) into the extracellular space or synapse. The action of neurotransmission ends when the presynaptic terminal or surrounding **glial cells** reuptake or reabsorb the neurotransmitters (see Figure 3.4). Specialised proteins called transporters aid the reabsorption process, and the density and availability of these transporter proteins determine the speed of the reuptake process. In certain instances, enzymes destroy the neurotransmitters instead of being reabsorbed back into the presynaptic neuron, a process we call *catabolism*.

Acetylcholine

Acetylcholine was the first neurotransmitter to be identified. It is a neurotransmitter we find in both the peripheral and central nervous systems in many living species, including humans. It is the only neurotransmitter used in the motor division of the somatic nervous system. In the autonomic nervous system, acetylcholine is the neurotransmitter in the preganglionic sympathetic and parasympathetic neurons. It activates muscles in the peripheral nervous system and is a major neurotransmitter in the autonomic nervous system. Inside the brain, acetylcholine acts as a neuromodulator, thus a chemical that alters the way other brain structures process information, rather than a chemical used to transmit information from point to point (neurotransmitter). Additionally, the brain contains several acetylcholine (cholinergic) pathways, each with specific functions. They play an important role in arousal, attention and motivation. There are three acetylcholine pathways in the CNS:

- pons to thalamus and cortex;
- magnocellular forebrain nucleus to cortex;
- septohippocampal.

Because of its role in muscle activation of the autonomic nervous system, as well as in brain function, many important medicines exert their effects by altering acetylcholine transmission. Also, many venoms and toxins from plants, animals and bacteria (e.g. black widow spider venom, nerve gas) can cause harm by inactivating or hyperactivating muscles via their influences on the neuromuscular junction.

There are two types of acetylcholine receptors. First, there are the muscarinic receptors, which have wide distribution throughout the brain, especially in the cortex, the thalamus, the hippocampus, the mesolimbic system and the basal ganglia. They play important roles in cognitive and motor functions, as well as opiate reward. The muscarinic receptors that we find in the VTA regulate the release of dopamine in the nucleus accumbens. The other acetycholine receptor subtype is the nicotinic receptors, which we find in all muscle cells at neuromuscular junctions. When acetylcholine binds to these receptors, they control calcium channels, which leads to muscle contraction.

Adrenaline

Adrenaline, also known as epinephrine, is an excitatory neurotransmitter and a hormone essential for the breakdown of fat. Adrenaline originates from the compound noradrenaline (norepinephrine). As a neurotransmitter, adrenaline regulates attentiveness and mental focus. As a hormone, it is secreted along with noradrenaline, mainly in the medulla of the adrenal gland directly above the kidneys. An increase in the secretion of adrenaline can occur in response to fear or anger, and will result in an increase in heart rate and the breakdown of glycogen to glucose. We commonly refer to this reaction as the 'fight or flight' response, and it prepares the body for strenuous activity. It is an evolutionary adaptation that allows the body to react to danger quickly. When an individual encounters a potentially dangerous situation, the hypothalamus in the brain signals to the adrenal glands to release adrenaline and other hormones directly into the bloodstream. The body's systems react to these hormones within seconds, giving the person a nearly instant physical boost. Both strength and speed increase, while the body's ability to feel pain decreases. We often refer to this hormonal surge as an 'adrenaline rush'.

We use adrenaline medicinally as a stimulant in cardiac arrest, as a vasoconstrictor in shock, as a bronchodilator and antispasmodic in bronchial asthma, and to counteract anaphylaxis. Commonly, adrenaline levels will be low due to adrenal fatigue (a pattern in which the adrenal output is suppressed due to chronic stress). Therefore, symptoms can present as fatigue with low adrenaline levels. Low levels of adrenaline can also contribute to weight gain and poor concentration. An increase in the levels of adrenaline can be one of the factors that contribute to restlessness, anxiety, sleep problems or acute stress.

Noradrenaline

Like adrenaline, noradrenaline (norepinephrine) is a hormone, as well as an excitatory neurotransmitter, that is important for attention and focus. Noradrenaline is made from *dopamine*. The levels of adrenaline in the CNS are only about 10 per cent of the levels of noradrenaline. The brain produces noradrenaline in closely packed brain cell neurons, and the most important of these nuclei is the *locus coeruleus*, found in the pons. They form an excitatory pathway to the cortex called the **reticular activating system (RAS)**. Noradrenaline binds to several different receptor subtypes that control widely different functions.

As a neurotransmitter, noradrenaline functions in the sympathetic nervous system by stimulating alpha- and beta-adrenergic receptors (both adrenaline receptors). The stimulation of alpha-adrenergic receptors causes vasoconstriction of the radial smooth muscle of the iris, arteries, arterioles, veins, urinary bladder and the sphincter of the gastrointestinal tract. Stimulation of the beta-1-adrenergic receptors causes an increase in heart contraction, heart rate, automaticity and atrioventricular (AV) conduction, while stimulation of the beta-2-adrenergic receptors leads to the breakdown of glycogen in the liver (hepatic glycogenolysis) and the pancreatic release of glucagon, which increases plasma glucose concentrations.

Noradrenaline functions mainly in the sympathetic nervous system near the spinal cord or in the abdomen. The adrenal glands release noradrenaline directly into the bloodstream. Regardless of how and where it is released, noradrenaline acts on target cells by binding to and activating noradrenergic receptors located on the cell surface. The noradrenergic system is most active when an individual is awake, which is important for focused attention. An increase in noradrenaline activity seems to be a contributor to anxiousness. Also, brain noradrenaline turnover increases in conditions of stress. Interestingly, *benzodiazepines*, which are the primary anxiolytic medicines, decrease the firing of noradrenaline neurons. This may partly explain why benzodiazepines induce sleep. Noradrenaline is rapidly removed from the synapse by two processes: reuptake and metabolism. The noradrenaline transporter protein in the synapse facilitates the transportation of noradrenaline back to the presynaptic axon terminal (reuptake). The enzyme monoamine oxidase (MAO) then facilitates the metabolism of the remaining noradrenaline.

Dopamine

Dopamine is an excitatory and inhibitory neurotransmitter, depending on the dopamine receptor type to which it binds. The dopamine D_2 type tends to show inhibitory effects while the D_1 type promotes excitatory effects (Keeler et al., 2016). It is formed from the dietary amino acid *tyrosine*. It is also the precursor to noradrenaline and adrenaline, which are all *catecholamines*, a group of amino acids. Dopamine has many functions but plays a large role in the pleasure/reward pathway, affecting addiction thrills, memory and motor control. In this respect, dopamine acts as an excitatory neurotransmitter. Like noradrenaline and adrenaline, it is stored in vesicles in the axon terminal. Dopamine plays a significant role in the cardiovascular, renal, hormonal and central nervous systems. Dopaminergic neurons have dendrites that extend into various regions of the brain, controlling different functions through the stimulation of adrenaline (adrenergic) and dopamine (dopaminergic) receptors. The key dopamine pathways in the brain are mesolimbic, mesocortical, nigrostriatal and tuberoinfundibular (see Chapter 8). Common symptoms with low dopamine levels are loss of motor control, addictions, cravings, compulsions and loss of satisfaction. When there is an increase in dopamine levels, symptoms may manifest in the form of anxiety, hyperactivity or psychosis. After use, the dopamine transporter protein quickly removes dopamine from the synapse back into the presynaptic axon terminal, where it integrates back into vesicles for reuse. In some intances, the enzyme MAO facilitates the breakdown or catabolism of dopamine.

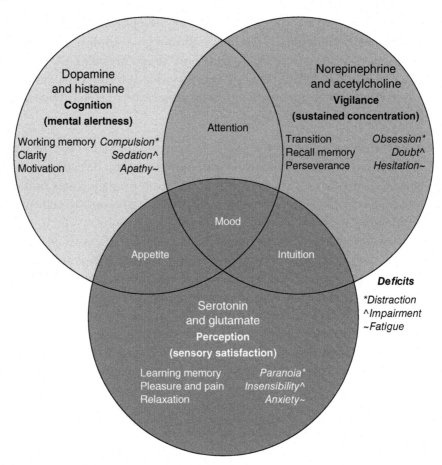

Figure 3.5   Classical neurotransmitters and function

Serotonin

Serotonin, or 5-hydroxytryptamine (5-HT), is a monoamine neurotransmitter made from tryptophan, a compound we primarily find in the gastrointestinal tract, blood platelets and the CNS. Approximately 80 per cent of the human body's total serotonin is in the gut, where its main use is to regulate intestinal movements. The remainder is made in serotonin neurons in the CNS, with the neurons of the raphe nuclei being the principal source of serotonin release in the brain. Because serotonin cannot cross the blood–brain barrier, the brain can only use serotonin that it produces inside itself. Depending on the receptor type, serotonin is both an excitatory and inhibitory neurotransmitter, and it targets for various functions. These include the regulation of mood, appetite and sleep. Serotonin also has some cognitive functions, including memory and learning. We believe that the control of serotonin at synapses is the major action of several classes of antidepressants.

The action of serotonin is terminated by transporting it from the synapse back to the presynaptic neuron. The serotonin reuptake transporter (SERT), a monoamine transporter, plays an important role in this regard. Various biochemical compounds can inhibit serotonin (5-HT) reuptake. These compounds include dextromethorphan and various classes of antidepressants, and there is comprehensive coverage of this in Chapter 5. Like dopamine and noradrenaline, the body can quickly degrade serotonin into its metabolites (5-hydroxyindoleacetic acid) using the enzyme MAO. The amount of 5-hydroxyindoleacetic acid is used as an indicator for serotonin activity. Dysregulation of serotonin can result in symptoms such as low mood, compulsions, anxiousness and headaches, as well as affecting appetite, sleep, muscle contraction and some cognitive functions, including memory and learning. Table 3.4 shows the effects of 5-HT receptor subtypes in relation to serotonin toxicity.

Table 3.4   Some serotonin receptor subtypes and their function

5-HT receptor	Main action relating to serotonin toxicity
5-HT$_{1A}$	Neuronal inhibition, regulation of sleep, feeding, thermoregulation, hyperactivity associated with anxiety, hypoactivity associated with depression.
5-HT$_{1D}$	Locomotion, muscle tone.
5-HT$_{2A}$	Neuronal excitation, learning, peripheral vasoconstriction, platelet aggregation.
5-HT$_{2B}$	Stomach contraction.
5-HT$_3$	Nausea and vomiting, anxiety.
5-HT$_4$	Gastrointestinal motility.

Glutamate

Glutamate is the most abundant excitatory neurotransmitter in the human nervous system, and it is necessary for memory and learning. Excitatory neurotransmitters increase the activity of signal-receiving neurons and play a major role in controlling brain function. Glutamate is made from glutamine, an abundant non-essential amino acid that we find in fish, eggs and dairy products. Approximately 70 per cent of the fast-excitatory CNS synapses use glutamate as a transmitter. In large quantities, glutamate can be neurotoxic and can lead to cell death.

Glutamate exerts its effects on cells, in part, by binding to at least four neuroreceptors: the kainite receptors, the alpha-amino-hydroxy-5-methyl-4-isoxazolepropionic acid receptors (AMPARs), the N-methyl-D-aspartate receptors (NMDARs) and the metabotropic glutamate receptors (mGluRs) receptors. Of these, the NMDARs play a particularly important role in controlling the brain's ability to adapt to environmental and genetic influences, which is important for learning and memory. The NMDARs have been studied extensively, especially when it was discovered that they play an important role in synaptic plasticity. These receptor types also play an important role in the origin of epilepsy. It is believed that this happens through the process of kindling, whereby repeated sub-threshold electrical stimuli of NMDARs in the limbic system leads to spontaneous seizure activity. When the person responds to stimuli with generalised convulsions, this signals the development of a permanent epileptic condition.

Therefore, activation of NMDARs, as well as their levels of function, is critical in kindling epilepsy. Selective NMDAR antagonists slow down kindling development, and at higher concentrations have an anticonvulsant effect.

The AMPARs are responsible for quick excitatory transmission within the central nervous system. AMPAR antagonists are anticonvulsant in nature.

Glutamate is also capable of exciting the mGluRs, of which there are currently eight subgroups that have been identified. Activation of mGluRs has been implicated in a variety of CNS functions, including different forms of synaptic plasticity, excitotoxicity and the release of other neurotransmitters.

Overall, an event or process that dramatically increases the activity of glutamate often increases the degree of neuronal excitation, and in extreme cases can induce the death of neurons. We believe that such a scenario takes place in conditions such as ischaemia, trauma, hypoxia, **hypoglycaemia** and hepatic encephalopathy. Milder but chronic dysfunction of glutamate systems may play an important role in many neurodegenerative diseases, such as Huntington's disease, Parkinson's disease, Alzheimer's disease, vascular dementia, and Tourette's and Korsakoff's syndromes. The **excitatory amino acid transporter (EAAT)** and **vesicular glutamate transporter (VGLUT)** facilitate several reuptake mechanisms responsible for the removal of glutamate from the synapse. We find these transporter family proteins (EAAT and VGLUT) either on the presynaptic axon terminal or the surrounding glial cells. Alterations in the function and/or expression of these carriers is implicated in a range of psychiatric and neurological disorders. For example, alteration in EAATs is implicated in cerebral strokes, epilepsy, Alzheimer's disease, HIV-associated dementia, Huntington's disease, **amyotrophic lateral sclerosis (ALS)** and malignant glioma, while alteration in VGLUTs is implicated in schizophrenia. Turn to Activity 3.6 to test your understanding of what you have read in this section.

Activity 3.6   Reflection

Name the classical neurotransmitters that are excitatory and inhibitory.

An outline answer is provided at the end of the chapter.

Gamma-aminobutyric acid

Gamma-aminobutyric acid (GABA) is the major inhibitory neurotransmitter of the brain, occurring in 30–40 per cent of all synapses. GABA concentration in the brain is 200–1,000 times greater than that of the adrenaline, noradrenaline, dopamine, serotonin or acetylcholine neurotransmitters. Essentially, GABA is made from the amino acid glutamic acid (glutamate) in the presynaptic neurons. The synaptic vesicles store the neurotransmitter until its release into the synapse during inhibitory neurotransmission.

GABA helps to induce relaxation and sleep, as well as balancing the brain by inhibiting over-excitation of the neurons, contributing to motor control, vision and many other cortical functions. GABA is one of several neurotransmitters that regulate anxiety, and some medicines that increase the level of GABA in the brain are used to treat epilepsy and to calm the trembling of people suffering from Huntington's disease.

GABA also stimulates the anterior pituitary, leading to higher levels of human growth hormone (HGH), a hormone that contributes significantly to muscle growth and prevents the creation of fat cells. The presynaptic GABA transporter or reuptake pump (GAT) terminates synaptic action, and the enzyme GABA transaminase (GABA-T) terminates GABA into an inactive substance by breaking down GABA to succinic semi-aldehyde. To fully understand the role of neurotransmitters, we now need to turn our attention to their connection to receptors and ion channels.

Receptors and ion channels

After release into the synaptic gap, a neurotransmitter diffuses towards the postsynaptic membrane, where there are receptor sites made of specific proteins or chains of amino acids. Receptors have specific molecular structures, which determines which substance (neurotramsmitter) can temporarily bind to them. When a neurotransmitter binds to postsynaptic receptors, this alters the permeability of the postsynaptic membrane to ions. Ions are atoms or molecules that possess negative or positive electrical charges, and they can move through ion channels. The principal function of ion channels is to allow the movement of ions (gating) across the cell membrane (see Figure 3.6). Gating refers to the opening or closing of these ion channels. It is the movement of ions in and out of cells through ion channels that creates an electrical signal essential for cell-to-cell communication.

There are two major classes of ion channels: voltage-gated ion channels and ligand-gated ion channels, and we will discuss these next (see Figure 3.6). We will look at voltage-gated, or ionotropic, ion channels first as they are involved in the generation of an action potential.

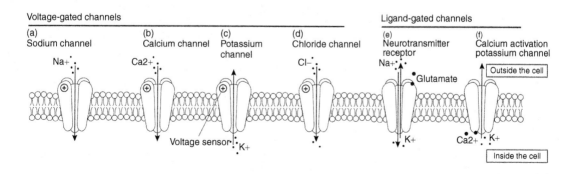

Figure 3.6 Voltage-gated ion channels (examples of voltage-gated ion channels include sodium, calcium, potassium, magnesium and chloride channels)

Voltage-gated ion channels, action potential and neurotransmission

Examples of voltage-gated ion channels are sodium, potassium, chloride, calcium and magnesium ions, and these are involved in classical neurotransmission. Voltage-gated ion channels are a class of channels we find across cell membranes (transmembranes) made from proteins. We find these along the axon and at the synapse, and they play a fundamental role in the generation and propagation of the nerve impulse (action potential). The difference in electrical charge between the inside and the outside of the cell membrane causes electromotive forces to drive ions inside or outside of the cell.

When a cell is in an unstimulated state, the concentration of sodium ions is greater outside the cell than inside. Simultaneously, the concentration of potassium ions is greater inside the cell than outside. We call this unstimulated state the *resting potential* of the cell, and its voltage is approximately −70 millivolts (mV). When a neuron cell is at its resting potential, it is *polarised* and its ion channels are closed (see Figure 3.6). This situation changes when we stimulate the neuron.

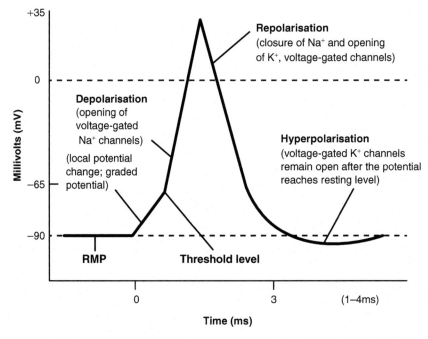

Figure 3.7 The generation of an action potential in a neuron

The stimulation of a neuron above a threshold will result in the opening of sodium channels, allowing positively charged sodium ions to rush inside the neuron, causing a brief positive charge. At this point, the electrical *membrane potential* (see Figure 3.7)

of the cell rapidly rises and falls, and we call this spike an *action potential*. The sodium channels then close; simultaneously, potassium channels open, allowing positively charged potassium ions to move out of the cell, therefore causing the membrane potential to go back to normal. The cell is now said to be *repolarised*. The potassium channels then close.

Before the membrane potential stabilises at -70 mV, there is a small undershoot called the *refractory period*. During this period, the neuron cannot fire another action potential. At this resting state (-70 mV), the excess sodium and potassium ions will slowly diffuse away from the membrane and the neuron is ready to fire another action potential. Once fired, the action potential quickly spreads along the axon like a wave until it reaches the axon terminal, where chemical neuro-transmission begins.

When an electrical impulse or action potential reaches the axon terminal, it causes the cell membrane to change its permeability and allows calcium ions (Ca^+) to enter the axon terminal. Calcium ion entrance into the axon terminal causes the neurotransmit-ter vesicles to migrate to the cell membrane and fuse. This results in the conversion of the original electrical message to a chemical message in the neurotransmitter. The amount of neurotransmitter released in the synapse depends on how many calcium ions enter the axon terminal. A more intense stimulation of the neuron allows more calcium ions to enter, resulting in the release of more neurotransmitters. The neuro-transmitters then travel to the postsynaptic neuron, where they bind to a receptor and initiate an action potential.

Ligand-gated ion channels, action potential and neurotransmission

The location of ligand-gated ion channels is on postsynaptic receptors, where the binding action of a neurotransmitter on to a receptor triggers the opening or closing of these ion channels. This transforms a presynaptic chemical message to a postsynaptic action potential (electrical message). In contrast to voltage-gated ion channels, where voltage differences initiate action, in ligand gated ion chan-nels it is the binding action of neurotransmitters to a receptor that is the initiator. Examples of ligand-gated receptors are GABA, serotonin ($5\text{-}HT_3$), nicotinic acetyl-choline and some of the glutamate family of receptors. Since these ligand-gated ion channels are also receptors, we sometimes call them ionotropic receptors or ion-channel-linked receptors. Some drugs, medicines and proteins can cause the ion channel to open to its maximum, allowing the maximum possible postsynaptic signal transduction. By contrast, other chemicals or drugs can cause the ion chan-nel to slow down and open infrequently, and some can put the ion channel into a closed and inactive state. Now that you have read this section, test your understand-ing by working on Activity 3.7.

Activity 3.7   Evidence-based practice and research

In a group or alone, research psychiatric illnesses that are a result of a shortage of one of the excitatory neurotransmitters. For each illness, list the neurotransmitter that is implicated.

An outline answer is provided at the end of the chapter.

Chapter summary

Contrary to popular belief, the brain is not an organ. It is the most complex structure in our body; and although our knowledge of the brain has increased thanks to new technology, there is a great deal we still do not know about this important structure. Currently, we know that the brain is divided into two hemispheres, which in turn are divided into the frontal, parietal, occipital and temporal lobes. In addition, the brain has two layers, namely the grey and white matter.

Neurons are the basic cells of the brain, and these are of many different shapes and sizes. They are involved in cell-to-cell communication, but at times the cells miscommunicate. The reason for this miscommunication is partly due to the wrong types of neurons making the wrong connections during a period of neural migration at the prenatal development level. Neural miscommunication can result in neurodevelopmental conditions or psychiatric symptoms.

Neural communication is aided by chemicals at the synapse called neurotransmitters. There may be thousands of different types of these in the body, but only seven are currently of pharmacological importance: acetylcholine, GABA, glutamate, dopamine, serotonin, adrenaline and noradrenaline. Most medicines used to treat mental health problems work on these neurotransmitters.

Activities: brief outline answers

Activity 3.1 Critical thinking (page 82)

If there is no electrical activity in the brainstem, it is possible to pronounce someone as clinically dead. The brainstem relays nerve impulses to the rest of the body. In particular, the medulla oblongata part of the brainstem is responsible for maintaining reflexes such as blood flow pressure, heart rate and breathing. If this is not happening, the individual is clinically dead.

Activity 3.2 Critical thinking (page 86)

Some of the causes of hypothalamic dysfunction include anorexia, bleeding, bulimia, genetic disorders, tumours, head trauma, infections and swelling (inflammation), malnutrition, radiation, and excess iron.

Activity 3.3 Research (page 87)

The cerebral cortex is divided into hemispheres, which in turn are divided into lobes:

- *Frontal lobe*: higher order functioning, critical thinking, memory including attention, planning, language and movement.
- *Parietal lobe*: processing of sensory information.
- *Occipital lobe*: vision.
- *Temporal lobes*: sound and language.

Activity 3.4 Evidence-based practice and research (page 90)

Illnesses associated with dysfunction of different areas of the brain are:

- cerebral cortex: depression, Huntington's disease, mania;
- amygdala: depression;
- hippocampus: Alzheimer's disease, mania;
- pons: sleep disturbance;
- substantia nigra: Parkinson's disease.

Activity 3.5 Critical thinking (page 93)

Most psychosis, especially schizophrenia, starts in the late teens and early adulthood. This coincides with higher rates of neural pruning, whereby new connections are being made at various synapses in the brain.

Activity 3.6 Reflection (page 100)

- Excitatory: glutamate, dopamine, serotonin, adrenaline, noradrenaline, acetylcholine.
- Inhibitory: dopamine, GABA, serotonin.

Activity 3.7 Evidence-based practice and research (page 104)

- Dopamine: depression/psychosis.
- Adrenaline: depression.
- Serotonin: depression/personality disorder/aggression.
- Glutamate: psychosis.

Further reading

Gibb, B. (2012) *The Rough Guide to the Brain*. New York: Rough Guides.

This is an accessible introduction to how the brain evolved and how it works.

Useful websites

www.neurogenesis.com/Neuroscience/index.php

This is a useful website that explains in very simple terms the concept of neural development.

www.neuroskills.com/brain.shtml

This is a useful website that explains in more detail the different parts of the brain and their function. It has useful colour diagrams.

www.waiting.com/brainanatomy.html

This is another useful website that explains brain anatomy and has very clearly annotated diagrams.

Chapter 4 Principles of pharmacology and medicine interactions

---

Chapter aims

By the end of this chapter, you should be able to:

- have an appreciation of how medicines are discovered and developed;
- understand the basic principles of pharmacology and their relationship with medicines management;
- understand the basic principles of pharmacodynamics and pharmacokinetics and their relationship with medicines management;
- describe the role of medicine interactions and genetic variation.

Introduction

Modern clinical psychopharmacology owes its origins to the discovery of antibiotics. The Second World War provided the incentive and the financial support to develop and mass-produce penicillin. Then the late 1950s saw a fast growth in the understanding of the way that our bodies metabolise neurotransmitters. This understanding was aided by our ability to isolate specific neurotransmitter receptors in test tubes. These developments allowed us to study the relationship between the structure and activity of receptors, thus preparing us for the next stage of modern clinical psychopharmacology in the 1970s and 1980s. During this era, scientists produced new molecules using theories and techniques developed in the 1950s and 1960s. These developments led to the discovery of first- and second-generation antipsychotics and antidepressants.

The need now is to develop truly novel CNS medicines that work by new mechanisms of action. Currently, the hope lies with the Human **Genome** Project and a better understanding of molecular neurobiology underpinning mental health problems. However, there are several problems that need to be solved first. One problem is that the Human Genome Project has many potential novel targets for medicines development, but currently there is not enough information to know which ones are likely to be the most fruitful for medicines development. This problem is further compounded by the fact that the blockbuster model of medicines development (i.e. one drug to treat a large part of the population) may no longer be viable. The main reason for this is that the improvement in molecular biology knowledge underlying mental illnesses is likely to result in the fragmenting of what currently appears to be one common syndromic illness (e.g. major depression or schizophrenia) into several distinct illnesses. This scenario has already occurred in oncology. This chapter will discuss the medicines discovery and licensing processes before discussing key principles of medicine interactions. Finally, the chapter will discuss the role of liver enzymes in medicine interactions before looking at the importance of ethnicity.

The medicines discovery process

Each year sees a couple of dozen new medicines licensed for use, but for every 10,000 potential medicines, the regulatory authorities approve only one medicine (see Figure 4.1 later in the chapter). The time from first compound development to medicine on the market typically takes 12–15 years and can cost around £1.15 billion. Importantly, when candidate medicines fail, they tend to do so in the later stages of clinical trials after a significant investment has been made. Overall, the probability of success in developing a new medicine is relatively low, but the reward of attaining such a success is disproportionately high.

For a medicine to work, it must interact with a disease target in our body and intervene in its own unique way. This can be likened to a lock and key mechanism, with the lock being the disease target and the key being the medicine. To treat the disease, the correct key must be found to open the lock.

The medicines discovery journey typically begins with research to understand the processes behind a disease. It is through better understanding of disease processes and pathways that we can identify new treatment targets. This might be a gene or a protein instrumental to the disease process with which a new treatment could interfere (e.g. blocking an essential receptor). An understanding of the status of genes and their associated proteins would help to pinpoint the cause of the disease and tailor medicines to attack the 'epicentre' of the disease. In this way, we can discover more specific medicines that are effective and have fewer side effects (i.e. they have a high therapeutic index).

Once researchers identify a potential target, they then search for a molecule or compound that acts on this target. Historically, researchers have looked to natural compounds from plants, fungi or marine animals to provide the basis for these candidate medicines, but increasingly scientists are using knowledge we have gained from the study of genetics and proteins to create new molecules using computers. The identified molecule or compound then enters preclinical development.

The preclinical stage of medicines development

After identifying a lead compound, the next stage is to confirm that the compound has an effect and that it is safe. This development stage includes pharmacological studies of the compound to get information on its toxicity, carcinogenicity, mutagenicity and reproductive development. The information is important in determining the safety and effectiveness of the compound as a potential medicine. An ideal medicine should be potent, efficacious and specific. That is, it must have strong effects on a specific targeted biological system (e.g. the brain) and should have minimal effects on the rest of the biological pathways to reduce side effects. No medicines are perfectly effective and safe. Many optimisation repetitions of the lead compound may be necessary to produce a potential medicine candidate for clinical trial.

Although pharmaceutical companies are increasingly using *in vitro* methods to evaluate pharmacological responses, some aspects of medicines development have no alternative but to use *in vivo* tests in animals to study the effects of a potential medicine. *In vitro* methods refer to experiments that are carried out on living organisms outside the biological context, colloquially referred to as a 'test tube'. *In vivo* methods refer to biological experiments that we conduct on whole, living organisms, usually animals, including humans. Where we use animals, the preferred models are mice and rats.

The use of animals for pharmacological and toxicological studies has produced important information for medicines development. However, many potential medicines fail in phase 1 and 2 clinical trials because the animal models (*in vivo*) are an insufficient representation of the human systems and functions for some medicines.

Ethical considerations in clinical trials

After establishing that the candidate compound has the potential to become a medicine, it is ready for clinical trial in humans. So, what is a clinical trial? According to the International Conference on Harmonisation (ICH GCP, 1994), the definition of a clinical trial or study is as follows:

> *Any investigation in human subjects intended to discover or verify the clinical, pharmacological, and/or other pharmacodynamic effects of an investigational product, and/or to identify any adverse reactions to an investigational product, and/or to study absorption, distribution, metabolism, and excretion of an investigational product with the object of ascertaining its safety and/or efficacy.*

Before a medicine goes for clinical trial, there are ethical and regulatory constraints that we must consider. The clinical trial must conform to the Medicines for Human Use (Clinical Trials) Regulations 2004 and the Declaration of Geneva of the World Medical Association. Further, there are at least seven ethical requirements, namely:

- *Clinical justification*: We should base our justification of clinical trials on scientific research that will result in improvements in health or the advancement of scientific knowledge. In other words, there must be social value to the research.
- *Scientific validity*: The clinical trial should have scientific validity. Thus, scientists should conduct studies that are methodical, with clear objectives and outcomes that can be verified statistically.
- *Fair subject selection*: Investigators should base their subject selection on scientific objectives, not on whether the subject is privileged or vulnerable, or because of convenience.
- *Informed consent*: Investigators should inform their subjects about the aims, methods, risks, and benefits of the clinical trial. They should explain the availability of alternatives and they should not pressure subjects into enrolling for the clinical trial. Rather, participants should voluntarily join in and be able to leave the trial at any time without pressure or penalty. For young and incapacitated people who are not able to understand the requirements and implications of the trial, researchers must obtain a proxy decision from their representatives (parents or guardians).
- *Favourable risk–benefit ratio*: Investigators should analyse the risk–benefit ratio, and – wherever possible – clinical trial subjects should be exposed to minimal risk and maximal benefit. The investigators should base the risk–benefit ratio on proven scientific data gathered at the preclinical stage. Investigators should not conduct a clinical trial if there is a doubt about the risk–benefit ratio.
- *Independent review*: There should be an independent review to ensure that an independent party assesses the clinical trial to address the question of conflict of interest. Members of the independent review body may consist of clinicians, scientists, lawyers, religious leaders and laypeople.
- *Respect for human subjects*: Investigators should take steps to protect participants and closely monitor the progress of the trial. They should also relay new developments in the trial without prejudice, including risks and benefits.

In addition to the ethical guidelines, the World Medical Association published the Declaration of Helsinki to describe the constraints on research involving human beings. Those countries that have signed this declaration are bound by the ethical principles. Now we can turn our attention to clinical trials.

Phase 1 clinical trials

In the UK, the Medicines and Healthcare Products Regulatory Agency (MHRA) approves the conducting of clinical trials before any testing on humans can occur. The investigators make a clinical trial application (CTA) that scientific experts review to determine whether enough preliminary research has been conducted to allow testing on humans.

After obtaining permission to conduct a clinical trial, the first clinical trial phase is phase 0, or the microdosing stage. At this stage, the investigators administer a single subtherapeutic dose of the candidate medicine to a small number of healthy partici-pants (usually between 10 and 15 people). Typically, the dosages are 100 times less than the intended therapeutic dose. The aim behind phase 0 trials is to gather preliminary information on the medicine's pharmacodynamics and pharmacokinetics. The trial should record information on the absorption, distribution, metabolisation and excre-tion of the medicine. It should also record the medicine's interactions within the body to confirm that these appear to be as predicted.

After microdosing (phase 0), the next stage is to screen for safety. This is done by conducting tests on a small group of healthy individuals (usually between 20 and 80 people). This stage is called a phase 1 clinical trial, and it aims to determine several fac-tors, including safe dosage ranges and the identification of side effects. A medicine's side effects can be subtle or long term, or may only be present in a subgroup of people. As previously mentioned, only healthy volunteers are normally recruited for the phase I trial, but in some situations patients who are critically ill or have a terminal disease can be given the option to be included in the trial after due consideration of the risk–benefit ratio. After the success of phase 1, the next stage is to establish the medicine's efficacy, usually against a placebo.

Phase 2 clinical trials

Phase 2 studies examine the efficacy of the potential medicine in volunteer patients who have the illness that the medicine aims to treat. This phase normally uses the fewest possible patients (usually between 100 and 500) to avoid unnecessarily exposing volunteers to a potentially harmful substance. The other aims of phase 2 studies are to determine the most effective dose and method of delivery (e.g. oral or intravenous), as well as the appropriate dosing interval, and to reconfirm product safety. Most medicines that fail clinical trials do so at phase 2 because the medicine may turn out to be ineffective, or have safety problems or intolerable side effects. The final stage before obtaining a licence is the confirmation of the safety and efficacy of the medicine.

Phase 3 clinical trials

After the success of the medicine at phase 2, the researchers test it on a much larger population (often between 1,000 and 5,000 participants) across multiple international sites. The aim of phase 3 trials is to reconfirm phase 2 findings in a larger population and to identify the best dosage regimen. The pharmaceutical company also needs to generate enough safety and efficacy information to demonstrate an overall risk–benefit ratio for the medicine to apply for a licensing application to the regulatory authority. Despite the rigorous testing that takes place, approximately 10 per cent of medicines fail at phase 3. If the medicine passes the phase 3 trial, it is ready for approval and mar-keting authorisation.

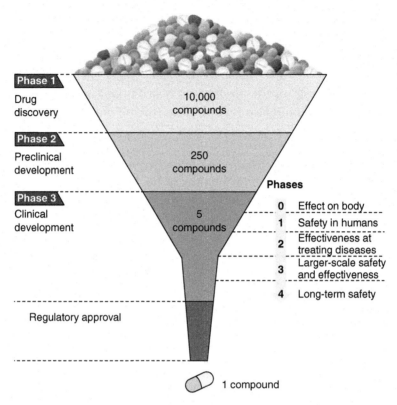

Figure 4.1 Stages of medicines discovery and development (adapted from Your Genome, 2016)

Marketing

The process of medicines development and marketing authorisation is similar across the world. In most countries, the pharmaceutical company submits a marketing authorisation application for medicines that have succeeded at phase 3 to the national regulatory authority. In the UK, the regulatory authority is the MHRA, and in the US it is the Food and Drug Administration (FDA). However, in Europe, pharmaceutical companies now opt to make a central application to the European Medicines Agency (EMA) to obtain marketing authorisation for the whole of Europe, and this avoids having to make multiple applications to individual countries. The submission contains preclinical and clinical information obtained during testing. This information includes the chemical make-up and manufacturing process of the medicine, the pharmacology and toxicity of the compound, human pharmacokinetics, the results of the clinical trials, and the proposed labelling.

The granting of a marketing licence is not the end of the process. In England and Wales, pharmaceutical companies need more than a marketing authorisation for most patients to access medicines on the NHS. They also need the National Institute of Health and Care Excellence (NICE) to recommend that the medicine should be made available through the NHS. NICE bases its decisions on the cost and efficacy of a treatment to determine if the cost–benefit is affordable to the NHS.

Phase 4 clinical trials

Clinical trials may also continue, as regulatory authorities may insist on phase 4 trials for post-marketing safety surveillance (pharmacovigilance) or the company may undertake more trials to allow them to target distinct markets. For example, they may conduct phase 4 in patients with complex medical problems or in pregnant women who are unlikely to have been involved in earlier trials in order to ensure that they do not interact with other medicines.

At phase 4, we usually watch the effects of medicines over a long time. Even after testing a new medicine on thousands of people, we may not know the full effects of the treatment for some time and there may still be questions to answer. For example, are there rare side effects that have not been seen yet, or are there side effects that only show up after a person has taken the medicine for a long time? These types of questions may take many years to answer, and phase 4 clinical trials often answer them. We can now turn our attention to the general principles of medicines action.

The general principles of medicines action

The 'principles of medicines action' refers to those general laws gathered from experience in the use of medicines. Medicines act on many different targets and in various ways, but they do not stimulate new responses; they only alter existing physiological activity. To understand medicine action, it is important to understand the physiological activity *before* the medicine was given (disease state) and the physiological activity *after* the medicine was given (treatment response). In depression, for example, the concentration of serotonin in the synapse is higher after treatment than before treatment with antidepressants.

Medicines work by interacting with the body in several ways. Usually, the medicine forms a chemical bond with specific sites that we call receptors. The bonding of medicines to these special sites was first proposed by scientists in the late nineteenth century, and this provided the foundation for the receptor site hypothesis of medicines action. According to these early ideas, if the medicine is to show an effect, it must first bond with a specific 'target molecule' or receptor on either the cell surface or on the surface of an organelle inside the cell.

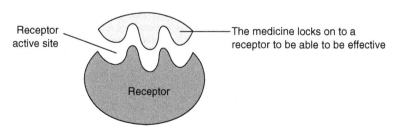

Figure 4.2 A schematic diagram showing the active site of receptor – the medicine fits or locks on to the receptor in a manner akin to a lock and key, forming a temporary bond

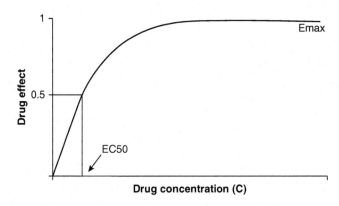

Figure 4.3 Graded medicine dose–response curves, showing the relationship between the medicine dose (x-axis) and the medicine effect or response (y-axis) – Emax denotes the highest possible drug effectiveness

It was soon realised that the medicine–receptor site interaction requires the 'right' chemical structure (see Figure 4.2). We call medicines that bind to a receptor and stimulate a response *agonists*, and *antagonists* are those that bind but do not produce a response.

We refer to the proportion of receptors that bind to medicines as *occupancy*. The relationship between occupancy and pharmacological response is usually non-linear (see Figure 4.3), and it forms the basis of pharmacodynamics.

In simple terms, pharmacodynamics is what the medicine does to the body. It is the study of where and how medicines act to produce their effects, including medicine actions on biological systems ranging from molecules to organisms.

The effects of medicines on a person vary from patient to patient, and this variation is due in part to medicine dosage and time. Different doses of the medicine result in different concentrations in various body tissues, producing a range of therapeutic and sometimes undesirable responses. Several factors, including pre-existing disease, age and genetic variability, may influence how the medicine acts on the body (pharmacodynamic response). In addition, factors such as temperature, pH, circulating ion and protein concentrations, levels of endogenous signalling molecules, and co-administration of other medicines may also alter pharmacodynamic responses to medicines. Medicines can interact with each other to produce an effect, and we will turn to this next.

The general principles of medicine interactions

Case study: Jamie

Jamie was 36 years old and suffered from depression. He was prescribed 200 mg of amitriptyline at night. He also used heroin and had been struggling to abstain. He was admitted to hospital to undergo a detoxification programme, and he was prescribed an initial dose of 60 mg of methadone. He was found dead early in the morning about a day after being admitted to hospital. The post-mortem report concluded that Jamie died from ventricular tachycardia, which was likely to have been caused by a higher than normal starting dose of methadone. More importantly, the interactive effects of methadone and amitriptyline are likely to have played a major contributory role in the ventricular tachycardia.

We can define medicine interactions as the modification of the action of one medicine by another. It can be beneficial or – as in Jamie's case – harmful, or it can have no significant effect. Put differently, medicine interactions are a change in efficacy or toxicity of one medicine by prior or simultaneous administration of a second medicine. Medicine interactions can also occur when food, drink or other environmental chemical agents alter the effects of a medicine.

Medicine interactions have been recognised for over 100 years. Because of the increasing availability of complex treatment options, the potential for medicine interactions is now enormous, and this is now an important cause of adverse drug (medicine) reactions (ADRs) and the the likelihood of treatment failure. Polypharmacy has been identified as an important cause of medicine interactions. Polypharmacy refers to the practice of prescribing several medicines to a person for different ailments. Unfortunately, polypharmacy increases the risk of unintentional adverse effects or *iatrogenic effects,* but importantly this is a preventable complication. Patients on polypharmacy and older persons are at the highest risk of **iatrogenic** effects due to medicine interactions, and they may require hospitalisation. However, patients usually do not report many medicine interactions. Moreover, most medicines currently in use in clinical practice are effective in only 25–60 per cent of patients because of adverse interactions. Adverse effects pertaining to medicine interactions are costly and can lead to serious illness and even death, as we have seen in the above case study. Accurate estimates of the incidence of medicine interactions are difficult to obtain. However, an early review reported that incidences of medicine–medicine interactions in hospital admissions ranged from 0 to 2.8 per cent (Jankel and Fitterman, 1993). Furthermore, a prospective study carried out in hospital inpatient settings reports that ADRs are responsible for hospital admissions in 6.5 per cent of cases, and medicine interactions cause 17 per cent of the cases (Pirmohamed et al., 2004). A related systematic review of 29 studies reports that the medicines most often involved in interactions are antiepileptics, antidepressants, corticosteroids and non-opioid analgesics. Commonly known clinical indicators of medicine interactions include sedation, respiratory depression, serotonin syndrome, neuroleptic malignant syndrome (NMS), delirium, seizures, ataxia, liver and kidney failure, bleeding, cardiac arrhythmias, and rhabdomyolysis (Kotlinska-Lemieszek et al., 2019). The risk of medicine interactions increases with the number of medicines the individual is taking.

Clearly, medicine interactions are a problem of which nurses and prescribers need to be aware. Our increasing understanding of molecular biology and the mechanisms involved in medicine metabolism and disposition support much of what we currently know about medicine interactions. In mental health, there are many psychotropic medicine interactions, but most are not clinically significant.

The main factors that determine medicine response are the blood concentration and elimination half-life of the active medicine. As previously mentioned, it is the biological and environmental factors that determine elimination half-life and medicine blood concentration. Biological factors include the amount of medicine administered, the extent and rate of absorption, the volume of distribution (determined by liver and kidney function, and body fluid balance), protein binding and localisation in tissue, biotransformation and excretion. Among the environmental factors, diet can influence medicine absorption and distribution. Smoking, concomitant uses of other non-psychotropic medications, herbal medicines, and some foods can each influence the metabolism of a medicine, and later sections will discuss these factors in more detail. One of the most important liver enzyme systems that plays a part in medicine metabolism is the cytochrome P450 (CYP450), which later sections will also discuss.

We usually classify medicine interactions as pharmaceutical, pharmacodynamic or pharmacokinetic. The following sections discuss the different types of interaction before focusing on the enzymes responsible for medicine metabolism.

Pharmaceutical interactions

Pharmaceutical interactions occur when we mix two or more chemically incompatible medicines outside the body before administration. An example is the incompatibility of phenobarbital with chlorpromazine or opioid analgesics when we mix these in the same syringe. Pharmaceutical interaction is the least likely of the three mechanisms to cause ADRs, and there are no known potentially hazardous interactions of this type with psychotropic medicines.

Pharmacodynamic interactions

Case study: Mark

Mark is a 28-year-old man who has used heroin in the past and is currently being maintained on methadone. He was found unconscious one morning, and all the indications were that he had taken an accidental overdose of opiates. To counteract the effects of an opiate overdose, he was given 2 mg of naloxone hydrochloride, administered intravenously. After a few hours, Mark's condition improved.

Pharmacodynamic interaction is the most common form of medicine interaction that we encounter in clinical practice. It occurs when different medicines have their effect in the body. This type of interaction occurs when medicines compete for the same receptor or produce antagonistic effects on the same target organ or system. An *antagonistic interaction* is when the medicine binds to a receptor but does not activate the receptor. Many instances of antagonistic pharmacodynamic interaction are beneficial. For example, naloxone is a specific antagonist that reverses the action of morphine by competing with it for occupancy of the μ-opioid receptor, as happened to Mark in the above case study. But often antagonistic pharmacodynamic interaction can be adverse. For example, antipsychotic medicines reduce the efficacy of levodopa in Parkinson's disease by blocking dopamine receptors, therefore preventing levodopa from activating the receptors.

In some cases, pharmacodynamic interaction is synergistic. *Synergistic interaction* means that the effect of two medicines taken together is greater than the sum of their separate effects at the same doses. Put simply, the effects of two medicines or more have an additive effect. Synergic pharmacodynamic interactions can produce harmful or beneficial effects on the same target organ or system. An example of beneficial synergistic interaction is the concomitant use of an antidepressant and lithium in treatment-resistant depression. The concomitant use of these two medicines is likely to be more effective than either lithium or antidepressants alone in the treatment of some forms of depression (Edwards et al., 2013). But some such interactions are harmful, as we see in the following case study.

Case study: José

José is a 56-year-old bank worker with a history of hypertension, hypothyroidism and depression. Currently, his daily medication regimen includes 150 mcg of levothyroxine and 200 mg of amitriptyline. He also takes 50 mg of a non-prescribed antihistamine medicine, diphenhydramine, to help him sleep. One day he went to the pub to celebrate a friend's birthday and drank three pints of beer. Afterwards, he went home and remembered to take his antidepressants and diphenhydramine. The next day, he could not be roused. An overdose was suspected and he was rushed to hospital.

It is important to warn patients of the effects of alcohol while taking antidepressants, as in the above case study. A good example of a harmful synergistic interaction is that of alcohol and tricyclic antidepressants (TCAs). Both substances – antidepressants and alcohol – have the synergistic effect of depressing the CNS. In José's case, the situation was complicated by his use of a hypnotic, diphenhydramine. Another useful example of a harmful synergistic interaction is between selective serotonin reuptake inhibitors

(SSRIs) and non-steroidal anti-inflammatory drugs (NSAIDs). SSRIs increase the risk of gastrointestinal bleeding when taken together with aspirin or other NSAIDs. This is due to the synergistic inhibition of platelet aggregation by these medicines. Before you move on to the next section, try Activity 4.1.

Activity 4.1   Critical thinking

You are working in a mental health clinic and notice that the doctor frequently prescribes both fluoxetine and amitriptyline for depression in the same patient.

- Is there any advantage in this?
- What is the ADR that is likely to result from taking two antidepressants concomitantly?

An outline answer is provided at the end of the chapter.

Pharmacokinetic interactions

In the previous section, we discussed how pharmacodynamics deals with the way that a medicine affects the body. We are now going to look at pharmacokinetics, which we define as the effect the body has on the medicine. Pharmacokinetics includes the study of the mechanisms of absorption, distribution, metabolism and distribution of an administered medicine. It also examines the rate at which a medicine begins to work, the duration of the effect and the chemical changes of the substance in the body. In short, we can define pharmacokinetics as the action of the body on the medicine. Pharmacokinetic interactions are more common and readily predictable than pharmacodynamic interactions. The most serious pharmacokinetic interactions are those in which one medicine changes the rate of metabolism and elimination of another. As we look at the different aspects of pharmacokinetics, we will examine the various possible types of medicine interactions.

Absorption

In pharmacokinetics, absorption is the movement of a medicine into the bloodstream, and it involves several phases.

First, the medicine needs to be introduced into the bloodstream via some *route of administration* (e.g. skin, oral, intravenous or intramuscular injection) and in a specific dosage form (e.g. tablet, capsule, liquid). The second stage involves *dissolution*, where a medicine, say an ingested tablet, dissolves into the stomach or small intestines. The rate of dissolution is a key target for controlling the duration of a medicine's effect. As such, several dosage forms that contain the same active ingredient may be available, differing only in the rate of dissolution. For example, some medicines are prepared as slow release, sustained release or enteric-coated, and these all affect the dissolution rate of the medicine. If a medicine is supplied in a form that does not readily dissolve, then the active ingredient of the medicine may be absorbed into the bloodstream more gradually over time, resulting in a longer duration of action. Before you proceed further, try Activity 4.2.

Activity 4.2 Critical thinking

You are the registered nurse administering medication on the ward and you see a patient's medicine administration chart indicating 800 mg of lithium carbonate SR, BD. You have run out of high-denomination lithium carbonate tablets and decide to give four 200 mg tablets. You repeat this at supper time. Late in the evening, another nurse reports to you that the patient looks disoriented and confused and has problems with coordination.

• What do you think might be the problem with the patient?

An outline answer is provided at the end of the chapter.

The small intestine (duodenum, jejunum and ileum) is the major site for medicine absorption. In oral administration of medicines, absorption takes place through the mucous membranes of the gastrointestinal tract. It is a physical process whereby atoms, molecules or ions enter a bulk liquid, or a solid material enters the gastrointestinal tract. The first part of the gastrointestinal tract that a medicine encounters is the stomach, which contains many digestive enzymes, but the stomach absorbs very few medicines because of its acidic environments (pH 1.5–3.5). Several factors affect the rate or extent of absorption (i.e. the total amount of medicines absorbed) in the gastrointestinal tract, and we discuss these below.

Changes in the gastrointestinal pH: The absorption of medicines across the mucous membrane depends on the extent to which the medicine exists in a non-ionised, fat-soluble form. In turn, the ionisation state depends on the pH of the absorption environment. The stomach is acidic or has a low pH (3.5), and this facilitates the absorption of medicines that exist in non-ionised, fat-soluble form. Weakly acidic medicines such as salicylates (aspirin) absorb better in acidic environments because they exist in non-ionised form at low pH. If the gastric pH alters due to antacids, histamine H_2 antagonists or proton-pump inhibitors, this can cause poor absorption of acidic medicines because of the alkalinising effect of these antacids on the gastrointestinal tract. However, changes in gastric pH tend to affect the speed of absorption rather than the amount of absorption. The alkalinising effect of antacids on the gastrointestinal tract are temporary, and we can mimimise the potential for interaction by leaving an administration interval of two to three hours between the antacid and the potentially interacting medicine.

Another point of consideration is that older persons readily absorb medicines that are destroyed by gastric acid because older adults tend to have higher pH due to an age-related inability to produce gastric acids. For example, in older persons, there is a poor absorption and a lower serum concentration of medicines that depend on low pH, such as aspirin and phenytoin.

Adsorption, chelation and other complex mechanisms: Some medicines react directly within the gastrointestinal tract to form chelates and complexes that the gastrointestinal tract cannot readily absorb. A chelate is a complex compound made of a central metal atom and a large complex molecule or ligand surrounding the metal (see Figure 4.4). The medicines we associate the most with this type of interaction include tetracyclines and quinolone antibiotics that can form large complex molecules. Antacids containing calcium, magnesium and aluminium also form chelates and therefore can reduce the absorption of medicines. Adsorbents (chemicals that attract other molecules or particles on to their surface) such as colestyramine can reduce the absorption of some medicines, such as digoxin, warfarin, propranolol levothyroxine and antidepressants.

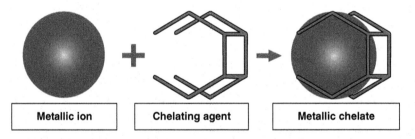

| Metallic ion | Chelating agent | Metallic chelate |

Figure 4.4 The formation of a chelate involving a metallic ion and a chelating agent. With courtesy from Transport phenomena and processes. *http://gruppotpp.unisa.it/en/.* No copyright required.

Effects of gastrointestinal motility: Since the upper part of the small intestines absorbs most medicines, those medicines that alter the rate of stomach content emptying can affect absorption. Medicines with anticholinergic effects, such as TCAs, phenothiazines, procyclidine and some antihistamines, decrease gut motility and delay gastric emptying. Motility refers to an organism's ability to move food through its digestive tract. The reduction in gut motility can either concomitantly increase or decrease the blood serum level of the medicine given. In the management of movement disorders, for example, anticholinergic medicines reduce the bioavailability of levodopa by as much as 50 per cent. Additionally, opioids such as diamorphine and pethidine strongly inhibit gastric emptying and reduce the absorption rate of paracetamol. By contrast, metoclopramide increases gastric emptying and increases the absorption rate of paracetamol, an effect that we use to therapeutic advantage in the treatment of migraines to ensure a rapid analgesic effect. To a lesser extent, metoclopromide also accelerates the absorption of propranolol and lithium.

From a gender perspective, women generally empty stomach solids more slowly than men and may have greater gastric acidity, thus slowing down the absorption of certain types of medicines.

Induction or inhibition of medicine transporter proteins: The oral bioavailability of some medicines is restricted by the action of medicine transporter proteins. This is because some medicine transporter proteins eject medicines that diffuse across the gut lining back into the gut. Currently, the most well-described medicine transporter protein is P–glycoprotein. This transporter protein is a substrate of digoxin, and medicines that inhibit P-glycoprotein – such as verapamil – may increase digoxin bioavailability with the potential for digoxin toxicity.

Malabsorption: Some medicines, such as the antibiotic neomycin, may cause malabsorption syndrome, leading to a reduction of absorption of other medicines such as digoxin. Malabsorption syndrome refers to a disorder in which the small intestine cannot absorb enough medicines or certain nutrients and fluids. Another useful example of malabsorption is that of orlistat. Orlistat inhibits gastric and pancreatic enzymes that break down fat (lipases). Therefore, taking orlistat can theoretically lead to an increase in undigested fat in the gastrointestinal tract. This increase in fat (lipids) reduces the absorption rate of fat-soluble medicines when we co-administer them with orlistat.

Special considerations: In neonates, an important and unique source of medicine absorption available until birth is the placenta. But after baby delivery, this route can no longer eliminate medicines in the neonatal circulation and the baby must use its own systems. Important examples of maternal medicines that may adversely affect the baby are pain relief during labour and beta blockers given to reduce pregnancy hypertension. In addition, the mother may be given the medicine with the intention of treating not her, but the foetus. An example of this is the use of corticosteroids such as bethamethasone to promote foetal lung maturation in preterm delivery. Before proceeding further, consider the following case study.

Case study: Denise

Denise, a 30-year-old solicitor who suffers from bipolar disorder, was brought to A&E in a state of stupor after taking an overdose of 40 capsules of valproic acid (500 mg each) several hours earlier in an apparent suicide attempt. On admission, her blood pressure was 95/50 mmHg, her pulse was 120 bpm, and her body temperature was 36.5°C. Blood analysis revealed lactic acidosis, an indication of hypoxia. The concentration of blood serum valproic acid was 4,678 mmol/L (normal therapeutic range 350–690 mmol/L).

Denise was immediately given activated charcoal by nasogastric tube and intravenous L-carnitine and sodium bicarbonate. **Haemodialysis** was then started, and by the next morning her valproic acid blood serum levels were back to normal.

In some situations, the way that medicines interact with each other at the absorption stage can be advantageous. The above case study is a case in point: we give activated charcoal following an overdose of TCAs or valproic acid. Charcoal absorbs the antidepressant or valproic acid in the gut, thereby reducing its absorption into the bloodstream and the effects of the overdose. However, in some situations, the absorption of medicines can have an adverse effect. For example, when an individual takes a phenothiazine medicine such as chlorpromazine concomitantly with an antacid, the antacid inhibits the absorption of the antipsychotic, which leads to a reduction of the antipsychotic effect. Once a medicine is absorbed, it will be distributed to tissues in various parts of the body.

Distribution

Following absorption, a medicine undergoes distribution to various tissues in the body, including its site of action (see Figure 4.5). Distribution refers to the way in which circulating body fluids transport medicines to the sites of action (receptors). How efficiently the body distributes a medicine between tissues is dependent on the permeability between tissues, the rate at which the tissues receive nutrients, and the amount and rate of blood flow to the tissues. It also depends on the ability of the medicine to bind to plasma proteins and tissue. Medicines are easily distributed in organs that receive high levels of blood and nutrients (i.e. they are highly perfused), such as the liver, the heart or the kidneys. By contrast, organs or tissues that receive low levels of blood and nutrients, such as muscle, fat and peripheral organs, have poor medicine distribution.

The most frequently recognised mechanism of distribution-related medicine interaction is *altered protein binding*. Many psychotropic medicines bind to plasma proteins, particularly to albumin, which act as a carrier for non-water-soluble medicines. Albumin is

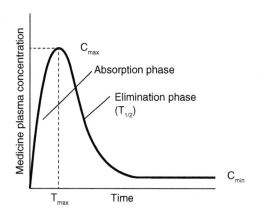

C_{min}
Minimum concentration
of the medicine

C_{max}
Maximum medicine concentration
after taking one dose

T_{max}
Time it takes for the medicince
to reach maximum concentration

$T_{1/2}$
Time it takes to eliminate half the
medicine concentration from the blood

Figure 4.5   Medicine distribution and elimination against time

also the main plasma protein that acidic medicines such as warfarin bind to, while alkaline medicines such as TCAs generally bind to α-acid glycoprotein. Medicines that bind to proteins are pharmacologically inactive because the large size of the medicine protein complex keeps it in the bloodstream and prevents it from reaching the sites of action, metabolism and excretion. However, it is the free, non-protein-bound portion of the medicine that is free to diffuse into tissues, interact with receptors, and either produce a therapeutic effect or be metabolised. If there is a reduction in the protein binding of the medicine, this increases the free medicine **fraction**, therefore increasing the effect of the medicine (see Figure 4.6). Medicines that bind highly to protein, such as phenytoin, are most prone to interactions mediated by this mechanism. For example, diazepam displaces phenytoin from plasma proteins, resulting in an increase in the plasma concentration of free phenytoin and an increase in the risk of adverse effects. Before you move on, try Activity 4.3.

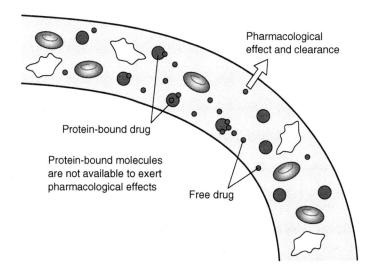

Figure 4.6   How binding to proteins affects medicine interactions

Activity 4.3 Decision-making

Errol is a 54-year-old man who suffers from diabetes, hypertension and bipolar disorder. He is currently taking 500 mg of metformin twice per day, and 40 mg of propranolol and 20 mg of olanzapine nocte (i.e. at night).

- How would you ensure that Errol is safe from the effects of medicine interactions?

An outline answer is provided at the end of the chapter.

Most medicines reach the CNS via the brain capillaries and the cerebrospinal fluid. Despite the brain receiving as much as one-sixth of cardiac output, medicine penetration to the brain is restricted because of its permeability characteristics. Although some fat-soluble medicines can enter the brain readily, many medicines do not. The reason is the blood–brain barrier. Because the brain requires a very stable environment with protection to function effectively, substances cannot easily pass between small gaps in the capillary membrane.

The capillaries that circulate blood in the brain are constructed differently from other tissue capillaries. Brain blood capillaries are constructed of cells with tight junctions that allow only very small molecules to pass. Additionally, glial cells (astrocytes) surround the capillary walls, and these glial cells provide an additional barrier by tightly adhering to the capillary endothelial membrane. This arrangement provides a highly selective, semipermeable border separating the circulating blood from the brain and the extracellular fluid in the CNS. We call this impermeable construction the blood–brain barrier. This arrangement slows down the diffusion of water-soluble medicines and protects the brain from disturbances in the chemical environment of the bloodstream. Additionally, the blood–brain barrier protects the brain from potentially toxic substances, including most viruses and bacteria. However, with ageing, the blood–brain barrier may become less effective, allowing an increase in the passage of compounds into the brain.

Metabolism

In pharmacokinetics, metabolism is the chemical process that changes or transforms a medicine into another chemical to facilitate its degradation and eventual elimination from the body. The liver is the principal site of medicine metabolism, although this process involves other organs, such as the gut, the kidneys, the lungs, the skin and the placenta. Whether a medicine has therapeutic (beneficial) or toxicological (harmful) effects largely depends on the rate of its metabolism, which consists mainly of two phases. Phase 1 metabolism consists of reactions such as *oxidation hydrolysis* and *reduction*. Phase 2 metabolism primarily involves the joining of the medicine with substances such as **glucuronic acid** and **sulphuric acid**. Most pharmacokinetic medicine–medicine interactions occur in phase 1, where alterations in metabolism or biotransformation generally involve the enzymes *CYP450*.

A person's genes (one gene–one enzyme) controls the production of CYP enzymes, and gene mutation gives rise to different versions of a CYP enzyme. We call this gene variation pharmacogenetic *polymorphism* (literally, 'many forms'), and it partly explains why medicine response varies between people.

This variation of medicine response and metabolism divides the population into at least three types. The first group is those people with a form of the gene (allele) that is not working or is missing. We call such individuals *poor metabolisers*. Poor metabolisers biotransform medicines more slowly than average, resulting in higher blood serum levels of the medicine. In practice, they require lower doses of medicine to achieve a therapeutic effect and they are prone to adverse side effects (see Figure 4.7a). The second group is those people with an allele that is functioning normally, and we call these individuals *extensive metabolisers*. Extensive metabolisers biotransform a medicine at the expected rate, and therefore – in practice – require the recommended dose of medicine to achieve a therapeutic effect (see Figure 4.7b).

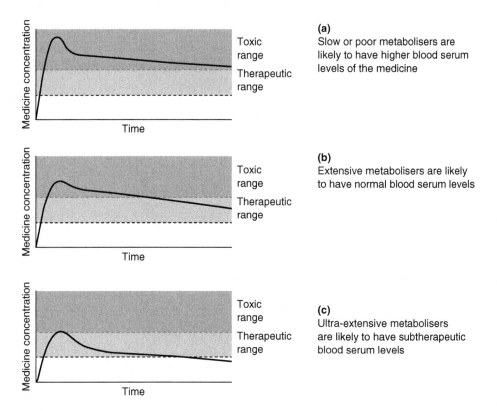

Figure 4.7 Graphs of slow, extensive, and ultra-extensive metabolisers of medicines

The third group is those people with an allele that is very fast at metabolising a medicine, and we call these individuals *ultra-extensive metabolisers*. These individuals biotransform medicines at a much higher rate than most people, and – in practice – will need a higher medicine dose to achieve a therapeutic effect (see Figure 4.7c). As mentioned earlier, the CYP450 enzymes play a key role in medicine metabolism, and we will focus on this in more detail next.

The CYP450 enzymes

There are as many as 57 individual CYP enzymes in humans, but many of these play a minor role in medicine metabolism. Six enzymes are responsible for more than 90 per cent of human medicine metabolism: 1A2, 3A4, 2C9, 2C19, 2D6 and 2E1. The enzymes themselves are denoted by 'CYP' followed by the numeral that denotes the enzyme family. The numeral is then followed by a capital letter that denotes a subfamily, and the last numeral denotes the individual gene. Thus:

2 = family;

D = subfamily;

6 = individual gene.

A CYP enzyme metabolises a medicine to a compound that the body can readily excrete. The medicine binds to the enzyme's active site (see Figure 4.2 earlier in the chapter) and departs as a changed molecule that we call a metabolite. However, the situation is slightly different when there is an inhibitor involment. An inhibitor is a chemical or substance that stops or slows down the enzyme's rate of metabolising the medicine. In other words, an inhibitor stops or slows down biotransformation. Some medicines act as inhibitors to the metabolism of other medicines.

Table 4.1   Clinical management of commonly encountered psychotropic medicine–medicine interactions

Medicine (class)	Concomitant offender (ex.)	Mechanism	Clinical management
Benzodiazepines (diazepam, alprazolam, midazolam, lorazepam)	Fluvoxamine Nefazodone Indinavir Clarithromycin Azole antifungals Grapefruit juice	Pharmacokinetic inhibition by: CYP3A4	Decrease dose of benzodiazepines by 50 per cent; monitor for excessive CNS effects
	Thiazolidinediones (pioglitazone, troglitazone)	Pharmacokinetic induction of CYP3A4 r	Consider increase of benzodiazepine dose; monitor for efficacy

Medicine (class)	Concomitant offender (ex.)	Mechanism	Clinical management
Tricyclic antidepressants (amitriptyline)	Paroxetine Fluoxetine	Pharmacokinetc inhibition of CYP2D6	Reduce dose of tricyclics; consider checking tricyclic levels; monitor for CNS effects
First-generation antipsychotics (phenothiazines, haloperidol)	Fluoxetine Fluvoxamine	Pharmacokinetic inhibition of CYP2D6 and CYP1A2 n	Increased risk for extrapyramidal side effects; consider reducing dose of haloperidol or phenothiazine
	Smoking	Pharmacokinetic induction of CYP1A2	Consider increasing antipsychotic dose in smokers; monitor therapeutic medicine level to help in monitoring of ADRs
Second-generation antipsychotics (clozapine, olanzapine, risperidone, quetiapine)	Fluvoxamine Paroxetine Fluoxetine Ketoconazole	Pharmacokinetic inhibition of CYP1A2, CYP2D6 and CYP3A4 i	Monitor clozapine concentrations; consider SSRI change; consider dose reduction of antipsychotic; monitor for extrapyramidal side effects; monitor for excessive CNS effects
	Smoking	Pharmacokinetic induction of CYP1A2 inducer	Monitor for clozapine or olanzapine efficacy
	Oral hypoglycaemics and anti-lipidemics	Pharmacodynamic: antipsychotic alterations of glucose and lipids	Patients may require additional or increased doses of medications to manage hyperglycemia and/or hyperlipidaemia
SSRIs (paroxetine, sertraline, citalopram) and SNRIs (duloxetine)	MAOIs	Pharmacodynamic: decrease metabolism of serotonin	Monitor for serotonin syndrome risk; consider 14-day washout prior to starting SSRI
	Triptans	Pharmacodynamic: enhancement of serotonin	Monitor for serotonin syndrome risk; consider avoiding combination
	Hydrocodone	PK: CYP2D6 inhibition	Reduction of analgesic effect due to CYP inhibition; may require increased doses of analgesic or switch to non-CYP2D6 metabolised analgesic

For example, fluvoxamine slows down (inhibits) the biotransformation of olanzapine, clozapine and zotepine if the metabolism of these medicines is via the CYP1A2 enzyme. In other words, the comcomittant administration of fluvoxamine with olanzapine or clozapine slows down the catalytic effect of the CYP1A2 enzyme, resulting in an increase in the blood serum level of these antipsychotics. In turn, an increase in the blood serum level could result in the patient experiencing side effects, or – at worst – toxicity can develop. In the case of clozapine, the blood serum levels may sufficiently elevate to cause seizures. In practice, the prescriber may need to lower the therapeutic dose of clozapine if the patient is taking fluvoxamine concomitantly. The CYP2D6 enzyme catalyses clozapine and olanzapine, and several antidepressants are inhibitors of this enzyme, so – in theory – these antidepressants can cause elevation of blood serum levels of clozapine and olanzapine.

Case study: Christine

Christine, a 46-year-old woman who suffers from bipolar disorder and epilepsy, was admitted to a general ward following an infection. Before admission to hospital, she was maintained on 800 mg of sodium valproate per day. To control the infection, she was prescribed the antibiotic ertapenem, but 21 days later she had an epileptic seizure. Her blood serum level for valproic acid was well below therapeutic levels. Ertapenem was discontinued in favour of a different class of antibiotic. After 14 days, Christine's valproic acid levels increased and were within therapeutic levels.

Conversely, an *inducer* allows the rapid metabolism of a medicine by making the enzyme act more quickly. For example, the CYP3A4 enzyme catalyses the metabolism of several antipsychotics such as clozapine, quetiapine and aripiprazole, but carbamazepine can induce this enzyme. Thus, concomitant administration of carbamazepine with any of these antipsychotics will lead to a reduction in the blood serum levels of the antipsychotic, therefore leading to a loss of efficacy. So, in practice, the prescriber should give higher than normal doses of the above antipsychotics to achieve efficacy if there is concomitant administration with carbamazepine. Other powerful CYP inducers are phenytoin, St John's wort, cigarette smoking and the antibiotic rifampicin. It is important to explain to the patient about the possibility of a reduction in efficacy of antipsychotics due to interaction. Christine's epilepsy was stable on an 800 mg dose of sodium valproate, but her blood serum levels of valproic acid were reduced substantially after she started taking the antibiotic ertapenem. The ertapenem acted as an inducer in this respect, helping to speed up the metabolism of valproic acid. Had the interaction between sodium valproate and ertapenem been checked prior to prescribing, this could have prevented Christine from suffering an epileptic seizure. It is therefore important to check medicine interactions in the *British National Formulary* (BNF) or to check credible government websites on the internet (see **www.bnf.org**). A way of solving this type of interaction is to prescribe medicines that have little potential for interaction or to administer the substrate (sodium valproate) and inducer (ertapenem) medicines at different times, allowing an interval of at least two to three hours between administration.

An important inducer of olanzapine is smoking. Smoking is an inducer of the CYP1A2 enzyme, which speeds up (catalyses) the metabolism of antipsychotics such as olanzapine. In this regard, the prescriber may need to increase the doses of olanzapine in those who smoke. It is important to inform patients of the effects of smoking on certain types of antipsychotics.

Another important area of pharmacokinetic medicine interactions is excretion, which we will turn to next.

Elimination

Elimination or excretion of a medicine is any one of several processes by which the body eliminates the medicine, either in its unaltered form (free and unbound to proteins) or modified as a metabolite (biotransformed). Excretion of the medicine takes place in the kidneys via the process of glomerular filtration. During this process, blood vessels retain larger molecules such as plasma proteins and blood cells. The blood then flows to other parts of the kidney tubules, where the tubular filtrate removes, secretes or reabsorbs medicines and their metabolites by active and passive transport systems. The body also eliminates medicines through other methods, such as the liver, the skin and the lungs, or tears, saliva, respiration, faeces or bile. Medicine interactions can occur when medicines interfere with kidney tubule fluid pH, active transport systems or blood flow to the kidney, thereby altering the excretion of other medicines.

Changes in urinary pH: Passive reabsorption of medicines in kidneys depend on the degree to which the medicines exist in non-ionised, fat-soluble form. Only the non-ionised form of the medicine is fat-soluble and can diffuse back into the blood capilaries. Thus, at relatively high pH (alkaline), weakly acidic medicines exist as ionised and fat-insoluble, which are unable to diffuse through the glomerular tubular wall, and therefore will be lost in the urine. Thus, at alkaline pH, weakly acidic medicines exist in ionised, fat-insoluble form, which is unable to diffuse into the tubule cells, and therefore will be exreted in the urine. However, this method of interaction is of minor clinical significance as medicines that cause large changes in urinary pH are rarely in use.

Changes in active renal tubule excretion: Renal elimination of medicines is the result of three concurrent processes occurring in the nephron: glomerular filtration, tubular secretion and tubular reabsorption. Glomerular filtration is a passive process while tubular secretion, and sometimes reabsorption, is an active process involving several protein transporters. These transporters are predominantly in the proximal tubule, and they work in tandem to eliminate medicines from the blood circulation to the urine. Medicines that use the same active transport system in the kidney tubules can compete with one another for excretion. This competition can be therapeutically advantageous. For example, we may give **probenecid,** a medicine that competes for the same protein transporters with penicillin, to increase the plasma concentration of penicillin. We now know that probenecid inhibits the renal secretion of many other medicines, including indomethacin, ketoprofen, naproxen, penicillins, ganciclovir and lorazepam.

Changes in renal blood flow. The production of renal vasodilatory prostaglandins partially controls the blood flow through the kidneys. Prostaglandins are hormone-like substances that take part in a wide range of bodily functions, including dilating blood vessels (vasodilatory), blood pressure and the modulation of inflammation. If we inhibit the production of prostaglandins with medicines such as non-steroidal anti-inflammatory drugs (NSAIDs), this reduces the renal excretion of medicines such as lithium, resulting in a rise in plasma levels, though the mechanism underlying this interaction is not entirely clear. In any event, we should closely monitor lithium plasma levels when an NSAID medicine is prescribed.

Biliary secretion and the enteral hepatic shunt. The bile excretes several medicines, either unchanged or as a conjugated compound such as glucuroride, to make them more water-soluble. The gut bacteria (gut flora) metabolise some of the conjugates to their parent compounds, and the bloodstream reabsorbs these. This recycling process prolongs the stay of the medicine within the body; but if the presence of antibacterial medicines diminishes gut flora, then the medicine is not recycled and is lost quickly from the body. This mechanism is proposed to be the basis of an interaction between broad-spectrum antibiotics and oral contraceptives. Antibiotics may reduce the **enterohepatic circulation** of ethyloestradiol conjugates. Ethyloestradiol is a semi-synthetic oestrogen medication in wide use as a birth control pill. However, there is considerable debate about the nature of this interaction as the evidence from pharmacokinetic studies is not convincing (Masters and Carr, 2009). Because of the potentially adverse consequences of contraceptive failure, most authorities recommend a conservative approach, including the use of additional contraceptive precautions, to cover the short-term use of broad-spectrum antibiotics.

Special case of lithium

In mental health, the clinically significant elimination medicine interactions involve lithium. The kidneys filter out lithium in the *distal tubule* and the *proximal renal tubule* reabsorbs some of the lithium. Incidentally, the proximal renal tubule also reabsorbs lithium and sodium concomitantly. This is particularly so if there is a sustained increase in sodium excretion, such as that which **thiazide** diuretics produce. Thiazides promote a compensatory reabsorption of sodium by the proximal renal tubule. Similarly, the reabsorption of sodium enhances the reabsorption of lithium. Because lithium has a narrow therapeutic window, this can increase the plasma lithium concentration to potentially toxic levels. Other medicines that increase lithium levels and lithium toxicity are NSAIDs, angiotensin-converting enzyme (ACE) inhibitors, furosemide and carbamazepine. By contrast, medicines that inhibit renal reabsorption of sodium at the proximal tubule (i.e. osmotic diuretics such as mannitol) result in a reduction of lithium concentration.

Generally, medicine elimination is proportional to the medicine's plasmatic concentrations, and this depends on the plasma half-life. The plasma half-life is the time that it takes for the plasma concentration of the medicine to fall by half from its maximum levels. One of the most important pharmacokinetic changes that influences medicine elimination is age. After the age of 30 years, the rate at which the kidney clears waste metabolites gradually slows, and this has implications for older people taking medicines. As we have seen, genetic variations also influence these processes, so it follows that racial or ethnic variations between people can affect medication efficacy and side effects profiles. A patient may prefer a medicine over another because that medicine has been very effective for a friend, but it does not follow that the same medicine will be as effective for themselves, as demonstrated by the following case study.

The importance of ethnicity in medicine response and interactions

Case study: Ming

Ming is a 28-year-old man of Chinese descent and he suffers from schizophrenia. For some time, he has been treated with olanzapine, but has continually complained that this medicine is not effective. Also, he forgets to take his medication some evenings, and has therefore asked if he could be prescribed a depot injection. He has asked for the Haldol decanoate injection because his friend, Jack, is on this medicine. Jack is very happy with Haldol and suffers no ill effects from the medicine. Ming's doctor explains to him about differences in medicine metabolism in different ethnic groups, and adds that there would be a high probability that Ming would develop sexual side effects as Haldol has been consistently associated with high prolactin levels in people of Chinese ethnicity. Having considered the doctor's explanation, Ming decides against Haldol and asks to explore other options.

It is well known that the frequency and even severity of disease may differ between races. Two simple examples include sickle-cell anaemia caused by a genetic mutation in people of African descent, while the genetic mutation that causes cystic fibrosis is seen primarily in individuals of white European descent. A key question is: Does an individual's ethnic or ancestral background determine their individual response to a medication? The answer is 'yes', and there is now robust evidence supporting the view that individuals from different ethnic groups experience variable responses to specific therapeutic agents. For instance, beta$_1$ adrenergic receptor blockers may be less effective in a subgroup of people of African origin for the management of congestive heart failure, and this may be due to the β1-adrenergic receptor (ADRB1) and G-protein receptor kinase 5 (GRK5) gene variants that are over-represented in this population (Dries et al., 1999). This creates problems because most medicines are developed and tested in North America and Western Europe. During development, these medicines tend to be tested on predominantly young, white patients. In addition, research conducted mainly in the West is extrapolated to all other parts of the world, and differences in treatment response from divergent ethnic and cultural backgrounds have often been minimised or assumed to be negligible. This has led to treatment decisions that inadvertently result in suboptimal patient care. Some argue that this unfortunately leads to a limitation in treatment success and questionable acceptance in many non-Western cultures because in any individual's response to pharmacological agents, cultural, racial and genetic factors are important (Lin et al., 1993).

From a genetic perspective, unique patterns exist in distinct ethnic groups, determining how the body metabolises the medicines and how the putative targets of medicines, such as neurotransmitter receptors, interact with the medicine. This pattern has been studied using modern laboratory techniques that allow us to identify genetic variants influencing medicine efficacy, and this forms the basis of pharmacogenetics. Pharmacogenetics is the study of the role of genetic variability in determining inter-individual (between-individual) variability in responses to a pharmacological therapy. The growth of pharmacogenetics has led to medicine regulatory agencies, such as the FDA and the EMA, to establish a wide variety of genetic polymorphisms as biomarkers for therapeutic recommendations or safety warnings (Fricke-Galindo et al., 2016).

In pharmacodynamics, pharmacogenetics evaluates the association of genetic polymorphisms in medicine targets with therapeutic outcomes or adverse effects. In pharmacokinetics, pharmacogenetics aims to predict medicine responses by identifying variants in genes associated with the metabolism of specific medicines. Such genetic variations affecting metabolism may lead to alterations in the bioavailability of certain medicines, resulting in a loss of efficacy (decrease in plasma levels) or an increase in toxicity (elevated plasma levels).

Many environmental factors, including diet and exposure to various substances such as tobacco, alcohol and herbal preparations, significantly modify gene expressions. In this regard, it is important to inform patients of the role that environmental factors such as diet play in medicine metabolism. Furthermore, it is important to know if the patient is taking other herbal medicines that might interact with a prescribed medicine. Ignoring culturally based environmental factors may lead the patient not to adhere to treatment fully, and this may lead to treatment failure.

Although different ethnic and cultural groups share biological and cultural characteristics, there is often a great danger of oversimplifying or over-interpreting results based on studies conducted in certain ethnic groups. For example, while people of Chinese ethnic backgrounds share similar cultural roots, northern and southern Chinese may diverge significantly in their genetic make-up, as well as in aspects of their lifestyles, which might impact significantly on medicine responses (Chen et al., 2008). Similarly, although Africans show a unique genetic variation as a group in medicine metabolism, they also show wide inter- and intra-ethnic variations in this respect (Masimirembwa and Hasler, 1997). Therefore, the use of pharmacogenetic biomarkers in clinical practice should consider ethnic, cultural and socio-economic variations, as well as genetic heterogeneity among regions and nations. During a discussion with the patient about medication, it is important to take these factors into account and advise patients accordingly. For example, in the above case study of Ming, the doctor rightly informed him about the high risk of sexual side effects. This allowed Ming to make an informed decision about his medication.

Ultimately, the goal of pharmacogenetics is to allow personalised medicine through genetic markers (individual genetic profiles) that would accurately predict which individuals with a particular condition would respond to a specific medical therapy, which would not respond to a therapy, and which would experience adverse effects, as in the case of Ming.

Differences in psychotropic medicine responses across ethnic minority groups

As already discussed, there is accumulating evidence that convincingly confirms significant cross-ethnic medicine response variations in practically all types of medications and psychotropics. For example, a series of studies demonstrated that in comparison to their Caucasian counterparts, Chinese patients are often successfully treated with lower dosages of haloperidol and other antipsychotic medications in inpatient settings (Chen et al., 2008). When given comparable doses of medication, Chinese patients with schizophrenia and Chinese normal volunteers exhibit plasma haloperidol concentrations that are approximately 50 per cent greater than their Caucasian counterparts (Lin et al., 1988). At the same time, this study also shows a greater prolactin response to haloperidol in Chinese people than in Caucasians. These studies, among many others, suggest that there may be pharmacogenetic influences in the way this population responds to antipsychotic treatment, and they may require lower doses of antipsychotics for similar therapeutic responses. This has important clinical implications for mental health nurses because of the need to monitor clinical responses and ADRs from ethnic populations. In the above case study, it would also be reasonable to inform Ming that should he be on Haldol, he will be at an increased risk of developing **extrapyramidal side effects**. Now we need to turn our attention to the role of ethnicity in medicine responses and with specific types of psychotropics.

Antipsychotics

From a prescribing perspective, there is considerable racial variation in the use of antipsychotics in people with schizophrenia, as reported by a relatively recent meta-analytic review (Puyat et al., 2013). With regard to black patients, it was previously thought that this disparity may be due to this population being significantly more likely to be on polypharmacy (Taylor et al., 2004), but later evidence seems to challenge this view (Connolly et al., 2011; Zai et al., 2013). Some authorities have argued that this disparity may contribute to increased rates of adverse effects, lower rates of adherence, and more frequent visist to A&E and psychiatric hospitalisations (Chaudhry et al., 2008), a finding supported by others (Herbeck et al., 2004).

Overall, evidence seems to suggest that Chinese and Hispanic patients need lower doses of antipsychotics to attain similar treatment responses (Chaudhry et al., 2008; Fleeman et al., 2011) and they are more sensitive to extrapyramidal side effects. With respect to movement disorders, they are more likely to have significantly higher proportions of movement disorders in comparison to Caucasians, despite the use of lower therapeutic doses (Strickland et al., 1995).

In the UK, clozapine is used much less among patients of African origin than with other ethnic minorities (Mallinger and Lamberti, 2006). Lower normal ranges for white blood cell counts in these patients may partly explain this discrepancy, and this has also been observed in Middle Eastern ethnic groups. Ashkenazi Jews also appear to have an increase in susceptibility to clozapine-induced agranulocytosis (Whiskey and Taylor, 2007).

There is a high prevalence of Type 2 diabetes in people of Indian subcontinent and African descent. All atypical antipsychotic medicines can induce diabetes, but medicines such as olanzapine and clozapine are known to induce diabetes more often than other medicines. Some ethnic minority patients, including Asians and those of African descent, are already predisposed to develop diabetes, but antipsychotics increase the risk further. Such a situation poses a problem in treating mental health problems in this population. Ethnic-based responses to antipsychotic medication are also seen in those undergoing antidepressant treatments. Before moving on to the next section, try Activity 4.4.

Activity 4.4   Critical thinking

Dolores is a 24-year-old black woman on your ward who suffers from bipolar disorder. Currently, she is suffering from an acute episode of mania and is very restless and irritable. She has flights of ideas and is interfering with other patients, and several have lodged complaints about her manner. Attempts to divert her using psychological means of management have been unsuccessful. She is, however, agreeable to take medication to help her to 'slow down'. A doctor asks for your opinion of what medication to give Dolores.

- What will your response be, and why?

An outline answer is provided at the end of the chapter.

Antidepressants

Consistent evidence demonstrates that major depression has a strong genetic background (Lohoff, 2010). As with antipsychotic medication, it is therefore not surprising that some key differences exist between and across ethnic groups in terms of treatment responses and side effects profiles. For example, early studies report that Caucasians appear to have lower plasma levels of TCAs and attain plasma peaks later in comparison with Asians from the Indian subcontinent (Rudorfer et al., 1984). Although an individual's response to psychotropic medications is a complex interplay of many factors, including genetics, diet, age and smoking, many of the differences in antidepressant response have been attributed to a greater incidence of slow pharmacokinetics among Asians compared with Caucasians (Wong and Pi, 2012). In support of this assertion, a study found that lower therapeutic doses of TCAs and lithium are required in Asian populations (Wong and Pi, 2012). Other findings which support interethnic variability in antidepressant treatment are that Hispanic women require lower doses of antidepressants in comparison to Caucasians (Sramek and Pi, 1996) and that black patients need lower doses of TCAs to attain similar treatment responses to those of Caucasians (Varner et al., 1998). Overall, current available evidence supports the use of lower doses of antidepressants in people of Asian origin. This is because they appear to metabolise antidepressants at a slower rate than Caucasians. Therefore, we conclude from these findings that we should carefully individualise dosages of antidepressants over a prolonged period.

With respect to other psychotropics, a study that investigated the use of lithium in Iran concluded that Iranians should be treated with lower doses in comparison with Europeans and North Americans (Hashemi and Movahedian, 2006). A different study that examined the use of lithium in African American patients found that those with bipolar disorder are more susceptible to lithium side effects than Caucasian North Americans (Strickland et al., 1995). Another finding supporting ethnic variability in the use of psychotropic medications shows more pronounced mental and psychomotor depression in people of Chinese origin compared with Caucasians after repeated use of diazepam (Chaudhry et al., 2008).

Overall, despite the ongoing debate on whether ethnicity is an important factor in psychopharmacology – if ethnicity is defined as a shared genetic and cultural or environmental background – it is indeed an important influence on psychotropic medicine responses and interactions.

Chapter summary

Modern clinical psychopharmacology started when the discovery of antibiotics provided the incentive and basis for launching the pharmaceutical industry, which now collectively develops approximately 24 new medicines a year. For every 10,000 potential medicines, only one will be approved by the regulatory authorities and reach the

(Continued)

(Continued)

market. The time from first compound development to medicine on the market is typically 12–15 years and costs approximately £1.5 billion. Medicines development typically takes place in phases: phases 0, 1, 2, 3 and 4 trials. Medicines act in many different and diverse ways, but they do not elicit new responses; they only alter existing physiological activity. From time to time, medicines interact with each other to produce an effect.

Medicine interactions has become an important topic in medicines management, and there are at least three types of interaction: pharmaceutical, pharmacodynamic and pharmacokinetic. Pharmaceutical interaction is where two incompatible medicines are mixed before they are ingested by the patient, and this is the least harmful of all medicine interactions. Pharmacodynamic interaction can be defined as what the medicine does to the body; if you give two medicines that work on the same receptor to a patient, this can give rise to synergistic effects. Pharmacokinetic interaction can be defined as what the body does to the medicine. Pharmacokinetic processes can be divided into at least four phases: absorption, distribution, metabolism and excretion. Metabolism plays a crucial role in pharmacokinetic medicine interactions, and this involves CYP450 enzymes. There are approximately six main CYP enzymes that are responsible for catalysing the metabolism of most medicines. The metabolism of medicines differs across ethnic and racial lines, but there is also intra-ethnic variation that has a genetic base.

Activities: brief outline answers

Activity 4.1 Critical thinking (page 118)

- No, as polypharmacy is more likely to result in medicine interactions.
- Serotonin syndrome is likely to result because of a synergistic reaction.

Activity 4.2 Critical thinking (page 119)

Sustained-release (SR), sustained-action, extended-release (ER, XR, XL), time-release/timed-release, controlled-release (CR), modified-release (MR), and continuous-release systems are used in tablets that dissolve slowly and are to be released into the bloodstream over a longer time. The advantages of SR tablets are that they can be taken less frequently than instant-release formulations of the same medicine and they keep steadier levels of the medicine in the bloodstream. Ingestion of the quick-release form of lithium carbonate (200 mg) is likely to result in higher blood serum levels of the medicine. Hence, the patient is likely to be experiencing severe side effects if large doses are taken. The medicine has not been administered correctly and the nurse has not followed prescribed instructions. This will be classed as a medicine error, and you will need to follow medicine error procedures.

Activity 4.3 Decision-making (page 124)

Although Errol is hypertensive, he is also at risk of the effects of a medicine interaction. Olanzapine may potentiate the hypotensive effect of propranolol, and this may lead Errol to develop orthostatic hypotension and **syncope**. Errol should be advised to avoid rising abruptly from a sitting or recumbent position and to notify the nurse if he experiences dizziness or light-headedness. You should also advise him to avoid driving or operating hazardous machinery until he knows how the medications affect him.

Activity 4.4 Critical thinking (page 134)

Dolores is likely to experience extrapyramidal side effects from even relatively low doses of antipsychotic, because current evidence suggests that people from black ethnic backgrounds are prone to these symptoms, even on low doses. Therefore, she might benefit more from sedatives such as benzodiazepines (e.g. diazepam, lorazepam). If the doctor decides to prescribe antipsychotics, you should explain the likely side effects to Dolores, and you need to manage these side effects aggressively.

Further reading

Baxter, K. (ed.) (2011) *Stockley's Drug Interactions Pocket Companion*. London: Pharmaceutical Press.

This pocket-sized book on medicine interactions is easy to carry around in clinical areas.

Brølsen, K. and Naranjo, C.A. (2001) Review of pharmacokinetic and pharmacodynamic interaction studies with citalopram. *European Neuropsychopharmacology*, 11(4): 275–83.

This is a detailed review of studies that have investigated the interactions of citalopram.

Stargrove, B.M., Treasure, J. and McKee, D.L. (2008) *Herb, Nutrient, and Drug Interactions: Clinical Implications and Therapeutic Strategies*. St Louis, MO: Mosby.

This is a very good book that gives information on not only medicine–medicine interactions, but also food–medicine interactions.

Useful website

www.medscape.com/druginfo/druginterchecker

This very useful website allows you to enter two or more medicine names, including herbal medicines, to check interactions between them. It is user-friendly and gives very detailed information.

Chapter 5　Principles of prescribing and medicines administration

Chapter aims

By the end of this chapter, you should be familiar with:

- inter-professional team roles, especially those of prescribers, dispensers and administrators of medicines;
- the prescribing and medicines use processes;
- the medicines administration and treatment effectiveness monitoring processes.

Introduction

Prescribed medicines are the main intervention for the prevention and treatment of many health problems, including mental health problems. Therefore, it is important to prescribe medicines appropriately and to ensure that patients continue to get the most from medicines after taking them. Nurses can help patients get the optimum benefit from medicines through the medicines management framework.

Medicines management is one of the most complex parts of a patient's care delivery, and it is not unusual that it may involve different healthcare professionals, departments, facilities and processes. Without full coordination of care between the prescriber who orders the medicine, the pharmacy that dispenses the medicine and the person who administers it, the risk of potentially harmful medication errors increases. A good starting point in minimising these errors is to understand the roles of the prescriber, the dispenser and the administrator of medicines. This chapter discusses the role of each professional involved in the medication process before focusing on the administration of medicines in different formulations. First, let us look briefly at the dynamic nature of medicines management.

The changing nature of medicines management

The traditional model of medicines management suggests that this process consists of a series of stages:

- prescribing (ordering a given medicine and dose);
- dispensing (supplying medicines to individuals or to hospital wards);
- preparation (preparing a dose of medicine for administration);
- administration (administering the dose of medicine via the appropriate route and method);
- monitoring (checking the administration and effect of a medicine).

In the traditional model, doctors prescribed, pharmacists dispensed, and nurses administered the medicine. Now the picture is more complex. Every stage of the medicines process involves many professionals, and medication safety has become a multi-professional concern.

The role of the prescriber

Traditionally, doctors have been entrusted with the role of prescribing medicines. Access to prescription-only medicines (POMs) has, until recently, been dependent on the written order of a doctor or dental practitioner. Doctors are eligible to prescribe all items within the *British National Formulary* (BNF). Non-medical professionals, such as nurses, pharmacists, physiotherapists and podiatrists, can prescribe medication after appropriate training. The prescriber is responsible for consultation and making a diagnosis before prescribing a medicine. The Royal Pharmaceutical Society (RPS) has published a prescribing competency framework, which includes a common set of competencies that form the basis for prescribing, regardless of professional background. The competencies were developed to help healthcare professionals to be safe and effective prescribers, with the aim of supporting patients to get the best outcomes from their medicines (RPS, 2015).

Nurses, including mental health nurses who complete an approved course in prescribing, can prescribe medicines. Among other things, they should have an appropriate background knowledge of clinical pharmacology and therapeutics to be competent in prescribing matters. There is also a requirement that prescribers should train in some of the following areas:

- legislation (see Chapter 1);
- professional role and accountability;
- prescribing principles and procedures;
- economic aspects.

They should consider all treatment steps, including the option not to prescribe medication. If they decide to prescribe, they should prescribe the product or medicine that is effective, appropriate, safe and cost-effective. Before you proceed further, try Activity 5.1.

Activity 5.1   Team-working

Arrange to talk to a prescriber on your team about their role as a prescriber. Find out about the challenges of prescribing medication.

As this is an individual activity, there is no outline answer at the end of the chapter.

The general principles of prescribing

There is a general acceptance that good prescribing is based on several basic principles, and in 1999 the National Prescribing Centre (NPC) developed a seven-step pyramid model (NPC, 1999), shown in Figure 5.1. The NPC recommends that prescribers should carefully consider each step before moving up to the next. The first step is to consider the patient through effective health consultation.

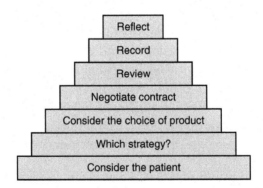

Figure 5.1   The seven-step pyramid prescribing model advocated by the NPC – a prescriber should carefully consider each step before moving up to the next

Health consultation is a two-way social interaction involving the prescriber and the patient. Typically, the prescriber draws out information from the patient, then offers a diagnosis or opinion, and may discuss treatment options. At this stage, the patient may choose what information to disclose and how to present it. The following case study demonstrates a consultation process.

> ## Case study: Martin
>
> ....
>
> Martin is a 23-year-old man who has suffered from schizophrenia since he was 18 years old. He is currently in hospital but generally keeps to himself and spends a lot of time in his room listening to music. He is prescribed olanzapine, which he takes regularly. One morning he approached his primary nurse complaining of abdominal pain and increased urinary output. The primary nurse thought that Martin was suffering from indigestion and gave him a dose of antacid. At lunchtime, Martin refused to eat his food, saying he was not hungry, and he continued to refuse food for the rest of the day.

In response to Martin in the above case study, the nurse treated him with an antacid, and he was provided with reassurance and monitoring of his condition. However, a nurse undertaking a consultation focuses on taking a clinical history and examination first, with the aim of reaching a differential diagnosis. A differential diagnosis is the distinguishing of a disease or condition from others that present with similar clinical features. In other words, for a set of symptoms, there is more than one possibility for a diagnosis or illness. If the primary nurse had sought a differential diagnosis in Martin's case, they would have typically gathered a detailed medical history and an in-depth exploration of the onset of the pain, its character, timing, and the factors that worsen it, as well as a physical examination of the abdomen.

Despite the advances in modern diagnostic tests, taking a patient's history is one of the most important aspects of the clinical consultation that a practitioner uses to formulate a differential or definitive diagnosis before starting a safe prescribing decision. A comprehensive history can provide more than 80 per cent of the information on which to base a diagnosis (Epstein et al., 2008). History-taking and clinical examination require a structured, logical approach to ensure that a prescriber obtains all the relevant information and does not overlook any important details. Consultation in mental health is like any other clinical consultation, with the exception that in mental health the prescriber also obtains the patient's social and developmental history. These skills are difficult to acquire, and importantly they require practice.

Although there are various recommendations for taking a history effectively, whichever way it is done, a systematic and structured approach is fundamental. Such an approach will improve the flow and time management of the consultation and is less likely to confuse the patient. Importantly, the prescriber should establish a rapport with the patient for a successful consultation (see Chapter 2).

Establishing rapport during consultation

Both good therapeutic relationships and clinical decision-making are the basis on which a good consultation depends. If consultation is to be successful, both elements need to be strong. According to Morris and Chenail (2013), the way in which the prescriber and the patient fulfil their respective roles, as well as the therapeutic relationship that arises, can influence outcomes (e.g. satisfaction, adherence, malpractice litigation). In other words, if the nurse is not able to communicate effectively with a patient, they will not be able to elicit enough and accurate information, without which the nurse's clinical decision will be fundamentally flawed and unsafe. The apparently simple process of one person talking to another is in fact a highly complex and subtle skill. As the nurse and the patient talk, a relationship develops where they acquire a greater sense of each other's perspectives, and a better appreciation of each other's individuality develops. Cohn (2007) suggests that it is good for the nurse to create a cognitive and emotional connection with the patient because understanding is valuable, especially when interpreting information gathered from the patient.

Just as important is the nurse's' own awareness of their own attributes, which is the first step towards understanding other people. It is only by being truly aware of the self that we can make an honest connection with a patient. During consultation, this rapport between the nurse and the patient, as well as involving the patient in decision-making, is associated with better health outcomes for the patient (Say and Thomson, 2003) (see Chapter 2). Although relationship growth or therapeutic alliance takes time – which is not always available – we also recognise that it is possible to see a patient once and gain their trust and elicit the necessary information (Elwyn et al., 1999). This suggests that time is not always a determining factor in successful therapeutic relationships, and therefore other factors must play a part (e.g. the actual act of communicating). Thus, a positive therapeutic communication can improve the consultation process, results in safer outcomes that reduce patient doubt (Thomson et al., 2005), and helps to reduce the possible burden of decision-making.

Practical steps during consultation

During consultation, the patient needs to believe that they are getting the nurse's full attention. For this reason, the patient is more likely to try to accurately answer questions and recall past events. To establish a rapport and to put the patient at ease, it is helpful to start the consultation by taking an approach recommended by Jevon (2016). The patient can ask questions that may influence the prescriber's perception of the problem, can make explicit requests, and – above all – can choose how to respond to the offer of advice or treatment prescribed. The choice and action of both the prescriber and the patient can affect the outcome of the consultation process. Put differently, a consultation involves interactive decision-making, an idea closely related to the idea of a therapeutic alliance (see Chapter 2).

Positive initial contact: Shake the patient's hand while introducing yourself.

Privacy: Reassure the patient that their privacy and dignity will be maintained.

Patient's name: Establish how the patient would like to be addressed (i.e. forename or surname).

Patient's physical comfort: Ensure that the patient is in a comfortable position, and position yourself so that the patient is not sitting at an awkward angle.

Confidentiality: Reassure the patient that all of their information will be treated as confidential.

Posture: Avoid standing up, towering over the patient. Ideally, sit down at the same level as the patient.

Effective communication skills: In particular, allow time to listen to what the patient is saying and avoid appearing to be rushed.

Appropriate language: Appropriate language and understanding are important aspects of history-taking. As the patient may not understand a particular word or phrase, always have an alternative available (e.g. 'sputum', 'phlegm').

Jevon (2016) suggests that the types of questions the nurse should ask during a clinical consultation depends on many factors, including the type of patient and the reason why the patient is seeking consultation. For example, has the patient been seen before? Is this a first contact care consultation? Should information be collaborated by a significant other? Below is a sequence of consultation process:

1. Introduction
2. Presenting complaint and history of current illness
3. Systemic enquiry
4. Past medical history
5. Family history
6. Social and personal history
7. Medication
8. Allergies
9. Patient's ideas, concerns and expectations

1. Introduction

It is important to introduce yourself to the patient (e.g. name, position). Confirm the identity of the patient, including their name and how they wish to be addressed. It is important to seek consent before history-taking and clinical examination. After obtaining consent, the prescriber should take history of the presenting complaint from the patient. Start off with open-ended questions and focus in on areas with more specific, closed questions, as necessary. This gives the patient a chance to talk about their experiences and concerns, while allowing the prescriber to get the information they need. In mental health consultation, it is not always appropriate to ask all of the questions all of the time. If the patient is suspicious, paranoid or acutely distressed, it is a better strategy to leave gaps that the prescriber can fill in later. The prescriber can gather history from old notes, as well as speaking to an informant such as the nearest relative or a carer. Over time, each clinician will develop their own style of interviewing and be comfortable with the style adopted so that questions do not seem awkward or forced.

2. Presenting complaint and history of current illness

During a new patient consultation, the prescriber should establish if the patient is ill, and – if so – what the diagnosis is. As previously mentioned, by far the most important part of consultation is the history of the patient's presenting complaint and the history of current illness. During history-taking, the prescriber is also trying to obtain information that usually helps to make a differential diagnosis, as well as providing important insight into the nature of the patient's complaints and concerns. Therefore, a significant part of taking the patient's history involves findings out about their presenting complaint(s) to determine the main symptom(s).

The patient may not be specific initially; but with gentle prompting and some echoing of their own words back, they are likely to elaborate on the problem and talk more freely. For example, a patient may complain of tiredness, and the prescriber could pick up on the complaint and ask about specific problems with sleep. The aim is to elicit symptoms of depression. The prescriber should allow the patient enough time to talk, and not interrupt (see Chapter 2). According to Shah (2005b), the prescriber should note the following during consultation:

- Who noticed the problem (e.g. patient, relative, caregiver, healthcare professional)?
- What initial action did the patient take (e.g. any self-treatment)? Did it help?
- When was medical help sought, and why?
- What action was taken by the healthcare professional?
- What has happened since then?
- What investigations have been undertaken, and what investigations are planned?
- What treatment has been given?
- What has the patient been told about the problem?

3. Systemic enquiry

In systemic enquiry, the prescriber asks a series of questions related to the bodily systems, which allows them to obtain more information that can then be linked to the presenting complaint. This is a safety net that can reduce the risk of missing out an important symptom or disease. However, the systemic enquiry can potentially cause confusion and misdirect the prescriber if the patient has multiple symptoms or is talkative. Therefore, the prescriber should undertake this systematically and carefully. The checklist for systemic enquiry should include cardiovascular, respiratory, skin, skeletal, endocrine, nervous and genitourinary.

4. Past medical history

It is useful to establish the patient's past medical history, because if the patient has a long-standing disease there is a strong possibility that any new symptom could be related to it. A long-standing medical illness such as thyroid problems could be related to depression, for example. Also, knowledge of the patient's past medical history could be useful in establishing the most appropriate treatment.

The prescriber should ask the patient if they have ever had any serious illness, been admitted to hospital previously, or had surgery. It is usual practice to ask if the patient has suffered or suffers from any of the following illnesses:

* jaundice;
* anaemia;
* tuberculosis;
* rheumatic fever;
* diabetes;
* bronchitis;
* myocardial infarction/chest pain;
* stroke;
* epilepsy;
* asthma;
* mental health problems (e.g depression, anxiety, psychosis).

5. Family history

A family history assessment is usually a good indicator of a person's family relationships. The prescriber should find out which members of the family the patient feels close to, and why. Equally, they should explore reasons for disharmony if present within the family. A recommended approach by Shah (2005a) should cover the following in taking family history:

* Find out who has the problem in the family. For example, is it a first- or second-degree relative?
* Determine how many family members are affected by the problem.
* Clarify what exactly the problem is. For example, 'a problem with nerves' could be several things (e.g. depression, anxiety, schizophrenia).

- Be exact as to the nature of the problem because several family members may have 'problems with nerves', but they may be completely different, and therefore not relevant to the patient's particular problem.
- Determine at what age the relative developed the problem. Obviously, early presentation is more likely to be important than presentation later in life.
- Find out if the patient's parents are still alive, and – if not – at what age they died and the cause of death.

6. Personal and social history

The personal and social history of the patient is important because it helps to understand what has led them to become the person they are. It is easier to work through personal history in chronological order, remembering that some of the information may have been gathered earlier. Things you need to ask about briefly include:

Premorbid personality: For mental health assessment, the prescriber may obtain information on premorbid personality from a third party or an informant. Premorbid personality information is particularly helpful because it helps us to understand how the illness has affected the individual.

Social history: The social history of the patient is important to understand, as well as the effect the illness might have on their life and the lives of their family.

Marital status and children: Ask if the patient is married or has a partner, and whether they have children. This is particularly important if the patient is frail or an older adult, because it will help to determine whether the family will be able to look after them if necessary.

Occupation: Establish the occupation of the patient (or previous occupation, if out of work). As certain occupations are at risk of illnesses, all past occupations should be noted. For example, construction and associated workers may suffer from asbestos-related diseases. Some occupations can be affected by certain diseases (e.g. taxi drivers diagnosed with epilepsy will need to give up their job).

Living accommodation: Determine where the patient lives and the type of accommodation (e.g. shared accommodation, bungalow, block of flats). This information may be relevant both as a contributing factor to the presenting complaint and as a consideration at patient discharge.

Travel history: In modern consultation, it is now important to ask a patient about their recent travel history, especially if there is a suspicion of an infection because of illnesses such as malaria, Ebola and Covid-19 (Shah, 2005b),

Hobbies and interests: If the prescriber has knowledge of the patient's hobbies and interests, this should allow for a better understanding, as well as determining what is important to the patient.

Smoking and alcohol: Because smoking and alcohol use are implicated in many illnesses, it is important to ask about the patient's past and present use of these. The prescriber should adopt a non-judgemental approach but get to the point. For example, when asking about alcohol, the prescriber might ask, 'Do you drink alcohol?' or 'How much alcohol do you normally drink?' If there is no clear answer, the prescriber might ask, 'How much did you drink in the last week/fortnight?'

7. Medication

The patient's beliefs about their medication can provide useful insight into what they believe is wrong with them. Before starting or adjusting medication treatment, be aware of what the patient is already taking (e.g. old medication could be ineffective or may interact with new medication). Remember to ask about side effects and adherence, as well as being mindful of possible medicine interactions. Medication side effects could be the cause of the patient's presenting complaint. The prescriber should establish if the patient is taking the following:

* prescription medicines;
* over-the-counter medicines (e.g. aspirin);
* herbal or 'natural' treatments;
* recreational drugs (e.g. cannabis).

If the patient is taking medications, find out about the dose, the route of administration, the frequency and the duration of treatment. The prescriber should explore the possibility of non-adherence to prescribed medicines by the patient. The patient may be unsure about what medication they are taking, and if this is the case it is worthwhile using their medical history to ask them if they are taking any treatment for each problem. For example, 'Do you take anything for your arthritis (or anxiety)?' (Shah, 2005a).

8. Allergies

The prescriber should record a detailed description of any past allergic reactions to medicines or other allergens by the patient. Specifically, the prescriber should ask the patient about allergy to penicillin. If this is affirmative, the next step is to find out what happened to differentiate between an allergy and a side effect (see Chapter 11). Once the patient complaint is established, the next step is to carefully evaluate to allow for appropriate investigations, as well as planning and reviewing treatment.

9. Patient's ideas, concerns and expectations

A good history-taking system will help the prescriber to identify the patient's ideas, concerns and expectations. This is possible only if the prescriber is methodical and effective in communication. One of the commonly identified reasons for patient dissatisfaction during consultation is a failure in communication on the part of the prescriber (Ford et al., 2005). To improve communication with the patient, it is helpful to thank patients for their cooperation and ask them if they have any questions to ask. To reduce the risk of misunderstanding, the prescriber should provide a short summary outlining the patient's problem or symptoms, as this will assist in confirming a mutual understanding.

An overview of clinical examination

Having completed history-taking, a differential diagnosis will be possible, which will help to direct the focus of the clinical examination. For physical examination, obtain the patient's consent before examining. A detailed treatise of physical clinical examination is beyond the scope of this book, and the reader is advised to consult an appropriate text. In mental status examination, a suggested approach to examination should include the following:

- appearance and behaviour;
- speech;
- mood;
- thought;
- perceptions;
- delusions;
- cognition;
- insight.

Conclusion

After a consultation, the prescriber makes a diagnosis, a differential diagnosis and a treatment plan. In formulating the treatment plan, the prescriber should decide if the patient requires treatment at the time; and if so, which problems and target symptoms the treatment should aim at, what kind of treatment or combination of treatments the patient should receive, and what treatment setting seems most appropriate. For instance, the prescriber should assess if the patient requires medication, inpatient or outpatient treatment, or psychotherapy. If the patient requires hospitalisation, the prescriber should specify the reasons for hospitalisation, the type of hospitalisation indicated, the urgency with which the patient must be hospitalised, and the anticipated duration of inpatient care. If either the patient or their family members are unwilling to accept the recommendation for treatment, and the prescriber believes that such as refusal may have serious consequences, then the patient should sign a statement of treatment refusal, or the prescriber should consider initiating a Mental Health Act application if the person is a risk to themselves or others.

The role of the pharmacist

The role of the pharmacist in medicines management is to promote and support the safe, effective and responsible use of medicines. The focus of a pharmacist's role is the medication needs of the patient. Recently, these patient-focused activities have evolved into the concept of *pharmaceutical care*, which we can define as 'the responsible provision of medicines with the aim of achieving desired treatment outcomes that enhance a patient's quality of life' (Hepler and Strand, 1990). In pharmaceutical care, pharmacists are directly accountable to patients for the outcomes of medicine therapies. In recent years, the role of the pharmacist has shifted from a focus on the preparation and supply of medicines to a focus on the sharing of pharmaceutical expertise and knowledge with doctors, nurses and patients (clinical pharmacy). Developments in pharmaceutical care are occurring in both the hospital and the community.

Pharmacy practice in the community

In the community, pharmacists help patients gain the maximum benefit from their medication, dispense medicines, and provide support to patients. In the management of long-term conditions, including many mental health conditions, pharmacists not only supply the medicines to patients, but are increasingly involved in the development of locally agreed shared care procedures that ensure patients use prescribed medicines to the best advantage to improve treatment outcomes.

Case study: Richard

Richard is a 26-year-old man who has been prescribed methadone replacement therapy by his doctor. He collected his medicine from his local community pharmacy. Before dispensing and administering the medicine, Satish, the pharmacist, spent some time with Richard to find out more details about his lifestyle. In particular, he asked Richard whether he felt that the dosage of methadone he was taking was enough. During the discussion, Satish was able to establish that Richard was still at risk of using illicit medicines while on methadone therapy. Satish explained to Richard the possible risks of taking these medicines in tandem with methadone.

In the management of common ailments such as allergies or flu, pharmacists play a vital role in supporting responsible self-medication by giving people advice and reassurance, as in the above case of Satish. They also supply non-prescription medicines when appropriate and refer people to other healthcare professionals where necessary.

In the promotion and support of healthy lifestyles, pharmacists help people to maintain good health by providing health screening, advice on healthy living, and other services. In the above case study, Satish was able to provide Richard with lifestyle advice after finding out more details about his life. Pharmacists now play a part in a range of such services, including blood pressure measurement, body fluid testing, cholesterol testing, pregnancy testing, smoking cessation advice and diabetes guidance. In the community, the pharmacist can – in special cases – supply POMs without a prescription on the request of a doctor or individual patient. Finally, pharmacists contribute their expert knowledge of medicines and their use for the benefit of other healthcare workers, including both doctors and nurses.

Pharmacy practice in the hospital setting

The hospital pharmacist's role has become more patient-focused, with emphasis on the provision of medicines for inpatients. Many hospital-based pharmacists supply medicines for outpatients together with advice and information about their use. Individual pharmacists now specialise in such areas as medicines information, formulary development and clinical trials. One of the most important developments of hospital pharmacy is the shift in their location from within the confines of the pharmacy to the ward or clinic setting. In many places, pharmacists visit wards to check prescription sheets and initiate supply, thus avoiding the need for prescriptions to be sent to the pharmacy and meaning that medicines should always be available on the ward. Pharmacists have become more involved on the wards, advising doctors on what they may prescribe and helping nurses with problems in medicine administration. Like the community pharmacist, the 'ward pharmacist' has evolved into a more patient-oriented 'clinical pharmacist'. By visiting the ward, the pharmacist can obtain detailed information on the medicines prescribed for each patient and contribute to areas such as the interpretation of prescriptions, checking dosage levels, and monitoring prescriptions for possible medicine interactions. By working at the ward level, the pharmacist has more access to information on a patient's clinical condition than would be the case if they were working solely in the pharmacy. Also, with respect to dispensing, they must ensure that medicinal products are properly labelled.

The labelling of medicinal products

The Medicines Act 1968 stipulates that medicines should be labelled and that the label must be clear, legible and comprehensible. It further orders that the information on the label includes:

- the name of the patient;
- the name of the medicine (usually its generic name rather than its brand name);
- preparation (e.g. syrup, tablets, capsules);
- strength of the medicine;
- quantity;
- storage instructions, if applicable;
- route of administration;
- expiry date;
- any special warnings about the product;
- batch reference number and instructions for use.

After dispensing medicines, they must be transported and stored in a safe place. Before you go any further, try Activity 5.2.

Activity 5.2   Reflection

Consider and then make a list of things that could go wrong if a medicine label is not clear.

An outline answer is provided at the end of the chapter.

Storage of medicines in the hospital setting

After ordering and transporting medicines to the ward, they should be stored in a secure locked cupboard. Separate locked cupboards should be used for clinical reagents, external medicines, internal medicines, disinfectants and antiseptics. In addition, some oral preparations require a refrigerator with a lock to separately store injections. In the case of controlled drugs, there should be a cupboard reserved solely for the purpose of storing these medicines. This cupboard should be secured to the wall and ideally fitted with a red warning light to identify when the door is open. These cupboards may be separate from others or inside other locked cupboards for use to store internal medicines. The lock must not be common to any other lock in the hospital. We store controlled drugs and keep records in accordance with local policy. Now we need to turn to prescribing, a process that starts with consultation.

The role of the nurse in medicines management

We can divide the role of the nurse in medicines management into the following areas, according to Luker and Wolfson (1999):

- to administer medicines to patients;
- to report any side effects and take action where appropriate;
- to give advice to the patient about medication and possible side effects;
- to promote patient adherence to medication;
- to provide alternative or supplementary care to medicines therapy;
- to adhere to procedures for the control of pharmaceutical products.

The role of the nurse is more than just performing tasks mechanically; there is a requirement for them to exercise professional judgement and apply their knowledge, skills and commitment. They must always be aware of the potential pitfalls of medicines administration, and therefore must always act in a way that promotes and safeguards the well-being of patients. For this reason, nurses are personally accountable for their own practice, and this applies to nurses in all fields of practice (see Chapter 1). Because nurses are accountable for their actions, it is important that they acquire practical skills supported by sound knowledge, because no matter how careful or competent the prescriber or the dispensing pharmacist, there may be adverse consequences if the nurse is not sufficiently prepared to administer medicines efficiently.

If the nurse is to advise patients and carry out the safe administration of medicines, they will need a good understanding of basic psychopharmacology. The nurse needs to understand prescribing, ordering and storage procedures, dosage levels, and routes or methods of administration, and will need to consult employer policies for detailed guidance. In addition to this, the nurse needs to know the mode of action of the medication, recognise side effects and signs of toxicity, and know how to manage cases of toxicity. There is also a need for knowledge of the interactions between medicines, as well as between medicines and certain foods.

Case study: Yusuf

Yusuf, a young man suffering from schizophrenia, is on a flupenthixol depot injection. He approaches Brian, a registered nurse, complaining of a dry mouth. Brian knows that dry mouth is a side effect of flupenthixol decanoate injections. Yusuf is prescribed 5 mg of procyclidine PRN (pro re nata/when required); but an hour after Brian administers to Yusuf, Yusuf approaches Brian saying that the medicine he has just given him does not work – if anything, it has made his problems worse.

Although Brian correctly identified that Yusuf is experiencing side effects due to flupenthixol, the administration of procyclidine in this case is incorrect. Procyclidine is for the alleviation of extrapyramidal side effects only. If anything, administration of procyclidine in this case is certain to make the dry mouth condition worse, as Yusuf correctly identified. By understanding the basic theory behind medicines and the conditions to treat, the nurse can act with precision and confidence in the exercise of their professional duties. For example, if you do not have good knowledge of the physiology of the very young or very old, you may put people in these age groups at risk, as they are more prone to adverse reactions from medicines than others. Before you read further, try Activity 5.3.

Activity 5.3   Critical thinking

George is 76 years old and is suffering from depression. He was referred by his GP to a psychiatric unit. George's condition has deteriorated since he started taking imipramine, a TCA. He is more confused and his appetite is now very poor. The older adult psychiatrist who interviewed him was convinced that George needed a change in medication. Therefore, he discontinued George's imipramine and prescribed citalopram for him instead.

- Why did the doctor do this?

An outline answer is provided at the end of the chapter.

The nurse should familiarise themselves with local policies and procedures that relate to medicines management. Above all, the nurse needs to understand the patient receiving the medicine. This information should include the patient's name, age and diagnosis. In addition, the nurse should be familiar with the patient's hypersensitivities, such as allergies or any history of adverse reactions to other medicines.

Above all, the nurse should master a variety of skills to be able to manage medicines in a clinical setting successfully. One important skill is that of good observation. By accurately observing a patient's condition before and after taking medication, the nurse should be able to assess whether treatment is indicated or is effective. The following case study adequately demonstrates this point.

Case study: Christine

Christine is 27 years old and takes 10 mg of diazepam three times per day for long-standing anxiety. Christine arrived on the ward after a day's home leave, and during medication administration time she asked for her medication. The nurse noticed that Christine's speech was slurred, and more importantly her breath smelled of alcohol. Upon further discussion with the nurse, Christine admitted that she had had a few glasses of wine while at home. The nurse informed Christine that she would not be able to administer medication to her until the effects of the alcohol wore off. The nurse further explained the role of alcohol and its interaction with medicines – in this case, with diazepam.

Nursing observations should always include the patient's mental state as well as the presence or absence of side effects. If the nurse had not been observant to Christine's slurred speech and the alcohol smell on her breath, she would have administered diazepam, which interacts synergistically with alcohol, with the likely consequence of depressing the respiratory system.

An additional important skill is good communication. Of all the skills that are relevant to mental health nursing, no skill is more important than the ability to communicate with people effectively, and this is a consistent theme throughout this book. During the early stages of treatment, the nurse should try to elicit information such as any history of allergies, previous medicines the patient used to take, any non-prescribed medicines that the patient is taking, any barriers that the patient might be experiencing in taking medicines as instructed, or their general attitude towards medication. The nurse should be able to communicate information to the patient, such as the name of the medicine, the dosage, the number of tablets to be taken at one time and the number of times a day, the likely duration before therapeutic benefits can be realised, and possible side effects and their management. The nurse should incorporate all of this knowledge and these skills into their practice of medicines administration.

Medicines administration

The National Patient Safety Agency (NPSA) estimates that each hospital in England and Wales administers around 7,000 doses of medication per day (NPSA, 2007). Clinical places of work have policies regarding medicines administration that are based on legal requirements, as well as codes of practice and standards of professional bodies, such as the Nursing and Midwifery Council (NMC). The NMC emphasises that competency in administration of medicines is an integral and essential entry criterion for its professional register, and it clearly states that nurses must not see medication administration as a solely mechanistic task, but as one that requires thinking and the exercise of professional judgement (NMC, 2010). Medicines administration is a complex role that encompasses several tasks, including:

- administering medication safely and efficiently by following the 'ten rights';
- assessing and monitoring the effects of medication;
- collaborating with other professions;
- monitoring the adverse effects of medication, and managing these.

Before the nurse administers medicines, they should do a mental check on the five factors we commonly refer to as the 'five rights' (5Rs). In recent years, another five rights (6–10) have been added, making a total of 'ten rights' (10Rs). Many textbooks, however, still refer only to the original 5Rs (1–5):

1. *Right patient.* In some instances, patient medicines administration charts bear the patient's photo. Ensure that you positively identify the patient.

2. *Right medicine.* Check the administration chart for the name of the medicine and compare this with the medicine on hand. As many medicines have similar spellings, there is a need to check this carefully. It is often recommended that the nurse does three checks of the medicine to be administered: (1) when reaching for the package that contains the medicine; (2) when opening the medicine; and (3) when returning the package to its storage area.

Scenario

A patient undergoing alcohol detoxification was prescribed chlordiazepoxide but was given chlorpromazine instead. Imagine the consequences of this error, for both the patient and the nurse.

---

3. *Right dose.* Compare the ordered dose to the dose on hand. At times, you may need to perform calculations to determine the correct dose. If you are at all unsure of your calculation, get someone to check it.

4. *Right route.* Check the medication record for how to administer the medicine, and the medicine label to verify the prescribed route. This is vitally important for medicines that are to be injected.

5. *Right time.* Verify the frequency of the dose, and that the time of day ordered matches the current time.

6. *Right documentation:* Document the dosage and the time the patient took the medicine. This supplements the information in the nursing notes. If you have given an injection, you need to document the name of the injection, the dosage and the site.

7. *Right patient education:* Inform the patient of the potential therapeutic and adverse effects of the medicine, and offer appropriate advice on overcoming the side effects.

8. *Right to refuse.* The patient has a right to refuse medication, though you must balance this right against the potential risk that can result from treatment refusal, particularly for those who show poor awareness of illness or lack capacity (see Chapters 1 and 2), in which case the Mental Health Act 1983 and the Mental Capacity Act 2005 should guide you. You should document all situations of treatment refusal.

9. *Right assessment.* Carry out the right assessment before or after giving medication. For example, for a patient on digoxin, you should only give the medication if the patient's pulse is over 60 bpm.

10. *Right evaluation:* Make sure you check for medicine allergies and interactions between different medications.

Scenario

A patient prescribed 40 mg of fluoxetine in the morning usually received his medication in the afternoon because he did not get up in time. Typically, his sleep pattern was disturbed and he was awake for most of the night.

It is important to handle all medicines in such a way that they do not encounter potentially contaminated objects or surfaces, including the nurse's own hands. The nurse should not leave any medicines unattended, and it is important to observe patients when they are taking medication. This avoids the disposal, hoarding, abuse or misuse of medication, as well as assuring the safety of the patient.

Documentation of medication administration is an important responsibility. The patient medicines administration chart tells the story of what substances the patient has received and when. Like other healthcare records, it is also a legal document. All institutions have policies and procedures on documentation. The administering nurse needs to initial the record and enter the time and date next to the appropriate prescription. The administrator may provide other information, such as the location, the severity of the ailment, or the pulse rate for medicines such as digoxin. The administrator should document patient refusals of medication and the reason, if possible, in the patient notes, as well as informing the prescriber.

Document all medicine errors and notify the prescriber. Most institutional policies require the administrator to file a separate form to document errors. Errors can include administering the wrong medicine or the wrong dose at the wrong time or via the wrong route. We consider omissions of medication due to administration as errors. If the nurse does not record errors, it becomes difficult to avoid such errors in the future, so it is your responsibility to complete this process.

Administration of controlled medicines/drugs

National health trusts normally draw up procedures relating to the prescribing, handling, storage and administration of controlled drugs against a background of the legal and professional responsibilities defined by the Misuse of Drugs Act 1971 (see Chapter 1) and the Misuse of Drugs Regulations 1973 and 2001, among others. As with all medicines, we administer controlled drugs in line with the principles and guidelines laid down by your professional body (NMC, 2010). For example, it clearly states that two people, one of whom must be a registered nurse or midwife, must witness the preparation and administration of all controlled drugs (standard 26). In cases where the nurse administers controlled drugs intravenously, two registrants ought to witness the event (standard 20). Apart from the administration of intravenous controlled drugs, a student nurse who has satisfied their practice or academic assessor of their knowledge and competence with medicines administration procedures may check controlled drugs with a registered nurse.

The administrator must complete every column in the controlled drugs register after administration, with the following details:

- the date and time of administration;
- the name of the patient;
- the dose administered and any doses discarded;
- the signature in full of the nurse administering the medicine, and the signature of the witness;
- the remaining balance of stock, on return to the cupboard.

If there is an incorrect entry or actual or suspected medicine loss, the nurse should report this to their line manager and the pharmacy immediately.

Under no circumstances should anyone alter an error in the controlled drugs register; instead, the entry should be correctly rewritten. We will now turn to the different routes and techniques of administration.

The routes and techniques of administration

> ## Case study: Ann
>
> Ann had been working on an acute admission ward since she had qualified as a registered nurse 18 months prior. At handover, she was informed that a patient under her care had been prescribed phenobarbital, which needed to be administered. Ann administered the medicine as per the medicine chart instructions, which stated 600 mg of phenobarbital BD. She dispensed ten 60 mg tablets. Although she thought that giving ten tablets at a time was excessive, she never queried this or checked in the BNF. About two hours later, the patient was found lying unconscious in the bathroom with depressed respiration. The patient was immediately transferred to the nearest general hospital. The prescriber was notified of the events, and a subsequent investigation revealed that the prescriber in fact meant to prescribe 60 mg of phenobarbital.

Prescribers, even if they are doctors or pharmacists, are not immune to making errors that we may detect easily or immediately. The administrator has a responsibility to ensure that patients under their care receive medicines that will produce the most benefits with minimum harm. Ann should have followed up on her instinct that ten tablets was not a sensible dose. If the administrator feels that a dose or medicine is not correct, they should contact the prescriber first without delay for clarification before giving the medicine. If Ann had contacted the administrator first before giving the medicine, she would have acted sensibly and in the best interest of the patient.

Even if the administrator contacts the prescriber to query a prescription, they should formulate their own judgement as to whether to give the medication or not, considering several factors, including the prescriber's experience. For example, the prescriber may consider an explanation given by a consultant psychiatrist with many years' experience more reasoned than an explanation given by a junior doctor who is coming to the end of a busy night shift. If the administrator is still unsure, they can elicit the views of the pharmacist and consult the BNF before committing to a decision. What is clear is that nurses protect patients every day by querying prescriptions that raise a concern in their minds, and failure to query a prescription when in doubt is a contributing factor that puts patients' lives at risk (Luker and Wolfson, 1999). In addition to ensuring that prescribed medicines and doses are appropriate, the nurse should take practical steps to ensure safe and effective administration.

Oral medication administration procedure

The oral route is the most common route of administration of medicines. This is because in comparison to injections, it is economically more viable and less time-consuming, it requires less equipment, and it is not associated with pain and anxiety.

Before the nurse starts administering medicines, they will need the following:

- an electronic prescription or paper prescription chart;
- a medication formulary to check medicine details (e.g. the BNF);
- the manufacturer's information (if required);
- a disposable medicine tray, cups and a spoon;
- a medicine trolley with the medicine and a tablet splitter/crusher;
- water;
- a pair of gloves.

The nurse must follow the local trust or employer policy for administration of medications as institutions may vary. Before administering medicines, the nurse should ensure that the treatment room doors are secure to avoid unauthorised entry. Avoid distractions and interruptions while making up and administering medications; this may involve the nurse letting other members of staff know that they will not be able to attend to other duties such as answering phone calls. Also, it is important to remember that although the Royal Pharmaceutical Society supports the single-checking of oral medication, within strict local policy guidelines and protocols a student nurse should not single-check medicines (RPS, 2019). However, student nurses are involved in medicines administration procedures during practice learning opportunities. If there is a requirement for double-checking, as in the case of controlled drugs, both nurses should carry out all aspects of preparation, administration and documentation from the beginning to the end. An important rule is never to administer medicines you have not checked yourself.

Stage 1

- *Read the prescription* carefully, and if there is a lack of clarity in the prescription, including the date and signature of the prescriber, you should not give the medicine. You should contact the prescriber without delay. Make any preliminary checks and necessary observations (e.g. blood pressure, pulse) prior to administration.
- *Check the prescription chart* to ensure that the right patient receives the right medicine. The prescription should be legible and should include:

  o the name of the patient;
  o the route of administration;
  o the approved name of the medicine;
  o the dose to be administered;
  o the frequency and time of administration and the duration of treatment;
  o any special instructions (e.g. with food or before food);
  o any medicine or food allergies, including alternative medicines.

If the nurse is in any doubt or feels that they need clarification, they should contact the prescriber or pharmacist before giving the medicine. If it is necessary to rewrite the prescription, it is the nurse's responsibility to contact the prescriber before giving the medicine.

Stage 2

- *Select the medicine required* and check the label against the prescription. Remove the medication from the box or bottle.
- *Prepare the medicine* and check again with the prescription for:

  o the name of the patient;

  o the name and form of the medicine;

  o the route of administration;

  o the calculation (if any);

  o the measured dose;

  o the correct date and time;

  o the time of the last dose;

  o the expiration date of the medicine.

Stage 3

Once the nurse is certain about the above, they need to ensure that they inform the patient about what the medicine is, what it is for, the number of times the medicine is to be taken per day, and potential side effects and how to alleviate these. The next step is to check for consent and offer the medicine to the patient. Once the nurse is sure that the patient has ingested the medicine, they must initial or sign the medicine chart. If the nurse does not give the medicine to the patient, for whatever reason, they should document this, both on the chart and in the patient's notes, and state the reason why the medicine was not given. If the nurse observes or is informed of any contraindications during or after administration of any prescribed medicine, they should contact the prescriber, after first taking the advice of the pharmacist where appropriate. See also the section on the administration of controlled drugs on page 156 and the overview of legislation concerning controlled drugs in Chapter 1. Before you read further, try Activity 5.4.

Activity 5.4   Evidence-based research

Spend some time identifying different types of medicines in the medicines storage cupboard. In your observation, note how medicines storage containers are designed and note aspects likely to induce administration errors.

An outline answer is provided at the end of the chapter.

Administration of injections

An injection is a parenteral route of administration (i.e. it does not pass through the digestive tract). There are several methods of injection, the most popular being intramuscular (IM), subcutaneous and intravenous. In mental health practice, we commonly administer IM injections, although their use in the general healthcare setting has decreased substantially over the last decade with the emergence of newer medication administration methods (Cornwall, 2011). However, in the mental health setting, nurses are expected to be highly skilled in administering IM injections to achieve quality outcomes.

Intramuscular injections

Giving injections is a regular and commonplace activity for nurses, and a good injection technique can make the experience for the patient relatively painless. However, mastery of technique without developing the knowledge base from which to work can still put a patient at risk of undesirable complications. For example, if we give an IM injection incorrectly, the medication may not reach the correct site and absorption of the medication may be incomplete, resulting in a suboptimal serum level of the medication, which may impact negatively on the patient's mental health outcome.

Depending on the chemical properties of the medicine, it may be absorbed either quickly or gradually, as in the case of IM depot injections, which are probably the most administered in mental health. Depot injections are pharmacological preparations that release their active compound in a consistent way over a long period. They are either solid (e.g. risperidone – Risperdal Consta) or oil-based (e.g. flupenthixol decanoate). The advantages associated with depot injections are listed in Chapter 8.

The administration of IM injections involves a complex series of considerations and decisions, including the volume of the injectate, the medication to be given, technique, the site to be administered, syringe and needle size, the patient's age, and the pre-existence of bleeding disorders (Malkin, 2008). The NPSA (2007) states that poor practices can create adverse risks for patients and healthcare workers. These can include haemorrhage in people with bleeding disorders (Plotkin et al., 2008), pain, sciatic nerve injury, injection fibrosis, and infection.

If we administer intramsucular injections properly, the medication should deposit under the muscle fascia, below the fatty subcutaneous layer of the skin. Site selection is based on the manufacturer's recommendations, the medication to administer, muscle density at the selected site, and – ideally – consumer choice. Tortora and Derrickson (2018) have recommended five sites that are potentially suitable for IM injection: the deltoid, dorsogluteal, ventrogluteal, vastus lateralis and rectus femoris muscles. Each site has advantages and disadvantages that should be considered when selecting a site.

Deltoid muscles are located at the lower edge of the acromial process (see Figure 5.2). We rarely use this site for IM injection, particularly for antipsychotic depot injections. Giving an injection at the deltoid site may be associated with discomfort and a risk of radial and branchial nerve damage. For this reason, only administer a maximum of 1 ml at any one time.

The *dorsogluteal* site, or the the upper outer quadrant (see Figure 5.3), is perhaps the most popular site. The enduring preference for the dorsogluteal muscle may be due to easier site access, larger muscle bulk, reduced pain and consumer request. However, the disadvantages of this site are that it is close to major nerves (sciatic nerve) and blood vessels. Moreover, there is slow medication absorption and there is a thick layer of adipose (fat) tissue on this site, making it difficult to inject medication into the muscle tissue using a standard needle. When there is an inadvertent deposit of medication into the subcutaneous tissue, this can alter the pharmacokinetics of the medicine, and there is an increase in granuloma, sterile abscess, ulceration of tissue or fat necrosis. Although CT scans show an average injecting site success rate of only 8–32 per cent using the dorsogluteal site, this site remains popular, despite the ventrogluteal site being increasingly recommended.

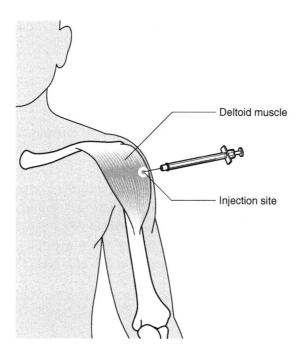

Figure 5.2 The intramuscular injection site on the deltoid muscle

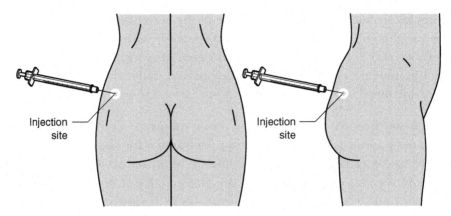

Figure 5.3   The dorsogluteal injection site

There is a preference for the *ventrogluteal* site injection for adults (see Figure 5.4). The advantage of a ventrogluteal injection is that it is reasonably free of major nerves and vascular branches. Other advantages include ease of location and a depth of muscle mass adequate for deep IM or Z-track injections. The use of the ventrogluteal site is now recommended with Z-tracking for IM use with antipsychotic medications, and pre-packed injecting kits now clearly advocate the practice. It has less variance of subcutaneous fat and research increasingly links it with safer practice. Further, we can administer injections in numerous patient positions: supine, lateral (left or right) and on the abdomen. A needle length of 3 or 4 cm is more than likely to penetrate muscle at this site. However, the use of the ventrogluteal site is infrequent, despite the compelling nature of the evidence for its superiority over other sites (Zimmermann, 2010). We can attribute the reluctance to use this site to nurses' perceived lack of confidence to perform the procedure or lack of knowledge regarding safe gluteal IM locations and rationale.

There is rare use of the *vastus lateralis* muscle as an injection site, but there are several advantages in using this method, the main one being that the muscle is normally well developed, even in children (see Figure 5.5). The injection can be given while the patient is lying flat, sitting down, or on their side, with the site pointing at the ceiling. Another advantage of this site is the potential for the self-administration of long-acting injectable (LAI) antipsychotics, which a small number of patients have learned to do. A disadvantage of using this site is the potential for the formation of a thrombosis in the femoral artery, especially if the landmarks are not located correctly.

There is rare use of the *rectus femoris* site, except for infants and self-administered injections.

The volume of an injectate that can be delivered to each muscle varies. This is based on muscle size, and there is little empirical evidence to support these recommendations. The maximum volume recommendation for an adult with a large muscle is 4–5 ml, and 1–2 ml in a smaller muscle (Workman, 1999). There are several factors that influence patient tolerance to injections, including whether the medicine is an oil-based formulation or not, the viscosity of the medicine, and the antibiotic or pH of the medicine. Therefore, the nurse should always use clinical judgement on what volume the individual is likely to tolerate; this can be based on the muscle size and the viscosity of the medicine. There is some evidence that smaller injected volumes help absorption and are less likely to cause a reaction (John and Stevenson, 1995). The Department of Health recommends dividing doses between two sites if there is a need to inject a volume greater than 3 or 4 ml (DoH, 2006). Table 5.1 gives the recommended injectate volumes for various injection sites.

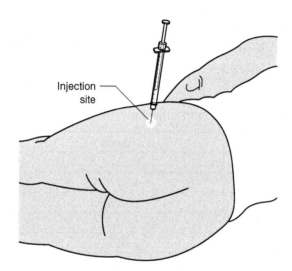

Figure 5.4   The ventrogluteal injection site

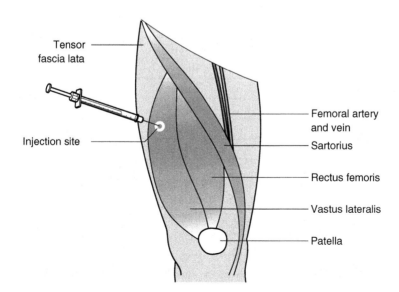

Figure 5.5   The vastus lateralis injection site

Choice of needle

Most needles for injection are made of stainless steel and the needle gauge (G) indicates the diameter of the needle. Needles are differentiated based on their length and diameter. The lengths of needles range from 16 mm ({5/8} inch) to 76 mm (3 inches). In general, we use long needles to give IM medications while we use shorter needles to give subcutaneous medications. The higher the needle gauge number, the smaller the needle's diameter, so a 25G needle has a smaller diameter than a 19G needle. Needles of the same length can have different gauge sizes.

We base the selection of needle gauge on the thickness of the medication that the nurse wants to give. If the medication is thick, as in the case of long-acting depot antipsychotics, the nurse could choose a needle with a small gauge and big diameter (e.g. 22G–19G). For each needle gauge, various needle lengths are available. Table 5.2 shows the colour codes of various needle gauges.

Table 5.1 Muscle types and maximum injectate volumes

Muscle type	Volume
Deltoid	1 ml
Dorsogluteal	4 ml
Ventrogluteal	2.5 ml
Vastus lateralis	1 ml
Rectus femoris – adults	5 ml

Table 5.2 Colour codes of needle gauges

Needle gauge	Colour code
26G	Brown
25G	Orange
23G	Blue
22G	Black
21G	Green
20G	Yellow
19G	White

In general, we give injections of liquid medicines, such as antibiotics, procyclidine or vitamin B_5, using a 22G needle. A 22G needle is also longer (25 mm) to enable it to reach deep into the muscle. If the medication is thicker (more viscous), as in the case of a long-acting depot injection (e.g. flupenthixol decanoate), we may use a 20G needle. Additionally, we use longer (5 cm) needles for those who have more gluteal fat, particularly women and those with a body mass index (BMI) greater than 30 kg/m².

The administration of an IM injection can cause complications and potential problems, including pain, anaphylaxis, and sterile and septic abscess formation if we administer large volume injections. In addition, needle phobia can develop into a long-term problem following a traumatic IM injection. Needle-stick injuries are also a serious concern for nurses, and risks from these injuries include the possibility of infection by blood-borne diseases such as hepatitis and HIV. For this reason, several measures have been introduced to minimise the risk and impact of needle-stick injuries, including the use of fixed-needle and auto-retractable safety syringes. Evidence suggests that using such devices can reduce the incidence of sharps injuries to nurses and patients, especially if they are combined with appropriate training and safe working practices (van der Molen et al., 2011).

Intramuscular injection technique

The first stage of an injection technique is to let the patient know that you will be administering an injection and obtain informed consent (see Chapter 1). This allows time for the patient to psychologically prepare for the occasion. The second stage is to gather all of the equipment you need for the injection, including the right needle, the right syringe, antiseptic pads and adhesive bandages (Band-Aids), on a disposable tray. Ideally, there is an emergency bag that contains equipment and materials to treat anaphylactic shock or cardiac arrest in case a patient suffers either of these during or soon after an injection. At the very least, medicines to treat anaphylactic shock should be available in every room where an injection is taking place. It is important to remember that cardiac arrest may develop because of anaphylactic shock, which can be caused by very small amounts of antigens. Once all the necessary equipment is available, the nurse should should follow the 10Rs (see page 154).

Before drawing the injection, the nurse should follow all basic infection control precautionary procedures, including washing hands and putting on disposable gloves. The next step is to draw the right amount of injectate and ensure that there are no air pockets in the injectate. Next, ensure the patient's privacy and explain the injection procedure, including any potential risks. The nurse should discuss with the patient their preferred injection site and follow the local standard operating procedure for the administration of the injection. Once the patient has consented and there is agreement on the preferred injection site, the nurse should clean the skin at the injection site thoroughly with an antiseptic pad (sponge with alcohol or Betadine).

Administering an injection using the Z-track technique

1. After you have cleaned the injection site, you allow the area to dry, then ask the patient to get into a comfortable position and relax the muscle to be injected. This may be lying down on the stomach, bending over a chair or counter, or sitting.

2. You need to use your non-dominant hand to pull the skin and subcutaneous tissue 3–4 cm to one side of the injection site (this prevents leakage or backtracking

of medication from the injection site) and then locate the site (see Figure 5.6). Pulling the skin and tissue before the injection causes the needle track to take the shape of the letter 'Z', which gives the procedure its name. This zigzag track line is what prevents medication from leaking from the muscle into surrounding tissue.

3. *Insert the needle.* Hold the needle at a 90-degree angle and insert it quickly (in a 'dart-like' motion) and deeply enough to penetrate the muscle but not to touch bone (see Figure 5.6). A quick insertion of the needle will minimise the pain for the patient.

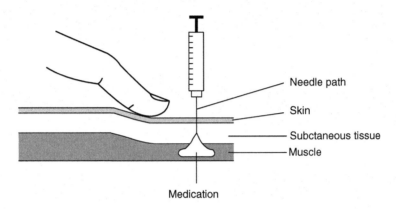

Figure 5.6 The Z-track technique during and after injection

4. *Check for blood.* Pull back the plunger and check the syringe for evidence of aspirated blood. If blood is present, it means a vein may have been pinched, so you must use a new site. This will involve a new needle and fresh medication. You should then explain your actions to the patient and select another injection site. There is ongoing debate on the necessity of aspirating when using the Z-track technique, so consult your local employer policy for guidance.

5. *Inject the medication.* If there is no blood in the syringe, push on the plunger to inject the medication slowly into the muscle.

6. *Create the Z-track.* Keep the needle in place for about ten seconds before taking it out. After you have removed the needle, release your hold on the skin and tissue. This disrupts the hole that the needle leaves in the tissues and prevents the medication from leaking out of the muscle.

7. *Apply pressure to the site.* Use gauze to apply gentle pressure to the site for a few moments. A small bandage may be used if there is bleeding. Please note that you should never massage the site of a Z-track injection as this may cause the medication to leak or cause irritation.

8. *Sign the chart and document.* You should sign the patient's medicine chart and record the administration of the injection in the patient's notes. The information you should record includes the medication, the dose, the route, the muscle site, and the date and time. If the injection is a repeat depot antipsychotic, you should state when it is next due.

After successfully administering the injection, cover the injection site by placing an adhesive bandage over it to protect clothes from possible bloodstains and to protect the injection site from infection.

Observe the patient for unusual reactions as any medication can cause anaphylaxis. Make periodic checks on the patient to ensure their safety and well-being after an injection – you should communicate this to the patient.

Subcutaneous injections

The subcutaneous route is the administration of medication into the tissue just below the skin; we commonly use this route in diabetes and with some vaccines. Examples of medicines we give via the subcutaneous route include insulin, anticoagulants, opioids and hormone treatments. Absorption of medication from the subcutaneous route is slower than from the IM route, and the rate of absorption varies depending on the site used. Potential injection sites include the abdomen, the buttocks, the hips, the lateral aspects of the thigh, and the upper outer arms. For the administration of insulin in people with Type 1 diabetes, we use the subcutaneous route. It is important that insulin is absorbed at the same rate and time every day, and ideally at the same injection site (e.g. the upper arm in the morning).

Subcutaneous injection technique

The technique is like giving an IM injection, except we use a much shorter 25G 19 mm or 27G 13 mm needle. The nurse should give the injection at a 90- or 45-degree angle, depending on the amount of skin that they can grasp between their thumb and first finger. If the nurse can grasp approximately 51 mm (2 inches) of skin, they can give the injection at a 90-degree angle. Alternatively, if the nurse can grasp only 25 mm (1 inch) of skin, they can give the injection at a 45-degree angle. There is no need to aspirate the needle to check if a blood vessel has been punctured as this is unlikely. The nurse should wash their hands and document in the same way as for other medication.

Rectal administration

We can also administer medication via the rectal route in the form of suppositories and liquids. The rectal route is particularly useful when a patient cannot tolerate oral medication due to nausea, vomiting or loss of consciousness.

Before starting the procedure, the nurse should observe infection control protocol to reduce the risk of cross-infection and explain the procedure to the patient. Be alert to cultural sensitivities, as people from other cultures may find rectal administration of medicines unacceptable, so in this regard it is important to obtain clear consent, which should be documented. The nurse should wear gloves and position the patient comfortably on one side with one leg flexed. Moisten the tip of the suppository or enema with water or a water-based lubricant (e.g. K-Y gel) before inserting. Insert the rounded end of the suppository into the anus and propel it forward. If possible, ask the patient to 'hold on' to the suppository for five minutes.

Sublingual administration

We administer sublingual (also known as buccal) medications to enable rapid absorption into the bloodstream through the mucous membranes of the mouth. When a medicine is in contact with the mucous membrane beneath the tongue (or the buccal mucosa inside the cheeks or lips), it diffuses into the profusion of connective capillaries under the epithelium and into the venous circulation. This contrasts with oral medication, which passes through the intestines and is subject to *first-pass metabolism* in the liver before entering the general circulation.

The sublingual method of administration has advantages over oral administration in that it is more direct, and there is little medicine degradation due to first-pass metabolism from hostile stomach acid, bile or gut enzymes. Additionally, oral medication must pass through the liver, which may chemically alter it before exerting its therapeutic effect. One disadvantage of using the sublingual method is that if we use acid or caustic medicines in the long term, it can cause tooth discolouration and decay. The nurse should not administer sublingual medicines in patients with inflamed mucous membranes or open sores. In mental health, one medicine we commonly administer via the sublingual route is buprenorphine, a replacement therapy for substance use disorder.

As with the administration of most types of medicines, the nurse should wash their hands first and wear non-sterile gloves. Then ask the patient to open their mouth with the tongue lifted. Place the medicine between the bottom part of the tongue and the lower gum (in buccal administration, place the medicine between the teeth and the cheek). Ask the patient to keep the medicine in position until it dissolves.

Medication errors

A medication error can be defined as 'a failure in the treatment process that leads to, or has the potential to lead to, harm to the patient' (Williams, 2007). In broad terms, they are errors in the prescribing, dispensing, storage or administration of a medicine, irrespective of whether such errors lead to adverse consequences or not (NPSA, 2007). Medication errors can cause unnecessary pain and harm to patients and can even lead to death. They rank among the most frequent failures in healthcare delivery, and they are the second highest category of errors reported (Cousins et al., 2012). Current estimates are that they are the fourteenth leading cause of morbidity and mortality in the world, placing them alongside tuberculosis and malaria (WHO, 2019). According to the NPSA (2007), medicines errors contribute to 25 per cent of adverse incidents litigation claims. Therefore, medicines errors have negative consequences not only for patient safety, but also for practitioners.

From an economic vantage point, the global cost associated with medicine errors is estimated to be US$42 billion, accounting for 0.7 per cent of global health expenditure (Aitken and Gorokhovich, 2013). In the UK, medicines errors cost the NHS at least £2.5 billion per year and £1.1 billion per year as a result of direct patient harm (Frontier Economics, 2014). Whatever the financial cost of mistakes, the real and lasting effect of medicines errors is on patients and their families.

Most serious incidents were caused by errors in medicine administration (41 per cent) and, to a lesser extent, prescribing (32 per cent). Medication errors involving injectable medicines represented 62 per cent of all reported incidents leading to death or severe harm. The NPSA further reports that medication is the third most frequently reported incident type after patient accident and treatment/procedure. Three medication incident types – unclear/wrong dose or frequency, wrong medicine, and omitted/delayed medicines – accounted for 71 per cent of fatal and serious harm. Whether they are mistakes, slips or lapses, the NPSA recognises that the majority of errors were not the result of reckless behaviour on the part of healthcare professionals, but occurred as a result of the complex nature of medicines management (NPSA, 2007). Medicine errors are the single most preventable cause of patient harm, and they can occur at all stages of the medication process.

Prescribing errors

In medicines management, prescription is the first stage of the process, and errors at this point can result in problems downstream. Prescribing errors usually include incorrect medicine selection for the patient, including dose, quantity, prescribing a contraindicated medicine, poor knowledge of the prescribed medicine and its recommended dose, and poor knowledge of the patient's details. Other contributing factors include illegible handwriting, inaccurate recording of medication history, confusion involving the medicine's name, inappropriate use of **decimal** points, and lack of a zero preceding a decimal point (e.g. .1 instead of 0.1). Similarly, tenfold errors in dosage have occurred because of the use of a trailing zero (e.g. 1.20). The use of abbreviations has also led to confusion (e.g. AZT for azathioprine and zidovudine, formerly called azidothymidine), as has the use of verbal orders.

Dispensing errors

Dispensing errors can occur at any stage of the dispensing process, from the receipt of the prescription in the pharmacy to the supply of a dispensed medicine to the patient, and include the selection of the wrong strength or product. This occurs primarily with medicines that have a similar name or appearance. Lasix (frusemide) and Losec (omeprazole) are examples of proprietary names that, when handwritten, look similar. This further emphasises the need to prescribe generically (Williams, 2007). Other examples of pairs of medicines with similar names include lorazepam and lormetazepam, and amiloride and amlodipine tablets. Other potential dispensing errors include the wrong dose, the wrong medicine or the wrong patient. The use of computerised labelling has led to typing errors, which are among the leading causes of dispensing errors. Methods for reducing errors include separating medicines with a similar name or appearance, keeping disruptions in the dispensing procedure to a minimum, and reducing the workload of the dispenser to a manageable level.

Administration errors

Administration errors are a result of a discrepancy between the medicine received by the patient and the medicine intended by the prescriber. In other words, administration errors occur when any of the 5Rs are violated (see page 154). Administration errors have long been associated with one of the highest-risk areas in nursing practice, and in most cases involve errors of omission where the medicine has not been administered for whatever reason. Other types of errors include the administration of incorrect or expired medicines.

Contributing factors to medicine administration errors include a failure to check the patient's identity prior to administration and the storage of similar preparations in similar areas. Environmental factors, such as noise, interruptions while undertaking a medicine round, and poor lighting, may also contribute to these errors. The likelihood of error increases where more than one tablet is required to supply the correct dose or where the nurse needs to make a calculation to determine the correct dose for the patient. Approaches to reduce medicine administration errors should include:

- checking the patient's identity, particularly older people with dementia;
- ensuring independent checking of dosage calculations by another healthcare professional before administering the medicine;
- ensuring that the prescription chart, the medicine and the patient are in the same place in order to check one against the other;
- ensuring that the medication is given at the correct time;
- minimising interruptions during medicine rounds.

Clinical pharmacists are important in the safe use of medicines; and if a system exists whereby pharmacists visit the wards daily, it places them in a good position to recognise particular training needs that can be addressed (Williams, 2007).

Chapter summary

The management of medicines is now a complex procedure that involves many professionals. In many cases, medicines management involves the prescriber, the dispenser and the administrator of the medicine. The traditional model is that the doctor prescribes, the pharmacist dispenses, and the nurse administers medicines.

Recent changes in medicines management have changed this approach. Many professionals, including nurses, midwives, physiotherapists, dentists and psychologists, can prescribe medicines after additional training. The role of the prescriber remains that of making a diagnosis, prescribing medicines and reviewing the effects. The pharmacist's role in modern medicines management is more complex: apart from dispensing medicines, they are also involved in providing expert advice on the usage of medicines to other professionals as well as patients. Pharmacists have become increasingly ward-based. In mental health, the administration of medicines requires that nurses are familiar and competent in several methods, including oral, IM, subcutaneous, sublingual and rectal. Medicines management gives rise to medicines errors, some of which can be fatal, so steps to minimise errors should be put in place.

Activities: brief outline answers

Activity 5.2 Reflection (page 151)

If the medicine's label is not clear, this could result in a variety of errors, including giving the medicine to the wrong person, giving the wrong preparation, using the wrong route of administration, or storing the medicines inappropriately.

Activity 5.3 Critical thinking (page 152)

TCAs are not particularly suitable for older people because they are more prone to adverse side effects such as dry mouth, constipation and cardiotoxicity.

Activity 5.4 Evidence-based research (page 159)

You are likely to observe that different dosages of a particular medicine (e.g. olanzapine) have very similarly designed containers, and this is a common source of error.

Further reading

Lawson, E. and Hennefer, D. (2010) *Medicines Management in Adult Nursing.* Exeter: Learning Matters.

O'Brien, M., Spires, A. and Andrews, K. (2011) *Introduction to Medicines Management in Nursing.* Exeter: Learning Matters.

These two books in the same series cover many topics that are relevant to mental health nursing.

Useful website

www.nmc-uk.org/Nurses-and-midwives/Advice-by-topic/A/Advice/Covert-administration-of-medicines

This NMC website offers advice on the covert administration of medicines.

Chapter 6   Management and treatment of major depression

Chapter aims

By the end of this chapter, you should:

- understand the main features of depression aetiology and the biological mechanism that may explain major depression;
- understand the main classes of antidepressants and their mechanism of action;
- have a knowledge and understanding of antidepressant side effects and their management.

Introduction

Case study: George

George, a 52-year-old who was made redundant six months ago, has visited his GP complaining of intermittent headaches, fatigue and generalised lower back pain during the previous eight weeks. He has also reported that he has been sleeping a lot but that his sleep pattern is fractured. As a result, he does not feel refreshed after sleeping and he wakes up very early in the morning. He admits to having experienced stress some years back but does not acknowledge that he suffered from depression then. He does not feel sad but lately finds it increasingly difficult to cope with the behaviour of people around him. He denies abusing alcohol and reports that his drinking patterns and amounts of alcohol consumed have not changed. However, his wife reports that for at least four months, her husband has been extremely irritable and difficult to rouse in the morning. She notices a definite increase in his alcohol consumption, estimating that he now has a few shots of whisky every night. The GP has suggested to George that he might be suffering from depression, and has prescribed antidepressants and referred George for counselling.

Written records by healers, philosophers and others show that major depression has always been a health problem for humankind throughout the ages (Nemade, 2017), even as far back as biblical times. According to the Old Testament, King Saul suffered from major depression and committed suicide as a result. To better understand our current attitudes towards mental illness, it is necessary to look back at prevailing attitudes during ancient times. At that time, it was believed that major depression was caused by supernatural forces. Indeed, ancient human skulls have been found with large holes in them caused by drilling into the skull to let evil spirits out. Thankfully, nowadays there is treatment for this illness; but before discussing the treatment of depression in detail, it is important to understand that not all forms of major depression require antidepressants. For that, we need to distinguish between different forms of depression, as well as which types of depression will benefit the most from pharmacological strategies.

The mildest form of low mood is *reactive sadness*, which is when a person is emotionally reacting to some event that has happened in their lives. This can last for a few hours or a few days. Second in terms of severity is the concept of *grief*. This is a reaction to a major loss in a person's life, and this response is normal. Situations that can cause grief range from divorce or separation from a loved one to bereavement. Grief usually lasts for months, but it is common for some people to experience grief for several years. The third type is *clinical* or *major depression*, which is a pathological condition characterised by loss of normal function in society, among other symptoms. It is this type of depression that we are concerned with in this chapter. Major depression is without doubt a leading global cause of disability, affecting at least 2–4 per cent of the population at any given point in time. The burden of major depression has increased worldwide since 1990, particularly in low- and middle-income countries, where most of the world's population resides. In these countries, healthcare services are generally less able to meet patient need. Major depression is associated with social disadvantage, a broad range of physical diseases, and shortened lifespan (Chesney et al., 2014). In contrast to many diseases that receive greater research funding, depression has occupied a higher rank over time in the global burden of diseases (Woelbert et al., 2019), and its persistence is a major source of individual and family distress.

This chapter starts with an overview of several hypotheses that underlie major depression, before listing common physical disorders and medication that may induce major depression. Different classes of antidepressants, as well as their modes of action and side effects, are covered in slightly more detail, followed by an overview of side effects management. The final sections deal with common treatment errors to avoid and what the patient needs to know about their treatment. You will need to understand these theories as they form the bedrock of understanding how antidepressants work.

The biological mechanism that may explain depression

Despite its well-defined symptoms, major depression appears to be a diverse mental health disorder whose pathophysiology is currently unclear (Rahe et al., 2014).

People's personal and social factors, in addition to their biological vulnerabilities, seem to play a significant part in triggering and sustaining the illness. This view finds support from a meta-analysis of studies examining the etiology of major depression, which concludes that the illness is complex and results from an interaction of biological and environmental influences (Menard et al., 2016). Early life traumatic events can contribute to the development of individual differences in the ability to react and cope with subsequent stressful events. For example, victims of childhood abuse or parental neglect have significantly higher probabilities of developing depression (Anacker et al., 2014). It has not been possible to establish precisely how these factors interact over time, but recent insights into the structure and function of distinct brain regions offer an opportunity to describe the neural basis of major depression and its unique course, clinical presentation, and how a person with the illness may respond to treatment. In this respect, there are now several hypotheses that seek to explain the foundations of depression. These include the hypothalamic-pituitary-adrenal (HPA) axis dysfunction theory, cognitive and behavioural theories, the neurogenesis hypothesis, the inflammatory theory, also known as the cytokine model, and the monoamine hypothesis. All of these hypotheses share a common biological backdrop and are being drawn together (Zunszain et al., 2011). For example, depression is highly prevalent in people with infectious, autoimmune and neurodegenerative diseases, and at the same time depressed patients show higher levels of pro-inflammatory cytokines. Since communication occurs between the endocrine, immune and central nervous systems, an activation of the inflammatory responses can affect neuroendocrine processes, and vice versa. Therefore, HPA axis hyperactivity and inflammation might be part of the same pathophysiological process. However, the theory that has direct relevance to current antidepressant treatment is the monoamine hypothesis, and we will discuss this next. But before we do so, please complete Activity 6.1.

Activity 6.1   Critical thinking

Do the neurotransmitters implicated in depression work in an excitatory or inhibitory manner?

An outline answer is provided at the end of the chapter.

The monoamine hypothesis of depression

Scientific studies have found that numerous brain areas show an alteration in activity in patients with major depression. From a biological viewpoint, it has so far not been possible to determine a single area of the brain that causes depression. Research on the brains of people with depression usually shows disturbed patterns of interaction between multiple parts of the brain. The areas that are most strongly affected are the raphe nuclei, the suprachiasmatic nucleus, the HPA axis, the ventral tegmental area

(VTA), the nucleus accumbens and the anterior cingulate cortex. There is a hypothesis that major depression is due to neurotransmitter malfunction in some or all of these parts of the brain.

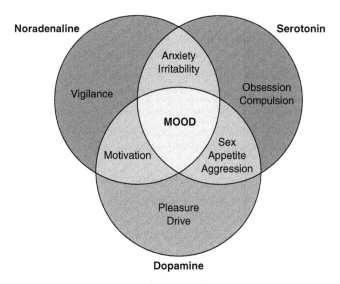

Figure 6.1   The three monoamine neurotransmitters implicated in depression

There are at least three classical neurotransmitters that play a key part in depression: noradrenaline, serotonin and dopamine (see Figure 6.1). We call these three neurotransmitters *monoamines*. Initially, there was some debate about which of these neurotransmitters is the most important in depression, but there is now a general acceptance that all three are important.

The classical monoamine hypothesis of depression in its simplest form states that depression is due to low concentrations of these three monoamine neurotransmitters in the brain. The origins of this theory come from the observation that certain drugs, such as reserpine, that reduce the concentration of monoamine neurotransmitters in the brain can induce clinical depression. Mood elation, in contrast, may have an association with an excess of monoamine neurotransmitters. Evidence supporting this hypothesis includes data from pharmacological studies, mainly in animals, suggesting that the actions of both major classes of antidepressant medicines work via the monoamines. The monoamine hypothesis comes under challenge mainly from the discovery that not all patients with depression have a reduction of monoamine neurotransmitter levels. Moreover, some people who have no depression but show violent or impulsive behaviour tend to have reduced levels of monoamines, especially serotonin. But most importantly, antidepressants can raise the levels of monoamine neurotransmitters very quickly in some brain areas, resulting in symptom alleviation, but in many cases antidepressant effects can take weeks. Therefore, the relationship between monoamine neurotransmitters and depression does not appear straightforward, and this has stimulated a search for better explanations. The monoamine hypothesis has therefore been modified to include the changes we see in neuroreceptor density during episodes of major depression.

The monoamine hypothesis and the role of glial cells

As stated above, the monoamine hypothesis of depression simply suggests that low concentrations of monoamine neurotransmitters lead to low activity levels in the brain. In turn, this results in an increase in the number of postsynaptic receptors as a way of compensating for the reduced activity. We call this increase in receptor numbers *receptor upregulation*. Receptor upregulation coincides with the emergence of clinical symptoms of major depression. When an individual with depression responds to antidepressant treatment, the number of postsynaptic receptors decreases back to normal, a process we call *receptor downregulation*. Receptor downregulation normally accompanies reduction in receptor sensitivity. Despite its better explanatory power, direct evidence in support of the monoamine hypothesis is largely weak.

In search of a better explanation for depression, the astrocyte hypothesis is increasingly gaining currency. There is a potential role for glial cells in the understanding of the mechanisms of depression and action of antidepressant medicines. Despite being the most abundant cell type in the brain, their full role in brain function was not fully appreciated, and they were thought of as just the glue that hold more important brain cells (neurons) together. It is now apparent that glial cells, especially astrocytes, are not merely silent spectators of neuronal activity, but are active participants in brain function. Astrocytes secrete molecules that are essential for dendritic growth and synaptogenesis during development. They also provide trophic (nutritional) and metabolic support to neurons, which is essential for their normal functioning. Importantly, astrocytes appear highly responsive to changes in extracellular monoamine concentrations. They express transporters for both norepinephrine (NET) and serotonin (SERT), which are the targets of several classical antidepressant medicines. This raises the possibility that antidepressants can have direct effects on astrocytes by blocking the reuptake of monoamines by astrocytes. Astrocytes also express $5HT_{1A}$, $5HT_{2A}$ and $5HT_{2B}$ receptors of serotonin, in addition to $5HT_{5A}$, which is a predominantly astrocyte-specific receptor. In people with depression, there is a degeneration of astrocytes, especially in the prefrontal cortex (Smialowska et al., 2013). Studies over the past two decades point to dysfunctional astrocytes as the potential root cause of some forms of major depression, and this has led to a shift from a neuron-centric to an astrocyte-centric cause of major depression (Wang et al., 2017a). To further complicate matters, there is now compelling evidence that there is an association between depression and deficits in other neurotransmitter systems, including GABAergic (Luscher et al., 2011), glutamatergic (Mitchell and Baker, 2010) and cholinergic (Mineur and Picciotto, 2010) systems. Whatever the hypothesis underlying major depression, established understanding of antidepressants is that they achieve their efficacy by increasing the concentration of monoamine neurotransmitters in the synapse. During the development of major depression, the patient develops a variety of symptoms, and these are outlined in the next section.

Symptoms of depression

The symptoms of depression are many and varied, but the most encountered symptoms are shown in Figure 6.2. For details of these symptoms, consult a textbook on psychopathology (several are listed in the further reading section at the end of the chapter). Apart from the social factors that trigger depression, there are some physical illnesses that are associated with depression, and it is those that we discuss next.

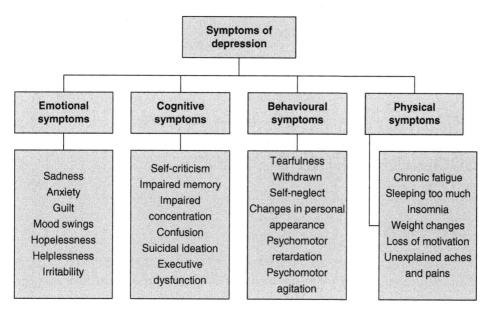

Figure 6.2 Symptoms of major depression in adults

Common disorders known to be associated with depression

Some medical conditions, in certain situations, can trigger biochemical changes that can ultimately affect neurotransmission of the identified monoamines in a way that may cause depression. Conditions such as influenza and thyroid disorder (**hypothyroidism**) are clear examples. For this reason, it is good practice to screen for thyroid function when a person presents with a mood disorder, as approximately 10 per cent of all people with major depression is a result of low levels of thyroxine. The list in Table 6.1 of common physical disorders associated with depression is not exhaustive, but provides you with an overview.

Table 6.1 Physical conditions that may cause depression in adults

• vitamin B deficiency	• cerebrovascular disease
• vitamin D deficiency	• hepatitis
• zinc deficiency	• syphilis
• selenium deficiency	• porphyria
• magnesium deficiency	• Parkinson's disease
• influenza	• systemic lupus erythematosis
• HIV/AIDs	• multiple sclerosis
• inflammatory conditions	• diabetes
• **Cushing's syndrome**	• chronic pain
• thyroid disorders	• Addison's disease
• asthma	• chronic fatigue syndrome
• cardiovascular disease	• post-partum hormonal changes

Medicines and drugs that are associated with depression

Case study: Fred

Fred is a 27-year-old gym instructor who was referred to a psychiatrist by his GP because his depression had not shown any improvement despite his being on fluoxetine for 12 weeks. During his interview with the psychiatrist, Fred revealed for the first time that he was taking anabolic steroids to aid muscle-building. The psychiatrist informed him that the anabolic steroids may have played a significant part in his depression, and therefore advised against taking them. Fred stopped taking anabolic steroids and his mood gradually improved. He continued to take antidepressants for six months and gradually weaned himself off them. He has not had a recurrence of depression since.

Some therapeutic and non-therapeutic medicines unfortunately may play a part in inducing depression as a side effect. Recreational substances, such as alcohol and the drugs that Fred used in the above case study, are known to alter mood, and therefore it is important for nurses to routinely elicit information about the use of drugs or alcohol when assessing a patient. It is common for people with depression to use alcohol as a mood stimulant, but this is only a temporary measure as alcohol usually worsens mood. Also, it is common for people suffering from depression to increase their caffeine intake as a way of overcoming fatigue; caffeine has some mild but transient antidepressant properties. This might sound like a good idea initially, but excess caffeine causes sleeplessness, which in turn will retard recovery from depression. Some of the drugs and substances known to cause depression are listed in Table 6.2.

Table 6.2 Drugs that may induce major depression in adults

• antihypertensives	• antibacterial and antifungal drugs (e.g. fluoroquinolones, beta-lactams)
• corticosteroids and other hormones	• analgesics
• anti-Parkinson's drugs (e.g. levodopa, carbidopa)	• alcohol
• anxiolytic drugs (e.g. diazepam)	• sedatives (e.g. Z-drugs, benzodiazepines)
• birth control pills	• barbiturates
• antineoplastic drugs	• appetite suppressants

Classes of antidepressants and their side effects

In many respects, we can regard the discovery of antidepressants as accidental. Researchers carrying out trials on new medication to treat tuberculosis in the 1950s found that the medication had mood-elevating effects. This initial discovery led to the creation of two classes of first- generation antidepressants: monoamine oxidase inhibitors (MAOIs) and tricyclic antidepressants (TCAs). More recently, selective serotonin reuptake inhibitors (SSRIs) form the second generation and selective noradrenaline reuptake inhibitors (SNRIs) the third generation of antidepressants introduced during the 1990s.

Tricyclic antidepressants

TCAs have an important place in the treatment history of major depression as they were the second group of such medicines to be discovered after MAOIs. It is their mode of action that helped to formulate theories of depression, and for many years TCAs were the first-line treatment for major depression. TCAs are effective in the treatment of depression even at low doses (75 and 100 mg per day), according to an early systematic review of 39 studies with a total of 2,564 participants (Furukawa et al., 2003). Although they are still considered to be highly effective, they have been increasingly replaced by SSRIs and other newer antidepressants. Nonetheless, we still use TCAs occasionally for treatment-resistant depression that fails to respond to treatment with newer antidepressants. We also use TCAs to treat secondary depression in other illnesses such as psychosis, cancer, HIV, dementia and post-stroke depression. They are not addictive and are somewhat preferable to MAOIs from a safety perspective.

Mode of action of TCAs

TCAs work by preventing the transportation of monoamine neurotransmitters from the synaptic cleft back into the presynaptic neuron. This therapeutic action of antidepressants is entirely consistent with the monoamine hypothesis of depression (see page 176). Most TCAs tend to act mainly as SNRIs by disabling the mechanism that transports serotonin and noradrenaline back to the presynaptic neuron. These mechanisms are known as the serotonin transporter (SERT) and the noradrenaline transporter (NAT), and are described elsewhere (see page 176). The disabling of these protein transporter systems results in the accumulation of serotonin and noradrenaline in the synapse, therefore enhancing the chances of neurotransmission. Although monoamine dopamine has been implicated in depression, TCAs have very little action on the dopamine transporter (DAT), and therefore have very little efficacy as dopamine reuptake inhibitors (DRIs) (see Table 6.3).

The best way to prescribe TCAs is by starting the medicine at a low dose and increasing the dose every three to five days. Most TCAs have a linear pharmacokinetics profile (i.e. a change in dose will lead to a proportional change in the blood serum level). Once the blood serum level reaches **steady state**, we can give TCAs as a single dose before bedtime because they have a relatively long half-life. They show therapeutic effects within 7 to 28 days. However, at times, patients may lose response to antidepressants after several months, a condition we call the *poop-out syndrome.*

Side effects of TCAs

Apart from their role in inhibiting neurotransmitter transport systems, many TCAs also have a high affinity as antagonists at specific receptor sites, such as the various serotonin and alpha-1 (α_1) adrenergic receptors, some of which may contribute to their therapeutic efficacy as well as to their side effects profile. For example, TCAs have varying but typically high affinity for antagonising the histamine (H_1 and H_2) receptors, resulting in weight gain and drowsiness. For this reason and others mentioned previously, it is best to prescribe TCAs as a single large dose at night after dose titration for those with sleep problems. This avoids drowsiness interfering with a person's daily activities during daytime. For those who have depression accompanied with agitation, we can give TCAs during daytime to help the individual to settle and prevent overexhaustion. Because TCAs induce weight gain, it is important to exercise caution in those who are overweight or obese. TCAs also antagonise the muscarinic acetylcholine receptors, and this leads to adverse side effects such as constipation, dry mouth, blurry vision, dry nose, urinary retention and cognitive impairment. In this respect, their use in the elderly is not advisable. Most, if not all, TCAs are potent inhibitors of sodium channels, which accounts for their adverse cardiac effects, but which can also explain their beneficial effects on neuropathic pain.

Table 6.3 Tricyclic antidepressants, showing the types of neurotransmitters they act on (the more plus signs, the greater the action)

Generic name	Noradrenaline	Serotonin	Monoamine oxidase	Dopamine
Imipramine	++	+++	–	0
Desipramine	++++	0	0	0
Amitryptiline	+	++++	0	0

Generic name	Noradrenaline	Serotonin	Monoamine oxidase	Dopamine
Nortriptyline	+++	++	0	0
Trimipramine	++	++	0	0
Doxepin	+++	++	0	0
Clomipramine	+++	+++++	–	–

Other common side effects of TCAs include anxiety, emotional blunting (apathy/ **anhedonia**), confusion, restlessness, akathisia, hypersensitivity, sweating, sexual dysfunction, muscle twitches, weakness, nausea and vomiting, tachycardia, and – rarely – irregular heart rhythms. TCAs can cause rhabdomyolysis, or muscle breakdown, in very rare cases. Tolerance to some of these adverse effects can often develop if there is treatment continuation. Side effects may also be less troublesome if treatment is initiated with low doses and then gradually increased (titration), although this may also delay the beneficial effects.

One of the most important side effects of TCAs is an irregular heart rhythm (arrhythmia), so they can – in theory – stop contraction of heart muscle fibres, decrease cardiac contractility, and increase collateral blood circulation to the ischaemic heart muscle. Naturally, in overdose, they are cardiotoxic, prolonging heart rhythms and increasing myocardial irritability. This makes TCAs unsuitable for those with a heart condition or with a family history of such conditions. Antidepressants in general may produce a *discontinuation syndrome*. This is not the same as drug withdrawal, and will be explained in later sections.

Monoamine oxidase inhibitors

MAOIs were the first type of antidepressants to be developed. There is a restriction on their use because of the availability of many other options and the relative lack of understanding about the safety profile of these medicines. For a variety of reasons, there is now a downgrading of these MAOIs to the role of third- or even fourth-line treatments for depression. They have mostly been replaced by the newer and safer SSRIs and other safe non-SSRIs or atypical antidepressants (see later sections).

Mode of action of MAOIs

The monoamine neurotransmitters, namely serotonin, noradrenaline and dopamine, are released into the synaptic cleft, where they transmit chemical messages by binding to the postsynaptic receptors. After transmitting messages, some of these monoamine neurotransmitters are reabsorbed back into the presynaptic neuron. The enzyme monoamine oxidase (MAO) destroys some of the monoamine neurotransmitters. Therefore, MAOIs work by simply disabling this enzyme from catalysing the destruction of neurotransmitters, resulting in the accumulation of monoamines in the synaptic cleft.

There are two types of MAO enzymes: type A and B. The MAO-A subtype metabolises serotonin, dopamine and noradrenaline neurotransmitters, as well as tyramine. We find this enzyme mainly in the brain, the gut, the liver, the placenta and the skin. On the other hand, the MAO-B subtype metabolises trace dopamine and trace elements such as tyramine and phyenylethylamine. We find this enzyme subtype mainly in the brain, the platelets and the lymphocytes. Therefore, the effect of combining MAO-A and MAO-B may have a robust antidepressant effect because they not only increase serotonin and noradrenaline, but also dopamine.

Both MAO-A and MAO-B have another role in the body; they control levels of *tyramine*, a chemical that can cause high blood pressure and headaches in sufficiently high levels. When an MAOI medicine inhibits MAO enzyme activity, it can cause higher levels of tyramine, which in turn causes high blood pressure if the patient has a diet rich in tyramine. The body normally has a huge capacity for processing tyramine, and the average person can handle roughly 400 mg of ingested tyramine before there is elevation in blood pressure. A high-tyramine diet is unlikely to contain more than 40 mg of tyramine. However, when a person takes MAOIs, it may take as little as 10 mg of dietary tyramine to increase blood pressure (Stahl, 2013). At times, a high spike in tyramine can lead to a sudden jump in blood pressure, called a *hypertensive crisis*, which can lead to stroke or even death.

The most significant risk associated with the use of MAOIs is the potential for interactions with over-the-counter and prescription medicines, illicit drugs or medications, and some herbal medicines such as St John's wort (*Hypericum perforatum*). For this reason, many users carry an MAOI card, which lets emergency medical personnel know what medicines to avoid. For example, if you are prescribing or administering adrenaline to someone on MAOIs, then there should be a reduction of the adrenaline by at least 75 per cent, as well as extending the duration for administration. Also, be aware that MAOI medications interact with other medicines or certain foods, and this can be particularly dangerous (this will be dealt with in other sections). Examples of foods and drinks with potentially high levels of tyramine include fermented substances, such as Chianti and other aged wines, and aged cheeses. Liver is also a well-known source of tyramine, and some meat extracts and yeast extracts, such as Bovril, Marmite and Vegemite, contain extremely high levels of tyramine and should be avoided with these medications.

One method of reducing the risk that tyramine poses is to use reversible inhibition of monoamines-A (RIMAs), a subclass of MAOIs that selectively and reversibly inhibit MAO-A. RIMAs are relatively new in comparison with MAOIs, but they have had much less impact on clinical practice than SSRIs despite their favourable safety profile. RIMA medicines include meclobomide, brofaromine, metralindole, minaprine and pirlindole.

MAOI medicines tend to bind to the enzyme tenaciously and irreversibly for the lifetime of the enzyme (i.e. 14–28 days), thus stopping the enzyme from ever functioning, and enzyme activity only returns after the synthesis of a new enzyme. RIMAs, on the other hand, do not bind to the enzyme for the duration of its life and the binding is reversible. This reversibility allows the reuse of the enzyme to destroy noradrenaline, the offending neurotransmitter that causes a hypertensive crisis. Before reading the next section on the safety profile of these medicines, try Activity 6.2.

Activity 6.2   Evidence-based practice and research

Consult a textbook or research on the internet the different types of foods that a patient should avoid eating while on MAOI therapy.

An outline answer is provided at the end of the chapter.

It is important not to combine MAOIs with other psychoactive substances, antidepressants, painkillers or stimulants, either legal or illegal. Certain combinations can cause lethal reactions, and common examples include SSRIs, TCAs, meperidine, tramadol and dextromethorphan.

Common side effects of MAOIs

As mentioned earlier, MAOIs interact with foods that contain tyramine, and eating these foods can cause a hypertensive crisis. Take emergency action if a patient on MAOIs reports or exhibits any of the following symptoms: severe chest pain, severe headache, stiff or sore neck, enlarged pupils, fast or slow heartbeat, increased sensitivity to light, increased sweating (possibly with fever or cold, clammy skin), or nausea and vomiting.

Other common side effects of MAOIs are blurry vision, urinary retention, sexual dysfunction, mild dizziness or light-headedness, especially when getting up from a lying or sitting position, drowsiness, mild headache, appetite increase followed by weight gain, increased sweating, muscle twitching during sleep, restlessness, shakiness or trembling, tiredness and weakness, or trouble sleeping. Other side effects that are less common with MAOIs are chills, constipation, appetite decrease and dryness of mouth.

Selective serotonin reuptake inhibitors

Currently, SSRIs are perhaps the most widely used antidepressants, and their clinical use extends far beyond the treatment of major depression. Their wide usage is partly due to their favourable safety profile, and they are at least as effective as the older TCAs. Like TCAs, it was initially thought that SSRIs exert their function by increasing the concentration of monoamines in the synaptic cleft by inhibiting their reuptake, but this mode of action may be too simplistic.

According to the monoamine hypothesis of depression, there is a deficiency of serotonin (5HT) and receptor upregulation of postsynaptic receptors at the axonal end of the neuron. Recent revisions of the hypothesis now involve the role of serotonin autoreceptors. The serotonin deficiency we see at the presynaptic axonal end of the serotonin neuron is also present at the somatodendritic **autoreceptors** ($5HT_1$). When we administer an SSRI, it immediately blocks the serotonin reuptake pump, causing serotonin to increase initially only in the somatodendric (presynaptic) area of the neuron. Increasing serotonin in the somatodendritic area desensitises or downregulates $5HT_1$ autoreceptors, triggering the release and flow of serotonin into the axon terminal end of the neuron and the synapse (Stahl, 2013). In turn, the increase in serotonin in the synapse results in a therapeutic effect.

Although all current SSRIs share the common property of inhibiting the reuptake of serotonin, individual patients may react very differently to one SSRI versus another. Some patients may experience a therapeutic effect from one SSRI and not another, or they may tolerate one SSRI and not another. This is because each SSRI has a varying degree of selectivity for the other monoamine transporters, with pure SSRIs having only weak affinity for the noradrenaline and dopamine transporters (see Table 6.4).

In addition to blocking the serotonin and – to an extent – noradrenaline and dopamine reuptake pumps, SSRIs have a secondary pharmacological action. Indeed, no two SSRIs have identical secondary pharmacological actions, which might include serotonin $5HT_{2c}$ antagonism, muscarinic cholinergic antagonism, and sigma$_1$ receptor actions. It is plausible that the secondary binding profile of SSRIs can account for differences in efficacy and tolerability in different patients. Serotonin actions at serotonin $5HT_{2c}$ receptors inhibit the release of both dopamine and noradrenaline. However, we know that medicines which block $5HT_{2c}$ receptors, such as fluoxetine, have the opposite effect, disinhibiting the release of dopamine and noradrenaline into the synapse. This may explain why many patients, even from the first dose, detect an energising and fatigue-reducing effect of fluoxetine that is accompanied by an improvement in concentration and attention. A disadvantage of $5HT_{2c}$ antagonism is that its energising effect can be a troublesome side effect, particularly for those who have agitation or insomnia. Some possible daily dosages of SSRIs are shown in Table 6.5.

Table 6.4 SSRIs, showing the types of neurotransmitters they act on (the more plus signs, the greater the action)

Generic name	Noradrenaline	Serotonin	Monoamine oxidase	Dopamine
Fluoxetine	0	+++++	0	0
Paroxetine	+	+++++	0	0
Sertraline	0	+++++	0	+
Fluvoxamine	0	+++++	0	0
Citalopram	0	+++++	0	0
Escitalopram	0	+++++	0	0

Table 6.5 A selection of SSRIs and possible daily dosages

Generic name	Recommended daily dose
Citalopram	10–60 mg
Escitolapram	5–20 mg
Fluoxetine	20–80 mg
Paroxetine	20–50 mg
Fluvoxamine	50–300 mg
Sertraline	50–200 mg

Common side effects of SSRIs

This section discusses the general side effects of SSRIs. It is important to note that most side effects are present and subside during the first four weeks of treatment, at a time when the body is adapting to the new medicine. The only exception to this is the occurrence of sexual side effects that persist for longer than two weeks. It is also during the first four weeks that the medicine begins to reach its full potential in terms of efficacy. In general, most SSRIs can cause one or more of the following symptoms: anhedonia, apathy, nausea and vomiting, drowsiness or headache, extremely vivid or strange dreams, dizziness, fatigue, pupil dilation (mydriasis), urinary retention, weight loss/gain, increased risk of bone fractures and injuries, increased feelings of depression and anxiety (which may sometimes provoke panic attacks), tremors (and other symptoms of Parkinsonism in vulnerable elderly patients), autonomic dysfunction, including **orthostatic hypotension**, increased or reduced sweating, akathisia, renal impairment, suicidal ideation (thoughts of suicide), photosensitivity and changes in sexual behaviour.

Sexual side effects

SSRIs can cause various forms of sexual dysfunction, such as the inability to achieve an orgasm, erectile dysfunction, and diminished sexual appetite. Recent evidence suggests that such side effects occur in 17–41 per cent of patients (Landen et al., 2005). Side effects of these antidepressants are due to the stimulation of postsynaptic 5-HT$_2$ and 5-HT$_3$ receptors. The stimulation of these serotonin receptor subtypes leads to a decrease in dopamine and noradrenaline release from the substantia nigra, leading to sexual dysfunction. The incidence of sexual dysfunction, particularly in men, appears to be much lower with medicines whose primary mechanism of action involves adrenaline or dopamine systems. There is accumulating evidence suggesting that sexual dysfunction tends to persist after SSRI discontinuation, a condition known as post-SSRI sexual dysfunction (PSSD), but its prevalence is unknown. Though there is no definitive treatment, low-power laser irradiation and phototherapy have shown some promising results (Bala et al., 2018).

SSRI discontinuation syndrome

Case study: Megan

Megan is 43 years old and suffers from depression. She has been taking 60 mg of paroxetine per day for eight weeks. Because she felt much better, she asked her doctor to be on a lower dose and the doctor tapered off the dose in 20 mg decrements. Within a couple of days of dose reduction, she started to experience severe flu-like symptoms: headache, diarrhoea, nausea, vomiting, chills, dizziness, fatigue and insomnia, agitation, impaired concentration, vivid dreams, depersonalisation, irritability, and suicidal thoughts.

SSRI discontinuation syndrome is a condition that can occur following dosage reduction, discontinuation or interruption of mainly SSRI or SNRI antidepressants. The condition typically starts from the time of reduction in dosage or complete discontinuation, depending on the half-life of the medicine and the patient's metabolism. In the case study above, Megan shows symptoms of SSRI discontinuation syndrome. Currently, there is no universally acceptable definition of SSRI discontinuation syndrome, but Schatzberg et al. (1997) have noted that:

SSRI discontinuation symptoms … may emerge when an SSRI is abruptly discontinued, when doses are missed, and less frequently, during dosage reduction. In addition, the symptoms are not attributable to any other cause and can be reversed when the original agent is reinstituted, or one that is pharmacologically similar is substituted … Physical symptoms include problems with balance, gastrointestinal and flu-like symptoms, and sensory and sleep disturbances. Psychological symptoms include anxiety and/or agitation, crying spells, irritability, and aggressiveness.

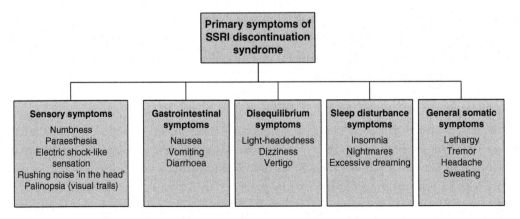

Figure 6.3 Key symptoms of SSRI discontinuation syndrome, but many other symptoms are reported in different combinations

Most antidepressant discontinuation reactions are of short duration, resolving spontaneously between one day and three weeks after onset, but in a minority of cases they can be severe, last several weeks and cause significant morbidity. The three common features that facilitate diagnosis of the condition are: (1) abrupt onset within days of stopping the antidepressant; (2) a short duration when untreated; and (3) rapid resolution of symptoms if we reinstate the antidepressant. There may be as many as 50 different symptoms of the syndrome (some are listed in Figure 6.3). The precise nature of SSRI discontinuation syndrome is uncertain, but suggestions include electrophysiological changes in the brain and the body, as well as dopamine dependency or an overexcited immune system. SSRI discontinuation syndrome has a potential for misdiagnosis, as either a physical or a mental health disorder, leading to the offer of inappropriate management for the 'incorrect' diagnosis. The condition may be mistaken for a relapse or recurrence of the underlying depression for which the antidepressant was originally prescribed, so it is important for you to be familiar with the symptoms of this condition and its presentation to avoid misdiagnosis. SSRIs with a short half-life, such as paroxetine in the above case study of Megan, are more likely to cause discontinuation syndrome. Those SSRIs with a long half-life, such as fluoxetine, are associated less with the syndrome. Also, because of its long half-life, fluoxetine is used in the treatment of the discontinuation syndrome by either prescribing and administering a single 20 mg dose or by starting the patient on a low dose and then slowly **titrating** (Stahl, 2013).

Serotonin syndrome

Case study: Jane

Jane is a 54-year-old woman with a history of depression who was on a high dose of fluoxetine. Because she was still experiencing acute symptoms of depression after eight weeks of treatment, the doctor decided to prescribe venlafaxine in addition to fluoxetine. Within 24 hours of starting venlafaxine, Jane became confused and agitated, with periods of unresponsiveness. Her vital signs were a temperature of 38.5°C and a pulse of 115 bpm. She also complained of nausea and abdominal pain. A neurological examination revealed **myoclonus** in all limbs with any stimulation. The venlafaxine was discontinued and Jane was given intravenous fluids to decrease the risk of renal failure. She was also administered 1 mg of lorazepam intravenously every four hours, resulting in decrease in tachycardia, hypertonicity, and clonus.

Serotonin syndrome is a potentially life-threatening adverse reaction that may occur following therapeutic use of antidepressants. It is not an idiosyncratic medicine reaction, but is predictable if there is an excess of serotonin in the central nervous system, which will in turn excessively stimulate the $5HT_2$ receptors. Numerous medicines and medicine combinations produce serotonin syndrome. Most types of antidepressants, serotonin-releasing agents such as amphetamines, opioid analgesics and SSRIs, as in the above case of Jane, can cause the condition.

Serotonin syndrome or toxicity starts within hours of ingesting medicines, such as SSRIs, that work on the serotonin neurotransmitter. In the above case study, Jane's symptoms started within 24 hours. The patient may experience hyperthermia and tachycardia. In addition, the patient may experience an alteration in mental state such as agitation and confusion. In severe serotonin toxicity, there is a rapid rise in temperature and muscle rigidity (see Figure 6.4). Other effects can include coma, seizures and cardiac toxicity, and – as you can see from the above case study – Jane experienced most of the key symptoms of the condition.

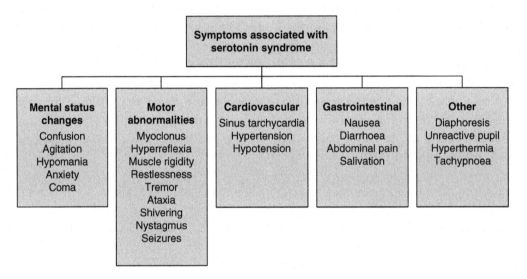

Figure 6.4   Common symptoms of serotonin syndrome

Serotonin syndrome can easily be mistaken for other conditions such as alcohol or drug withdrawal syndrome, non-convulsive seizures, and encephalitis. In particular, the classic clinical features of serotonin toxicity are like those of neuroleptic malignant syndrome (NMS) (see Chapter 12), and include neuromuscular excitation such as **hyperreflexia**, myoclonus and rigidity. However, patients with NMS are usually **akinetic** with rigidity, have decreased levels of consciousness, and are more likely to have mutism rather than the rambling speech that is associated more with serotonin toxicity. More importantly, the onset of NMS is slow, developing over days in contrast to hours, as in the case of serotonin syndrome.

Because the symptoms of serotonin syndrome overlap with those of other conditions, a thorough history of current and recent medication use is important, as is ruling out the use of illicit drugs and dietary supplements. In the diagnosis of serotonin syndrome, we need to consider pupil size and reactivity, skin colour, the presence of **diaphoresis**, dryness of the oral mucosa, and the presence or absence of bowel sounds.

Table 6.6 Signs and symptoms of serotonin syndrome

Seriousness	Autonomic signs	Neurological signs	Mental status	Other
Mild	• Afebrile or low-grade fever • Tachycardia • Mydriasis • Diaphoresis or shivering	• Intermittent tremor • Akathisia • Myoclonus • Mild hyperreflexia	• Restlessness • Anxiety	
Moderate	• Increased tachycardia • Fever (up to 41°C) • Diarrhoea with hyperactive bowel sounds • Diaphoresis with normal skin colour	• Hyperreflexia • Inducible clonus • Ocular clonus (slow, continuous lateral eye movements) • Myoclonus	• Easily startled • Increased confusion • Agitation and hypervigilance	• Rhabdomyolysis • Metabolic acidosis • Renal failure • Disseminated intravascular coagulopathy (secondary to hyperthermia)
Severe	• Temperature often more than 41°C (secondary to increased tone)	• Increased muscle tone • (lower limb > upper) • Spontaneous clonus • Substantial myoclonus or hyperreflexia	• Delirium • Coma	• As above

In its mild to moderate presentation, serotonin syndrome usually resolves in one to three days after stopping the offending medicine. By contrast, severe serotonin toxicity is a medical emergency, and the presence of severe hyperthermia and the breakdown of muscle fibres (rhabdomyolysis) may complicate the condition, therefore requiring intensive care support (see Chapter 11). It is likely that severe cases are due to medicine interactions, particularly MAOIs interacting with other antidepressants or with serotonin releasers such as amphetamines. Prompt recognition of toxicity and discontinuation of offending medications are most important as the mortality of severe serotonin syndrome is estimated to range from 2 to 12 per cent. Table 6.6 shows the different types of serotonin syndromes and their characteristics.

Suicidality in children and adolescents

Major depression among the young worldwide is a problem, and diagnoses have increased substantially, with prevalent rates of 2.6 per cent worldwide (Polanczyk et al., 2015). However, the treatment of adolescents and children with antidepressants has evoked lively debates about their safety in this population. There is a black box warning against their use in children and adolescents because of their purported tendency to induce suicidal ideation and behaviour. There is enough evidence that SSRIs can increase the risk of suicidality in children and adolescents, according to several meta-analytic reviews (Dubicka et al., 2006; Hammad et al., 2006; Sparks and Duncan, 2013). In support of this, in 2004, the US Food and Drug Administration (FDA) pooled studies and found a statistically significant increase of up to an 80 per cent risk of *possible suicidal ideation and suicidal behaviour* and an increase of up to 130 per cent of agitation in children and adolescents on SSRI medication. Also, in 2004, the UK Medicines and Healthcare Products Regulatory Agency (MHRA) judged fluoxetine (Prozac) to be the only antidepressant that offers a favourable risk–benefit ratio in children with depression, although it was also associated with a slight increase in the risk of self-harm and suicidal ideation.

In general, the risk–benefit ratio of antidepressants tends to favour those in the 25–64 age group, and less so for those in the below-25 age group. This is because of the tendency of antidepressants to increase suicidality in younger adults. In this regard, National Institute for Health and Care Excellence (NICE) guidelines advise prescribing SSRIs in children only in combination with a specific psychological treatment, and only if there has been no response to psychological treatment alone for over four to six weeks. Close supervision of children and adolescents on SSRIs is necessary, especially during the early stages of treatment and following dose changes (NICE, 2015a). In the UK, fluoxetine tends to be the first-line antidepressant, followed by sertraline and citalopram as second-line treatment, for major depression in children. The use of paroxetine, venlafaxine, TCAs and St John's wort is specifically prohibited for children (NICE, 2015a).

Atypical antidepressants

In addition to the antidepressants described so far, there is a range of antidepressants that work in increasingly more complex ways, including serotonin-noradrenaline reuptake inhibitors (SNRIs), noradrenaline reuptake inhibitors (NRIs), noradrenaline dopamine reuptake inhibitors (NDRIs) and serotonin antagonist reuptake inhibitors (SARIs). Of these classes, we will cover the SNRIs in more detail because of their increasing popularity.

Serotonin-noradrenaline reuptake inhibitors

SNRIs work by inhibiting the reuptake of serotonin and noradrenaline neurotransmitters. This results in an increase in the concentration of serotonin and noradrenaline in the synaptic cleft, and therefore an increase in neurotransmission. Most SNRIs, including venlafaxine, desvenlafaxine and duloxetine, are several times more selective for serotonin over noradrenaline, while milnacipran is three times more selective for noradrenaline than serotonin. A property of SNRIs, which they share with older TCAs, is that they are effective against neuropathic pain. Further, they have action on the dopamine in the prefrontal cortex but not elsewhere in the brain. Thus, SNRIs not only boost noradrenaline and serotonin in the brain; they also boost dopamine in the prefrontal cortex. This last action may explain their purported marginal superiority over SSRIs in the treatment of major depression.

Because SNRIs were developed more recently than SSRIs, there are relatively few of them. However, SNRIs are among those antidepressants with wide usage because they have demonstrated slightly higher antidepressant efficacy than SSRIs (apparently owing to their dual mechanism) and because their side effects are slightly less severe. However, NICE guidelines assert that these compounds do not offer clinically important advantages over other antidepressants (NICE, 2015b).

Because the SNRIs and SSRIs both act similarly to elevate serotonin levels, it is not surprising that they share many of the same side effects, although to varying degrees. The most common include loss of appetite, weight and sleep. There may also be drowsiness, dizziness, fatigue, headache, mydriasis, nausea and vomiting, sexual dysfunction, and urinary retention. There are two common sexual side effects: diminished interest in sex (libido) and difficulty reaching climax (anorgasmia), which are usually somewhat milder with SNRIs in comparison with SSRIs. Nonetheless, sexual side effects account for lack of adherence to both SSRIs and SNRIs.

Treatment and management of depression

NICE guidelines advocate a stepwise approach to managing depression. They recommend offering, or referring people for, the least intrusive and most effective intervention first. Therefore, non-pharmacological interventions such as talking therapies should be the mainstay of treatment for many people with depression (NICE, 2015b). A range of psychological and psychosocial interventions for depression have been shown to relieve the symptoms of the condition, and there is growing evidence that psychosocial therapies can help people recover from depression in the longer term (NICE, 2009b). However, not everyone responds adequately to psychosocial therapies. For those who do not, the use of antidepressants may be a viable alternative, and there is long-term recognition of their long effectiveness.

The severity of depression for which antidepressants show consistent benefits is at present poorly defined, but in general the more severe the symptoms, the greater the benefit. In this respect, the recommendation of antidepressants as the first-line treatment is for depression that is moderate to severe. Out of this group, approximately 20 per cent will respond with no treatment at all, 30 per cent will respond to a placebo, and 50 per cent will respond to antidepressant drugs (NICE, 2009b).

Until recently, we used to believe that antidepressants take about two to four weeks to begin to work. This view has come under challenge as evidence from clinical trials shows that symptom improvement can start immediately, with the greatest degree of improvement occurring in the first week. A meta-analysis of 47 studies found that 35 per cent of the improvement occurrs between weeks 0 and 1, and 25 per cent between weeks 1 and 2 (Posternak and Zimmerman, 2005). It is still important to emphasise to patients that antidepressants in general can take a long time to take effect. What we now know is that antidepressant effects can be immediate in some people, and they can take up to eight weeks or more in others. A large landmark study called Sequenced Treatment Alternatives to Relieve Depression (STAR*D) enrolled 2,876 patients, followed them for up to 12 weeks, and found that the average response time to antidepressants was 5.7 weeks. However, in some cases, the average response time for patients on antidepressants can be longer (Trivedi et al., 2006).

Choice of antidepressant

No antidepressant has been consistently proved to be superior to another, but they do differ in their side effect profiles, and this can usually be the determining factor in choosing an antidepressant. In this regard, it is important to discuss antidepressant treatment options with patients, which should cover the choice of antidepressant and any possible side effects, such as insomnia, sexual side effects, discontinuation symptoms or sedation. NICE guidelines recommend that the first-line antidepressant treatment should be an SSRI (NICE, 2009b). This recommendation is made partly due to these medicines' low-risk profile and because they are just as effective as other antidepressants. However, there is an association between SSRIs and an increase in the risk of bleeding, especially in older people or those taking other medicines that have the potential to damage the gastrointestinal mucosa or interfere with clotting. These include herbal medicines such as ginkgo biloba.

If the patient has been treated with antidepressants before, find out from them whether they were effective or not. In certain cases, patients may not show improvement with one class of antidepressant, and in such cases it may be preferable to switch to a different type.

Activity 6.3   Critical thinking

Bill is a 57-year-old man who presented to his GP with depression, complaining of low mood, loss of energy and concentration, and poor appetite. He was prescribed 50 mg of amitriptyline to be taken twice per day. After six weeks, Bill has approached a nurse to say that his depression has hardly changed, and if anything he feels worse. Bill is worried about the sedation and the lack of energy he has been experiencing. He asks you for your view regarding medication.

- What would you advise Bill to do?

An outline answer is provided at the end of the chapter.

We generally prescribe antidepressants in lower doses to start with and then gradually increase the dose. Adults between the ages of 16 and 55 should receive doses within the dose recommendation range, with adults over the age of 55 receiving lower doses.

The treatment of depression can be roughly divided into three phases: acute, continuation and maintenance treatment. Acute treatment will usually begin with the first dose and extends until the patient no longer has symptoms, and this may take up to eight weeks. The next phase is the continuation phase, during which treatment is maintained to avoid a relapse of symptoms, and this can last up to six months beyond the acute phase. Available evidence suggests that the antidepressant maintenance dose during this continuation phase should be the same as that used during the acute stages of the illness. Therefore, advise the patient to remain on the same dose for maximum effect.

In first-episode depression, it is possible to gradually reduce the dose at the end of the acute phase. Inform the patient that gradual withdrawal of antidepressants is very important to prevent discontinuation syndrome (see page 187). After the withdrawal of antidepressants, advise the patient to be alert for any signs of relapse, such as poor sleep, tiredness or poor appetite. In the event of these symptoms recurring, advise the patient to contact a member of the healthcare team.

Available evidence suggests that those people whose depression occurred before the age of 18 and who have a family history of mood disorders are likely to have a recurrence of the illness. In such cases, be alert to the possibility of recommending lifelong treatment to the patient to avoid that relapse. If these risk factors are absent, it is possible to discontinue antidepressants gradually. If a patient suffers three or more depressive episodes, lifelong medication treatment is recommended (NICE, 2009b).

Management of side effects

Chapter 12 discusses the management of common side effects. However, the nurse may notice that in people with depression, their feelings of hopelessness and pessimism are pervasive. When they encounter troubling side effects, they are likely to discontinue taking medication, particularly where these side effects occur long before the patient enjoys the positive therapeutic effect of the medication. It is therefore important to know how to manage common side effects. It is also important to know what to do in the case of a patient taking an overdose of antidepressants.

Overdose

When comparing with traditional antidepressants such as TCAs, SSRIs appear to be safer in overdose. Case studies of deaths per number of prescriptions support this relative safety. However, case reports of SSRI poisoning indicate that severe toxicity can occur, and deaths have been reported following massive single ingestions. In comparison to TCAs, this is uncommon because SSRIs have a wide therapeutic index, and therefore most patients will have mild or no symptoms following moderate overdoses. The most reported severe effect following SSRI overdose is *serotonin syndrome* (see page 187). Treatment for SSRI overdose is mainly based on symptomatic and supportive care. The patient may require medical care for agitation and maintenance of the airways, as well as treatment for serotonin syndrome. Electrocardiogram (ECG) monitoring is usually necessary to detect any cardiac abnormalities. With respect to TCAs, the initial treatment of an acute overdose includes gastric decontamination of the patient by performing *gastric lavage* using activated charcoal. Furthermore, it may be necessary to give the patient respiratory assistance, as well as administering intravenous sodium bicarbonate as an antidote to counter the effects of metabolic acidosis that can arise as a result of the overdose.

Common treatment errors to avoid

Prescribing SSRIs such as fluoxetine for patients with depression showing symptoms such as restlessness and agitation might worsen the symptoms. By contrast, it may be more appropriate to prescribe TCAs for agitated depression because of their sedative properties. Further, many SSRIs have a long half-life and have energising effects. Therefore, it is appropriate to give a single dose in the morning to reduce the risk of insomnia. By contrast, many TCAs are sedating, and we can give them at night as a single dose to aid sleeping and avoid daytime drowsiness. Many patients with depression are prone to non-adherence to medication, and therefore it is important to put in place strategies to improve adherence for those at risk. Be particularly alert for those patients using illicit substances as the use of such substances, particularly alcohol, is a common reason why antidepressants lose their efficacy. Antidepressants should be allowed enough time to work, and a patient can be on the same dose for up to eight weeks before review. Avoid abrupt or rapid withdrawal of antidepressants as this could result in the patient suffering from discontinuation syndrome. TCAs should be avoided in the elderly or those with a history of heart problems as they are cardiotoxic. The elderly are particularly vulnerable to developing heart conditions due to their use.

What the patient needs to know

- Tell the patient that although psychological symptoms of depression may take up to four weeks to begin to improve, physical symptoms may start improving soon after the commencement of treatment.
- Highlight to the patient subtle indicators of improvement if they are present during the early stages, such as being more relaxed, sleeping better, and appetite improvement. This should help the patient to feel positive.
- Tell the patient that they may experience side effects, and that these can best be managed by dose adjustment or by switching to another antidepressant.
- Advise the patient not to drink alcohol while on antidepressants as alcohol can inhibit their effects.
- Advise the patient that antidepressants are not addictive but should not be withdrawn abruptly as this leads to discontinuation syndrome.
- Advise the patient to take up exercise and refrain from taking stimulants such as alcohol or caffeine. These substances will impair sleep, and this leads to prolonged or poor recovery from depression.
- Patients on MAOIs should be given a list of foods rich in tyramine that they should avoid.

Chapter summary

The main symptoms of depression are loss of appetite, poor sleep and concentration, low mood, lack of energy, and suicidal feelings. Most types of depression subside without pharmacological treatment, but in many cases antidepressants are required.

Most antidepressants work by increasing the level of monoamine neurotransmitters in the synapse. TCAs achieve this by stopping the absorption of these neurotransmitters back in the presynaptic neuron. MAOIs achieve the same by inhibiting the enzyme that destroys these neurotransmitters, thereby increasing their concentration in the synapse. SSRIs are the first-line treatment because of their good safety profile, but other antidepressants can be used. All antidepressants are equally effective but differ in their side effect profiles. Therefore, the choice of antidepressants should consider safety and side effects. Antidepressants should never be stopped abruptly or discontinued too quickly for fear of discontinuation syndrome. MAOIs are restricted in their use because of their high-risk profile and because foods rich in tyramine should be avoided.

Activities: brief outline answers

Activity 6.1 Critical thinking (page 174)

In the case of depression, they are excitatory, therefore causing symptoms of depression.

Activity 6.2 Evidence-based practice and research (page 183)

Examples of types of food to avoid include banana peels, bean curd, broad (fava) bean pods, cheese, fish, ginseng, protein extracts, meat (non-fresh and liver), sausage, bologna, pepperoni, salami, sauerkraut, shrimp paste, soups and yeast.

Activity 6.3 Critical thinking (page 192)

It is very likely that Bill's lack of energy may have been exacerbated by the current medicine he is taking, amitriptyline. One of the side effects of this medicine is sedation, particularly if it is taken during the day, as in Bill's case. One option is for Bill to take a single dose of 100 mg at night-time, or you should inform Bill of an SSRI or SNRI as an alternative option. These medicines are unlikely to cause sedation, but you should warn Bill of the possibility of poor sleep, sexual dysfunction or serotonin syndrome.

Further reading

Preston, J.D., O'Neal, J.H. and Talaga, M.C. (2017) *A Handbook of Clinical Psychopharmacology*, 8th edition. Oakland, CA: New Harbinger.

This is a clearly written book that is particularly useful for those from a non-medical background. It explains non-pharmacological mental healthcare well.

Stahl, S.M. (2013) *Stahl's Essential Psychopharmacology: The Prescriber's Guide,* 4th edition. Cambridge: Cambridge University Press.

This is a comprehensive guide to psychopharmacology that is clearly written and has good illustrations.

Taylor, D.M., Barnes, T.R.E. and Young, A.H. (2018) *The Maudsley Prescribing Guidelines in Psychiatry,* 13th edition. London: Informa Healthcare.

This is a very useful, easy-to-understand, evidence-based prescribing and general medicines management manual. It is particularly useful for prescribers.

Useful websites

www.depressionalliance.org

This website provides information and support to depression sufferers.

www.mind.org.uk/help/diagnoses_and_conditions/depression

This website provides information and support to depression sufferers and carers of people with depression.

www.nhs.uk/Conditions/Depression

This is an NHS website that provides information to patients, carers and professionals.

Chapter 7 Management and treatment of bipolar disorder

Chapter aims

By the end of this chapter, you should be able to:

- outline the main clinical features of bipolar disorder and the pathophysiological mechanism underpinning the illness;
- identify different types of mood stabilisers and their mechanisms of action and side effects;
- communicate important treatment options to the patient and identify the most common mistakes to avoid in the treatment of bipolar disorder;

Introduction

Case study: Elizabeth

Elizabeth is a 29-year-old married mother of two young children who presented with a history of recurrent and disabling depression. A few weeks before presentation, she became severely depressed and had difficulty moving because of a loss of energy and appetite. She felt suicidal. At the time of presentation, she was prescribed 30 mg of the antidepressant paroxetine per day. In the past, she confessed to her mood lifting very quickly to the point of elation after being on a course of antidepressants for a relatively short time. For this reason, she found it unnecessary to continue taking her paroxetine, but relapsed very quickly; hence, she was admitted to hospital. On admission to the ward, she was seen by a doctor who was keen to take a more detailed

(Continued)

(Continued)

medical history of her and her family. She revealed that she fell off a horse and sustained concussion when she was 19 years old. She described a history of mood swings since the age of 13, and during her teens she had abused alcohol and recreational drugs. She also revealed that both her father and paternal grandmother suffered from mood swings. Her paternal grandmother was hospitalised for an unspecified illness that the family refuses to talk about.

The doctor was unsure about the diagnosis of major depressive disorder given the pattern of her response to antidepressants. She was prescribed fluoxetine, but this was discontinued because it worsened her underlying mood swings. The doctor suspected that Elizabeth was suffering from bipolar disorder and placed her on 800 mg of lithium carbonate per day. Within a week, she began to improve markedly, with clearer thinking, more productive work, less depression, fewer mood swings and more energy. Within five weeks of treatment with lithium carbonate, Elizabeth felt 'terrific'. She was referred for supportive psychotherapy, which helped her to settle down and gave her more confidence and a feeling of control over her life.

Mood or affective disorders have been recognised as early as the fifth century BC. Hippocrates was the first physician to recognise that mood disorders may be due to a 'brain disorder'. Nowadays, we know that mood disorders are categorised into at least three groups: mixed states, unipolar and bipolar disorder. They usually cause significant handicaps and problems in patients' lives, and in many cases lead to disability. In most cases, mood disorders are recurrent and are characterised by many episodes. The duration of each episode varies from several weeks to several months.

Bipolar disorders are generally characterised by four types of illness episodes: manic, major depressive, hypomanic and mixed states. A patient may have a combination of any of these episodes over the course of the illness. Thus, the presentation of mood disorders can vary widely. Major depression is the most common mood disorder, and this has been discussed in Chapter 6. Here, we will focus on bipolar mania, but first we need to examine bipolar disorder in more detail.

What is bipolar disorder?

Bipolar disorder is a mood disorder condition that is characterised by alternating periods of depression and mania. We classify bipolar disorder into four basic types: bipolar I, II, III and IV. Bipolar I and II are the most common types; the lifetime prevalence for bipolar I disorder is 1 per cent and for bipolar II is 4 per cent, with suicide rates ranging from 15 to 20 per cent. These disorders tend to be common in people from a higher socio-economic and educational grouping. There is an association between bipolar disorder and an increase in the risk of suicide and physical illness such as ischaemic heart disease, diabetes, chronic obstructive pulmonary disease (COPD), pneumonia and unintentional injury. Around two-thirds of people with bipolar disorder also experience another mental health disorder, usually anxiety, substance misuse or impulse control disorders.

Pathophysiological mechanisms underlying bipolar disorder are currently uncertain, but what seems clear is that the disorder is highly heritable. At least 65 per cent of sufferers have a positive family history of bipolar disorder, with a greater prevalence of the illness in women than in men. In addition to other factors, several genes may be involved in the aetiology of the disorder. One of the most consistent genetic findings implicates the calcium channel encoder gene CACNA1C and other genes such as ANK3 and ZNF04A. Specifically, the CACNA1C gene codes for pore formation of voltage-gated L-type calcium channels (LTCCs). The LTCCs play an important role in the development of dendrites, the survival of neurons, synaptic plasticity, memory formation, learning and behaviour (Bhat et al., 2012). The genetic association of the CACNA1C gene with mental disorders appears to extend beyond bipolar disorder, with recent studies showing its association with depression and schizophrenia (Moon et al., 2018). In this regard, bipolar I disorder is strongly genetically correlated with schizophrenia, whereas bipolar II disorder is more strongly correlated with major depressive disorder (Stahl et al., 2019). In addition to genetic factors, neuroimaging studies of bipolar disorder clearly demonstrate abnormalities in neural circuits supporting emotion processing, emotion regulation and reward processing (Phillips and Swartz, 2014). Neuroimaging studies of individuals with bipolar disorder indicate predominant patterns of abnormally elevated amygdala activity in response to emotional stimuli and in reward-processing neural circuitry. Further, structural imaging studies reveal that there is an abnormal volumetric reduction (grey and white matter volume) in the cortical regions of the brain in people with bipolar disorder. In addition, inflammatory markers, particularly of the tumour necrosis factor (TNF) superfamily and inflammatory cytokines (I-Ls), may have an association with the neuroprogression of the disease (Castano-Ramirez et al., 2018). A meta-analytic study of 13 studies with a total sample of 556 bipolar disorder patients and 767 healthy controls also supports this view. The study found that compared to healthy control subjects, people with bipolar disorder have elevated inflammatory markers, such as tumour necrosis factor-α (TNF-α), the soluble tumour or necrosis factor receptor type 1 (sTNF-R1) and the soluble inlerleukin-2 receptor (sIL-2R) (Munkholm et al., 2013).

From a presentation perspective, bipolar I patients have full-blown manic episodes or mixed episodes of depression and mania. The course of the illness can be characterised by *rapid cycling*, which means that the patient can suffer at least four episodes of mood switching in one year. In practice, many patients experience switches in mood more than four times per year. In some patients, this rapid cycling manifests as rapid cycling between depressive episodes and mania. During a manic episode, the patient may experience an abnormal elevation of mood with accompanying symptoms such as inflated self-esteem, pressure of speech, flight of ideas and an increase in risk-taking behaviour (see Figure 7.1 later in the chapter). Mania rarely occurs as a primary illness by itself; therefore, the presence of manic symptoms implies a bipolar disorder even if a history of depression is not apparent in the individual. Because bipolar disorder can combine mood and psychotic symptoms, it is difficult to classify the illness as belonging to psychotic illnesses such as schizophrenia or to other mood disorders.

Differentiating bipolar depression from unipolar or major depression

One of the most important recent developments in the field of mood disorder is the discovery that many patients who appear to be suffering from a major depressive disorder are in fact suffering from a form of bipolar spectrum depression, in particular bipolar II. In the past, this has led to many bipolar patients who might have benefited from mood-stabilising and antipsychotic treatment being treated with antidepressant monotherapy, which may increase mood cycling, mixed states and the conversion of hypomania to mania. The above case study of Elizabeth is typical of someone who was treated for unipolar depression when in fact she was suffering from the depressive phase of a bipolar illness. As much as it is important to distinguish those patients suffering from bipolar spectrum disorder from those suffering from major depression, in reality patients in the depressive phase of a bipolar illness present with identical symptoms to those suffering from unipolar major depression. To be able to make the distinction, we require additional information in the form of family history and treatment response. Familial history of bipolar disorder is a strong indicator that the patient has a bipolar spectrum illness, even though the symptoms presented are those of unipolar major depression. Patterns of past symptoms can also provide important clues, and include previous episodes of hypomania, early age of onset, high frequency of depressive symptoms, high proportion of time unwell, and acute abatement or onset of symptoms.

Current symptom presentation can also provide important clues, such as increased time sleeping, overeating, concurrent anxiety and psychomotor retardation. Also, changeable mood, psychotic symptoms and suicidal thoughts can suggest that someone is suffering from bipolar spectrum depression instead of unipolar depression. Therefore, when interacting with the patient, it is important to look out for these symptoms, particularly in those whose depression is difficult to treat.

For example, if a patient has tried several antidepressants that were not effective, this could be an indication that they are suffering from bipolar spectrum depression. Previous responses to antidepressants, such as insomnia, agitation and anxiety, can also be useful in distinguishing bipolar spectrum depression. Again, it is important to be watchful of the patient's response to medication as this can be a useful indicator as to whether a mood stabiliser is required or not.

Although these points cannot separate major depression and bipolar spectrum depression with absolute certainty, the point to emphasise here is to exercise vigilance to the possibility that what looks like unipolar depression might in fact be bipolar spectrum depression if we investigate it more carefully.

As mentioned, bipolar disorder consists of both depressive and manic symptoms. Depressive symptoms have been outlined in Chapter 6; therefore, this chapter discusses manic symptoms only before briefly reviewing common physical disorders and medicines that may cause mania. The final sections of the chapter discuss common treatment errors to avoide and what the patient needs to know. Now we turn to bipolar mania.

What is bipolar mania?

Case study: Gale

Gale is an 18-year-old A-level student who was admitted to hospital following a summer trip to the US after her final exams. During her last week on holiday, she was overly talkative, irritable and in an expansive mood. When she arrived back in the UK, her parents were very concerned about her behaviour, which was out of character. They contacted her GP, who in turn referred Gale to hospital for admission as she was threatening violence. On admission to the ward, she was overly cheerful, overactive, irritable, and overfamiliar with staff. She talked of being a 'star' and going to Hollywood. She changed clothes very frequently. The night staff reported that she did not sleep at all on her first night. After only two days on the ward, other patients were complaining about her interfering and overbearing manner. She was prescribed haloperidol and lithium carbonate on a regular basis and lorazepam when necessary. After ten days of treatment, her condition improved. She was able to reveal that before she became ill, she was under a great deal of pressure to do well in her A levels as she had been offered a conditional place at the University of Cambridge. She also revealed that her maternal grandmother suffered from bipolar disorder.

Bipolar mania is a state of mind and mood whose common characteristics are excessive energy along with other symptoms, such as extravagant behaviour, rapid speech, reckless spending and – in some instances – psychotic symptoms, as in the above case study of Gale. The person with bipolar mania experiences a sustained and abnormal elevation, expansive or irritable mood throughout the episode. The exaggeration in mood elevation is beyond what most people would experience, and it may not have any relationship to anything going on in the person's life. Gale's behaviour during the early stages of hospital admission is a typical example of how someone with bipolar mania might symptomatically present.

We can describe the manic phase of a bipolar spectrum disorder as a distinct period of abnormally and persistent elevated expansive or irritable mood lasting at least a week. The description of manic episodes can be mild, moderate or severe (see Figure 7.2). If the manic condition is severe, psychotic symptoms may be present – but not always (see Figure 7.1).

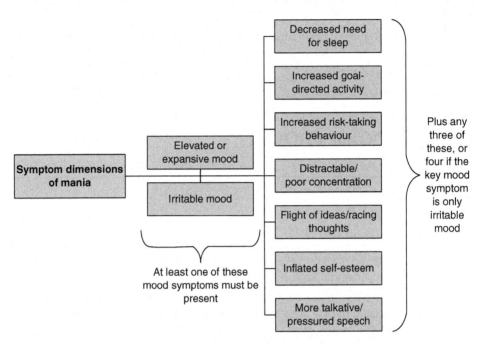

Figure 7.1 Key symptoms of mania according to the DSM-5 – the patient must show at least elevated or irritable mood symptoms in addition to at least three symptoms in the second cluster

Stage 1 Corresponds to hypomania	Stage 2 Frank mania	Stage 3 Shown by some patients with severe mania
1. Increased psychomotor activity 2. Emotional lability 3. Euphoria or grandiosity 4. Coherent but tangential thinking	1. Increased psychomotor activity 2. Heightened emotional lability 3. Hostility and anger 4. Assaultative or explosive anger 5. Flight of ideas, cognitive disorganisation 6. Possible grandiose or paranoid delusions	1. Incoherent thought process 2. Ideas of reference, disorientation, delirium 3. Frenzied psychomotor activity 4. Florid psychosis

Figure 7.2 The course of mania, which can be acute or gradual (according to Carlson and Goodwin, 1973)

For the diagnosis of mania, elevated/expansive or irritable mood must be present. In addition to these two symptoms, at least three of the following should be present: inflated self-esteem, grandiosity, pressure of speech, decreased need for sleep, increased risk-taking behaviour, increased goal-directed activity, and distractibility (see Figure 7.1).

Common disorders and medicines associated with mania

Many mental health disorders can simply be a secondary manifestation of an underlying physical illness and therapeutic drugs. The physical illnesses shown in Table 7.1 can present bipolar mania symptoms.

Table 7.1 Physical conditions implicated in the triggering of mania

Common physical disorders that may cause mania	
• Neurological disorders such as Huntington's disease, extrapyramidal disease and Wilson's disease (copper accumulation) • CNS infections, viral encephalitis • Cerebral trauma • Brain tumour • Cerebrovascular accidents • Temporal lobe epilepsy	• Pick's disease (chronic constrictive pericarditis) • Hyperthyroidism • Dialysis dementia • Pellagra (vitamin B_3 deficiency) • Vitamin B_{12} deficiency • Post-partum mania • Influenza • Multiple sclerosis

Medicines that can cause bipolar mania

There are numerous reports of substance-induced mood disorders dating back to the 1950s, when the association between reserpine and depression was first noticed. In addition to illicit drugs, several over-the-counter medicines are implicated in the onset of drug-induced mania. Drug-induced mania tends to occur when the person is using the drug, during intoxication or withdrawal. Table 7.2 contains a list of drugs known to cause mania.

Table 7.2 Drugs that have been implicated in causing mania

Drugs that are associated with bipolar mania	
• Procycline • Cocaine • Corticosteroids • **Hallucinogens** • Disulfiram	• Bromides • Isoniazid • Procarbazine • Opiates • Amphetamines • Cimetidine

The treatment of bipolar spectrum disorders

The risk of relapse in bipolar disorder after a first episode is particularly high in comparison with other mental health disorders. Relapse is approximately 50 per cent in the first year and greater than 70 per cent four years after a first episode. This has important implications for the long-term management of the disorder. For this reason, the treatment of bipolar disorder has at least two important goals: first, the reduction of symptoms; and second, the stabilisation of the illness through medicines and other psychosocial interventions.

Several medicines from different classes of compounds are in use for the treatment of bipolar disorder. During the depressive stage, antidepressants and mood stabilisers are usually the treatments of choice. However, treatment with antidepressants without concomitant use of mood stabilisers is associated with the development of bipolar mania and rapid cycling, so it is not recommended. National Institute for Health and Care Excellence (NICE) guidelines suggest that if a person develops mania or hypomania while taking an antidepressant monotherapy, then the patient should stop taking the antidepressant (NICE, 2014). If a person develops moderate or severe bipolar depression and is not taking a medicine to treat the disorder, fluoxetine in combination with olanzapine, or quetiapine on its own, are the treatments of choice, depending on the person's preference and previous response to treatment (for details of antidepressant and antipsychotic therapies, see Chapters 6 and 8, respectively).

In the manic phase, antipsychotics and mood stabilisers are the treatments of choice. The antipsychotics with proven efficacy in treating bipolar mania are olanzapine, risperidone, quetiapine, aripiprazole and asenapine. In exceptional cases, it is possible to prescribe antipsychotics as monotherapy, but it is their combination with mood stabilisers that shows the greatest clinical effect. With respect to children and adolescents with bipolar mania aged 13 years or older, the treatment of choice is usually aripiprazole (NICE, 2013). The following section discusses the use of mood stabilisers in the treatment of bipolar spectrum disorders.

Mood stabilisers

Mood stabilisers are the main medicines in use for the long-term management of bipolar disorder. Their role is to maintain a person's mood at a reasonable level and to help prevent future episodes of low mood (depression) or high mood (mania). There are several types of mood stabilisers, but the oldest medicine is lithium.

Lithium

Lithium is a naturally occurring metal that is water-soluble; it does not bind to plasma proteins and is able to cross the blood–brain barrier. It has been in use for the treatment of bipolar disorder since the nineteenth century, but interest in its use waned for a time before being revived in Australia after the Second World War. Even so, the rest of the world was slow to adopt this treatment, mainly because of deaths that resulted from its use. In the US, it was not until 1970 that lithium was licensed for the treatment of mania, but only under strict conditions of blood lithium monitoring to reduce the risk of lithium toxicity.

Although lithium has been in use for the treatment of bipolar disorder for a long time, it has a complex mode of action that is proving difficult to understand. One popular concept is that it works by altering sodium transport across cell membranes of both nerve and muscle cells.

Another theory is that lithium has multiple effects on neurotransmitter systems in the brain, including decreasing the release of noradrenaline and dopamine from nerve terminals and transiently increasing the release of serotonin, which may account for its mood-stabilising properties (Meyer, 2011). It also regulates responses of the cholinergic system at the neurochemical, electrophysiological and behavioural levels. Lithium also enhances the inhibitory effects of gamma-aminobutyric acid (GABA) in the brain and reduces the excitatory effects of glutamate neurotransmission.

Whatever the mode of action of lithium, its effectiveness in people suffering from certain mood disorders is beyond doubt. It is particularly effective in the treatment and prevention of manic episodes. A systematic review and meta-analysis of seven trials (1,580 participants) concluded that lithium is more effective than a placebo in preventing overall mood episodes (Severus et al., 2014). This is supported by an earlier head-to-head comparison of lithium and valproate. The study found that lithium alone, or lithium plus valproate, is more likely to prevent relapse than valproate monotherapy. Further, prophylactic treatment with lithium monotherapy may be as efficacious as lithium plus valproate (Geddes et al., 2010). Therefore, lithium remains a first-line option for the treatment and prophylaxis of bipolar mania. However, lithium is less effective in the treatment of bipolar depression and rapid cycling bipolar disorder (Malhi et al., 2012b). Despite its modest success in the treatment of bipolar depression, it is well established in the prevention of suicide and self-harm, and may have neuroprotective and immunomodulatory properties (Rybakowski, 2018).

Before a patient starts on lithium, it is important to explain to them that certain tests need to be carried out on thyroid and liver function. A very important test to carry out before prescribing lithium is renal function. We assess renal function by measuring the levels of urea and electrolytes along with the creatinine clearance rate from the kidneys. Creatinine is a product of muscle protein metabolism that we find in the blood circulation and is distributed in total body water. The rate at which the kidneys filter creatinine is proportional to its efficiency. If the creatinine filtration rate is low, then the kidneys are likely to excrete lithium slowly, resulting in lithium building up in the blood plasma, which causes toxicity. Lithium causes electrocardiogram (ECG) changes, with the most frequently reported changes being unspecific ST-T changes and wave flattening. The problem becomes more acute with advancing age. For this reason, it is important to carry out an ECG before prescribing lithium to patients above 50 years of age or those with a predisposition to developing a cardiac condition.

Clinically, we administer lithium in salt form as lithium carbonate, lithium sulphate, lithium chloride or lithium citrate. These lithium formulations differ in their absorption rate. An example of this is that the chloride and sulphate preparations reach peak plasma concentrations within one hour after oral administration, in comparison to four hours for the carbonate preparation. This is because lithium carbonate is the least water-soluble of the various lithium salts, and as such its absorption in the upper gastrointestinal tract is slower than for the other preparations. However, all lithium salts have similar pharmacokinetic properties with respect to volume of distribution, bioavailability and half-life.

Lithium is completely absorbed in the gastrointestinal tract without undergoing first-pass metabolism. Peak plasma levels of the medicine occur one to two hours after administration of an immediate-release preparation, but if we administer a slow-release preparation the peak time can increase to up to 12 hours. If the person is on a high dose of lithium, it is preferable to use a slow-release preparation to overcome the problems that an immediate-release preparation presents. In the brain, reaching peak lithium concentrations can take approximately 24 hours post-ingestion because of the lower permeability of lithium through the blood–brain barrier.

Therapeutic drug levels in the blood usually guide the dosing of lithium. During acute treatment, the average daily dose tends to range from 900 mg to 2,400 mg. The patient's lithium levels should be measured after one week of starting the medicine and one week after every dose change, and then weekly until the blood serum lithium levels are stable. Although there is some variability in the literature regarding target serum lithium levels, generally serum lithium levels should be within the range of 0.5–1.0 mmol/L and should not exceed 1.5 mmol/L. During the acute phases of the illness, the blood serum therapeutic levels should be 0.8–1.2 mmol/L, but the upper limit can be as high as 1.5 mmol/L in exceptional cases. This is because people in acute manic stages can have an increased tolerance to lithium (Girardi et al., 2016).

We see low toxicity at serum concentrations of 1.5–2.5 mmol/L, moderate toxicity at 2.5–3.5 mmol/L and severe symptoms at more than 3.5 mmol/L. Table 7.3 shows lithium serum levels and corresponding possible toxic symptoms.

Table 7.3 To be interpreted 12 hours after the last dose. Concentration range is indicative only and is based on patients subjected to chronic exposure to lithium. In acute ingestion of lithium, these ranges may not apply (Baird-Gunning et al., 2017)

Plasma lithium concentrations (mmol/L)	Severity (Hansen and Amdisen classification)
Grade 1 (low toxicity): 1.5–2.5	Symptoms include nausea, vomiting, tremor, hyperreflexia, agitation, ataxia, muscle weakness
Grade 2 (moderate): 2.5–3.5	Stupor, rigidity, hypertonia, hypotension
Grade 3 (severe): greater than 3.5	Coma, convulsions, myoclonia, collapse

In general, lithium has a narrow therapeutic index, which means the safe therapeutic and toxic serum levels are very close to each other. Despite this, lithium remains a cornerstone for the treatment of bipolar disorder. During the maintenance phases of the treatment, the average daily dose of the medicine should be between 400 and 1,200 mg per day. If a person develops moderate or severe bipolar depression and is already taking lithium, check the person's plasma lithium level. If it is inadequate, the dose should be increased. If the dose is at its maximum level, then the prescriber can switch the medicine to either fluoxetine in combination with olanzapine if the person is in the depressive phase, or quetiapine on its own depending on the person's preference and previous response to treatment (see later sections). Before you read further, try Activity 7.1.

Activity 7.1   Critical thinking

A patient is prescribed 400 mg of lithium carbonate slow-release tablets. During medicines administration, the nurse notices that the slow-release tablets are out of stock, and therefore gives the patient two tablets of lithium carbonate, each of 200 mg.

• Can you explain what the risk is with such an action?

An outline answer is provided at the end of the chapter.

Side effects

Well-known side effects of lithium include gastrointestinal symptoms such as indigestion, nausea and vomiting. Other side effects include hair loss, weight gain, acne, tremor, sedation, a reduction in glomerular filtration rate (GFR), impairment of cognition, weak muscular coordination, excessive urination, abnormal increase in white blood cells, blurred vision, sexual dysfunction, and oedema. The loss of sodium through vomiting or diarrhoea can induce a compensatory effect that will result in excessive lithium retention, which in turn can cause lithium toxicity. In this case, it is important to reduce the dose of lithium. Heavy sweating can also lead to increases in blood lithium levels. Concurrent rapid increase of lithium and an antipsychotic is normally discouraged as this may lead to neurotoxicity.

Both thyroid hormone secretion and renal function can decline with long-term lithium use, and can in some cases lead to hypothyroidism and stage 3 chronic kidney disease. Interestingly, these complications are more likely to occur earlier in women than in men during lithium treatment. In addition, long-term lithium therapy can also cause hypercalcaemia (i.e. high total plasma calcium concentration).

Special considerations

When we use lithium with the elderly, it is important to ensure that the person's kidneys can cope with lithium excretion. This is done by performing a kidney function test. It is important to ensure that the person is taking adequate salt and fluids as the ability to excrete lithium decreases with age because kidney function declines as we get older. Medical illnesses such as chronic heart failure and hypertension compromise kidney clearance and are also common as people age. This can result in longer elimination time for the medicine. Even at safe therapeutic levels, older people are prone to developing cognitive impairment and damage to nervous tissue. The patient should start lithium at a relatively lower dose but be aware that side effects can also occur at a relatively low blood plasma level of the medicine. Slow-release preparations may help to minimise side effects that occur because of peak plasma levels. Before reading further, try Activity 7.2.

Activity 7.2   Evidence-based practice and research

Alone or in a group, research medicine interactions that cause an increase in blood lithium levels.

An outline answer is provided at the end of the chapter.

If possible, avoid the use of lithium in pregnant women, particularly in the first trimester. Lithium use during pregnancy has been associated with an increased risk of foetal malformation and premature birth. Its use is also associated with severe infant toxicity, although this has been known to be reversible.

We also find lithium in the milk of breastfeeding mothers, and this causes symptoms such as involuntary movements, dehydration, hypothyroidism, cyanosis, heart murmurs, and lethargy in the child. If the mother wishes to breastfeed, it is important to inform her of the risks to the infant while she is taking lithium. It is also important to monitor the lithium levels and thyroid function of the infant.

It is important to observe the patient's behaviour before and after lithium initiation and be alert to the presence of adverse side effects and lithium toxicity. Report these to the prescriber and withhold administering the dose. Common signs and symptoms of lithium toxicity are given in Table 7.4.

Table 7.4   Organs affected and manifestation of lithium toxicity (adapted from Baird-Gunning et al., 2017)

Organ system	Manifestations
Cardiovascular	Wandering atrial pacemaker, sinus bradycardia, ST-segment elevation, unmasking Brugada syndrome, prolonged QT interval, Uncommonly, life-threatening arrhythmias
Neurological	Lethargy, ataxia, confusion, agitation, neuromuscular excitability (irregular coarse tremors, fasciculations, myoclonic jerks, hyperreflexia). Severe lithium toxicity can manifest as seizures, including non-convulsive status epilepticus.
Gastrointestinal	Nausea, vomiting, diarrhoea, ileus

The nurse should monitor fluid intake and adjust salt intake if there is any loss through vomiting, heavy sweating or diarrhoea. It is important to explain to the patient that they should expect generalised discomfort, thirst and frequent urination during the first few days of treatment initiation, but this will subside within weeks. Also, inform the patient to take lithium with meals to minimise gastrointestinal disturbance. Before reading further, try Activity 7.3.

Activity 7.3   Critical thinking

Steven, a 40-year-old man who is on 1,000 mg of lithium per day, has just informed you that he will not be able to fulfil an appointment scheduled for August because he will be on holiday for two weeks in Cyprus.

- What precautions should Steven take while on holiday?

An outline answer is provided at the end of the chapter.

Management of lithium side effects

For further details on the management of psychotropic side effects, refer to Chapter 11. The management of lithium side effects is outlined below.

- *Lithium poisoning:* One of the most serious side effects of lithium use is the potential for lithium poisoning; therefore, understanding the management of lithium poisoning is important. In the event of a patient taking excess lithium medication, the first step is to consider gastric lavage if they have ingested more than 40 mg per kg of body weight of lithium within the previous hour. In addition to treating symptoms, the second step is to correct fluid and electrolyte imbalance. In this regard, you may consider using sodium chloride intravenous solution (0.9 per cent). This solution is used because the kidneys' handling of lithium is like that of sodium. Where the patient has not sustained renal failure or congestive cardiac failure, the administration of up to 3 litres per day of an isotonic solution of sodium chloride (0.9 per cent) is recommended. In exceptional situations, you can use low-dose dopamine to increase lithium excretion, but the use of forced diuresis is not usually recommended. The third step is to regulate kidney function. In this regard, haemodialysis is the treatment of choice for rapid removal of lithium from the body. Patients who may benefit from haemodialysis are those who show severe poisoning and progressive clinical deterioration, and present during the first 8–12 hours following ingestion of the medicine. Haemodialysis reduces the serum half-life of lithium to 3–6 hours. It also reduces cellular concentrations and may shorten the duration of symptoms. After haemodialysis, be watchful for a rebound increase in the serum lithium concentration because of the slow diffusion of lithium from inside the cell (intracellular) to outside of the cell (Baird-Gunning et al., 2017).

- *Kidney problems*: Unlike many medicines, lithium relies on the kidneys for elimination from the body. Therefore, any slight interference or alteration of kidney function could lead to a build-up of lithium. Increased thirst (polydipsia) and excessive passing of urine (polyurea) are common side effects. Encourage the patient to drink plenty of fluids even if they are experiencing polyurea. Polyurea is common in about 60 per cent of people on long-term treatment. If creatinine increases sharply, withdhold the medicine and carry out a creatinine tolerance test or GFR before recommencing lithium. Alternatively, reduce the dose of lithium or discontinue altogether. Some patients may experience less polydipsia if they take the dose of lithium at bedtime.

- *Neurological and cognitive problems*: These include memory impairment, lethargy, weakness, postural tremors, and headaches. Nearly 50 per cent of patients experience fine hand tremors at some stage during treatment with lithium, but the symptom remits in 90 per cent of cases. Lithium may increase extrapyramidal side effects in patients taking antipsychotics. In rare cases, it can reactivate neuroleptic malignant syndrome (NMS) (see page 244). Reduce the lithium dose or increase the interval between doses. Advise the patient to reduce caffeine and other stimulant use. In some cases, you may prescribe beta blockers to help reduce tremors. Use low doses of lithium for the elderly and those with brain trauma. In some cases, worsening of tremors, confusion, stupor, and slurred speech may be signs of lithium toxicity, and to rule this out take blood lithium levels. It is important to note that although we can use various methods such as dialysis, there is no antidote for lithium toxicity.

- *Endocrine problems*: Hypothyroidism develops in 20 per cent of patients treated with long-term lithium; this usually affects thyroid hormones, but not to a clinically significant extent in most cases. A baseline thyroid function test (TFT) should be carried out and checked every six months. If there is an elevation of thyroid-stimulating hormone (TSH), consider adding levothyroxine (T4).

- *Cardiac problems*: These are minor changes in the ECG. Carry out a baseline ECG for those with a history of cardiac problems or over the age of 50 years. Monitor the pulse periodically and avoid medicines that cause bradyarrhythmias.

- *Dermatological problems*: These include acne, hair loss, psoriasis and pruritis. Consider a change in mood stabiliser if symptoms persist. Use anti-acne formulations, although these may be of limited effect.

Anticonvulsants

Several anticonvulsants have been established as a treatment option for bipolar disorder. They may constitute an alternative to lithium for prophylactic treatment; however, not every anticonvulsant acts as a mood stabiliser. Moreover, there are clear differences in their efficacy and tolerability. One anticonvulsant in common use in the treatment of bipolar illness is sodium valproate, or valproic acid.

Valproic acid

Valproic acid, or valproate, was first made in 1882, and it was mainly used as a solvent until French scientist Pierre Eymard discovered its anticonvulsant properties in 1963. There has been an increase in the use of valproic acid in the treatment of bipolar disorder, but – as with most anticonvulsants – its mode of action is not clear. One popular theory is that valproic acid works by reducing the level of excitation of neurons. It does this by reducing the flow of sodium into the neuronal cell through sodium channels. It has also been postulated that it works by interfering with calcium channels and indirectly blocks glutamate action. A third theory is that this medicine increases the concentration of GABA by a mechanism that is yet to be uncovered.

Research evidence seems to suggest that valproic acid is effective in the treatment of bipolar disorder (Bond et al., 2010). It is effective in the treatment of mania, in mixed states or for patients with secondary or rapid cycling disorder. Oral valproic acid can lead to rapid stabilisation of manic symptoms, though there is limited evidence to support its efficacy in long-term treatment of bipolar disorder according to a Cochrane review (Cipriani et al., 2013). Valproic acid can take anything from a few days to a few months to stabilise a bipolar condition.

Before valproic acid treatment, it is important to carry out several investigations, including a full blood count, coagulation tests and a liver function test. It is normally the responsibility of the prescriber to ensure that these tests are ordered, and the nurse is responsible for coordinating these tests within the multidisciplinary team (MDT). During the first few months of treatment with valproic acid, monitor liver function tests and platelet counts regularly; again, the prescriber is responsible for ordering the tests. Reduce the number of tests to two per year once the patient's symptoms have stabilised. Like lithium, valproic acid is associated with weight gain; therefore, monitor the patient's weight closely. If the patient is already overweight, with a body mass index (BMI) above or equal to 25, carry out a pre-diabetes test (fasting blood glucose). If the test is positive, you should refer the patient for weight management or nutritional advice to a specialist, usually a dietician. If a patient on valproic acid therapy gains more than 5 per cent of their initial weight, it is important to carry out a pre-diabetes or **dyslipidaemia** test.

The usual starting dose of valproic acid in the treatment of bipolar disorder is 750 mg per day in divided doses, gradually increased until reaching therapeutic levels or until side effects become intolerable. The dose range for valproic acid is between 750 and 2,000 mg per day in a single or divided dose. The gastric intestinal tract usually absorbs valproic acid rapidly, and time to peak concentration differs according to the formulation (i.e. regular-release, delayed-release, extended-released), but can range from 2 to 17 hours. The recommended therapeutic plasma level for valproic acid is 350–800 μmol/L. It is metabolised primarily in the liver and has an average half-life of 9–19 hours in a healthy adult.

Side effects

Common side effects of valproic acid are indigestion and/or weight gain. Less common are fatigue, swelling of tissues (usually in the lower limbs), acne, dizziness, drowsiness, hair loss, headaches, nausea, sedation, and tremors. Valproic acid levels within the normal range can cause an excess of ammonia in the blood, or hyperammonaemia, which can lead to brain damage. Rarely, valproic acid can cause blood abnormality (dyscrasia), impairment of liver function, jaundice, an abnormally small number of platelets in the blood (thrombocytopenia), and prolonged coagulation times. The medicine has one of the highest potentials to induce toxicity of the mitochondria. This usually worsens mitochondria-related disorders, such as **Alpers-Huttenlocher syndrome**, ataxia neuropathy spectrum, **Leigh syndrome** and lactic acidosis. Due to these side effects, most doctors will ask for blood tests initially and then as often as once per week, before reducing to once every two months. Temporary liver enzyme increase has been reported in 20 per cent of cases during the first few months of taking this medicine. Inflammation of the liver (hepatitis), the first symptom of which is jaundice, is found in rare cases.

There have also been reports of **cognitive dysfunction**, Parkinsonian symptoms, and even reversible shrinkage (pseudoatrophy) of the brain in long-term treatment with valproic acid.

Special considerations

The use of valproic acid should be avoided in pregnant women because of the incidence of baby malformation, which can be as high as 11 per cent. The Pharmacovigilance Risk Assessment Committee of the European Medicines Agency (EMA) published advice recommending not to use valproate in pregnancy unless the woman has a form of epilepsy that is unresponsive to other anti-epileptic medicines. The committee further recommended not using valproic acid in women of childbearing potential unless they follow a comprehensive 'pregnancy prevention programme' (Wieck and Jones, 2018), and the Medicines and Healthcare Products Regulatory Agency (MHRA) endorses this recommendation (Iacobucci, 2018). Despite these recommendations, the use of valproic acid in the treatment of bipolar disorder has been increasing, especially among women of childbearing age (Macfarlane and Greenhalgh, 2018). This may be due to the very difficult clinical issue of managing the mental health needs of the mother while minimising the teratogenic risk to the developing foetus. Our understanding of the mechanism of teratogenic effects of valproic acid is currently poor, but they may possibly involve epigenetic effects or oxidative stress.

In expectant mothers taking valproic acid, the serum levels of the baby are likely to be higher than those of the mother. Furthermore, the half-life of the medicine in the infant is likely to be longer than that of the mother, presenting considerable health problems for the infant. Some of the health risks for babies associated with maternal use of valproic acid include spina bifida, atrial septal defect, cleft palate, hypospadias, polydactyly, neural tube defects, neurological dysfunction, and general developmental deficits, which can involve as many as 70 per cent of children. Infants may be at a relatively higher risk of hypoglycaemia. Non-teratogenic associations include intra-uterine growth restriction, infant hepatic toxicity and foetal distress during labour.

No clear evidence of harm has been seen in infants of breastfeeding mothers taking valproic acid, even though the half-life of the medicine is higher for the baby than the mother (Uguz and Sharma, 2016). In exceptional circumstances where valproic acid must be prescribed, you should inform parents of the possible risks involved and monitor the liver enzymes of both the mother and the infant.

Management of valproic acid overdose

Excessive amounts of valproic acid can result in tremors, stupor, respiratory depression, coma, metabolic acidosis and death. Try to establish the following details to aid your intervention: the precise time of the overdose, the amount taken, any previous medical problems, and any other medication taken. There may be a need to carry out a physical examination to provide clues as to the nature of the toxicity. If a patient has valproic acid poisoning, a physical examination normally shows the following: hyperthermia/hypothermia, tachycardia, respiratory depression, confusion, somnolence, dizziness, hallucinations, irritability and headache. With respect to the treatment of valproic acid poisoning, consider decontamination methods, including the administration of activated charcoal to asymptomatic patients who have ingested valproic acid within the preceding hour. Only healthcare professionals should carry out pre-hospital activated charcoal administration, and only if no contraindications are present. Do not delay calling for emergency support to administer activated charcoal. In patients who have ingested valproic acid and who are comatose, consider administering naloxone for pre-hospital administration in the doses used for treatment of opioid overdose, particularly if the patient has respiratory depression (Manoguerra et al., 2008). For the management of other valproic side effects, see 'Management of lithium side effects' on page 209, as well as the general management of psychotropic medication in Chapter 12.

Carbamazepine

Carbamazepine was first discovered in Switzerland by the scientist Walter Schindler and was initially used to treat **trigeminal neuralgia**. It has been available in the UK as an anticonvulsant since 1965, but its use as a mood stabiliser started in Japan in the 1970s. Unlike lithium and valproic acid, the mechanism of action of carbamazepine is well understood. It works by blocking sodium channels, therefore making neurons less excitable. Furthermore, it has been hypothesised that it also works by blocking calcium and potassium ion channels, potentiating the inhibitory effects of GABA (see Chapter 3).

Carbamazepine is effective in the treatment of manic symptoms, rapid cycling and mixed bipolar states, and it normally takes a few weeks for the medicine to take effect. Overall, it is as effective as valproic acid and lithium in the treatment of manic symptoms; however, there is some evidence to suggest that carbamazepine is more effective in the treatment of major depressive disorder.

Full blood count, as well as liver, kidney and thyroid function tests, should be done before a patient starts carbamazepine therapy. Ensure that after the initiation of treatment, a blood count is done every two to four weeks for the first two months, and reduce this to every three to six months throughout the treatment. With respect to kidney, thyroid and liver functions, repeat these tests every 6 to 12 months.

In bipolar disorder, initial doses are normally 400 mg per day, and this can increase by 200 mg per week, usually in divided doses. In acute conditions, the daily dose can be as high as 1,200 mg, and in maintenance doses it can be between 800 and 1,200 mg per day. Note that carbamazepine liquid suspension reaches a higher blood serum peak level than in the equivalent tablet form. For this reason, we normally start carbamazepine suspension formulation at a lower dose and then titrate up slowly. Controlled-release formulations can significantly reduce side effects, and carbamazepine should be slowly titrated when the patient is taking other sedating medicines or anticonvulsants. However, the downside of slow titration is that it delays therapeutic effects. The recommended plasma level for carbamazepine is 17–54 µmol/L and its estimated half-life is about 30 hours after the first dose. Peak blood concentration appears between 6 and 24 hours after ingesting a therapeutic dose; however, a large overdose will take up to 72 hours after ingestion to reach a peak level.

Side effects

It is the excessive action of the medicine on the sodium channels that causes the side effects of carbamazepine, and these side effects include sedation, dizziness, confusion, unsteadiness, headache, nausea, vomiting, diarrhoea, dry mouth, blurred vision, menstrual disturbances, weight gain and skin rash. Carbamazepine also presents with rare but life-threatening side effects such as **aplastic anaemia**, **agranulocytosis**, cardiac problems, and activation of suicidal ideation and behaviour. It can also cause rare but severe dermatological conditions such as *Stevens–Johnson syndrome* and *toxic epidermal necrolysis*.

Stevens–Johnson syndrome is a life-threatening condition affecting the skin in which cell death causes the epidermis to separate from the dermis. Both Stevens–Johnson syndrome and toxic epidermal necrolysis are characterised by blisters arising on altered skin colour (purple). The patient develops widespread skin lesions, and these are usually predominant on the trunk of the body. Although the incidence of Stevens–Johnson syndrome is low, mortality rates are as high as 12.5 per cent, and 33.3 per cent for toxic epidermal necrolysis. Specific ethnic groups are more susceptible to developing Stevens–Johnson syndrome and toxic epidermal necrolysis because they have a high frequency of the gene variant human leukocyte antigen (HLA-B*1502). Such ethnic groups include the Han Chinese, Thai and Malaysian populations. The incidence of Stevens–Johnson syndrome and toxic epidermal necrolysis is ten times higher in these ethnic populations than in Caucasians, and carbamazepine is the most common cause. The screening of the HLA-B*1502 allele in patients requiring carbamazepine therapy in this population is important (Tangamornsuksan et al., 2013). For the management of Stevens–Johnson syndrome and toxic epidermal necrolysis, see Chapter 12.

Management of carbamazepine toxicity

Carbamazepine overdose is common and accounts for 30 per cent of all anticonvulsant overdoses (Spiller, 2001); the first overdose was reported in 1967. Significant toxicity occurs at levels higher than 40 mg/L; a common cause for carbamazepine toxicity is co-administration of other medications such as lamotrigine and levetiracetam. Furthermore, any inhibitors of cytochrome P450 (CYP450), such as grapefruit juice, will cause elevated levels of carbamazepine (Garg et al., 1998). An intentional overdose of carbamazepine is less common, and usually seen with a suicide attempt in a severely depressed patient during the initial stages of carbamazepine administration (Al Khalili and Jain, 2019). We can divide carbamazepine toxicity into the following three levels: (1) disorientation and ataxia with levels of 11–15 mg/L; (2) aggression and hallucinations with levels of 15–25 mg/L; and (3) seizures and coma with levels above 25 mg/L. There is usually a delay in the onset of acute symptoms of overdose because of the erratic absorption of carbamazepine in the gastrointestinal tract. It causes dizziness, imbalance, drowsiness, coma, and generalised seizures. Carbamazepine toxicity causes abnormal cardiac conduction that can lead to arrhythmia. It has been reported that acute carbamazepine toxicity could be associated with the presence of **spindle coma** on an electroencephalogram (EEG). Anticholinergic symptoms are common with carbamazepine toxicity. **Hyperchromic anaemia** and minor rhabdomyolysis, as well as resultant movement disorders, also have been reported.

The nurse should observe the patient closely and carry out a neurological examination if symptoms deteriorate. In any event, anesthesia and an **intubation** kit must be ready at the bedside, so that any worsening of symptoms – or anticipation of worsening – should prompt pre-emptive patient intubation. Additionally, it is important to carry out an ECG and obtain carbamazepine serum levels every four hours.

Treatment of carbamazepine toxicity ranges from physiological clearance, to the use of activated charcoal, to haemodialysis or **plasmapheresis**. Activated charcoal binds to carbamazepine and prevents its absorption from the gastrointestinal tract into the bloodstream. Activated charcoal also enhances the elimination of carbamazepine by interrupting the enterohepatic circulation of the medicine. Charcoal haemoperfusion is another technique that can improve clinical outcomes for carbamazepine overdose. Haemoperfusion is a method of removing toxins from the blood by passing the blood through a tube containing either treated charcoal or ion exchange resins. However, it has risks, such as hypocalcemia and thrombocytopenia. Charcoal will compete with plasma proteins for carbamazepine binding. Due to the risk of death in 13 per cent of cases of carbamazepine toxicity, it requires an aggressive treatment plan that includes haemoperfusion, hemodialysis and multiple doses of activated charcoal. However, if we manage symptoms well soon after the overdose, the outcomes for most patients with carbamazepine toxicity are good.

Special considerations

The elimination of carbamazepine is through the kidneys, and therefore patients with kidney impairment require lower doses. Also, the careful use of carbamazepine in those who have liver impairment is important as cases of liver failure have been reported. Normally, there is a restriction on the use of carbamazepine in those with cardiac problems.

Like lithium and valproic acid, we should restrict the use of carbamazepine in pregnancy because of reported incidences of foetal malformation. If we give carbamazepine to a pregnant person, we should monitor blood serum levels of the medicine throughout the pregnancy. The medicine can cause birth abnormalities and vitamin K deficiency. If the mother is breastfeeding while on carbamazepine, then it is important to monitor the blood serum levels of the infant and inform the mother of any signs and symptoms of liver dysfunction. For the management of the common side effects of carbamazepine, see Chapter 12.

Lamotrigine

Since 1994, lamotrigine has been used to treat partial seizures in epilepsy. It was not until 2003 that this medicine was used as a mood stabiliser in bipolar disorder. It is a well-established anticonvulsant but has also received regulatory approval for the treatment and prevention of bipolar depression in more than 30 countries worldwide. Like most mood stabilisers, there is a poor understanding of the mode of action of lamotrigine. Laboratory pharmacological studies suggest that lamotrigine inhibits sodium channels, thereby inhibiting the release of excitatory neurotransmitters such as glutamate. One interesting thing about lamotrigine is that while most mood stabilisers work mostly by controlling the manic phase of bipolar disorder, lamotrigine tends to be most effective in the treatment and prophylaxis of bipolar depression (Amann et al., 2011). Most importantly, it treats bipolar depression without triggering mania, hypomania, mixed states or rapid cycling. To date, there is little evidence for its efficacy in the treatment of the manic phase of the disorder. It is recommended as the first-line treatment for acute depression in bipolar depression as well as the maintenance. If lamotrigine is given at a **subtherapeutic** dose, it has a mild antidepressant effect.

Currently, there is no need to monitor blood plasma before commencing lamotrigine. Generally, the medicine should be initiated at very low doses to minimise the incidence of skin rash (see 'Side effects' below). The starting dose is usually 25 mg per day for the first two weeks. We can increase to 50 mg per day for a further three weeks. From the fifth week, we can increase the medication to 100 mg per day and then increase to 200 mg per day (maximum dose) in the sixth week. If the patient stops taking lamotrigine for five days or more, the best course of action may be to restart the drug with initial dose titration to minimise the incidence of skin rash. Also, patients should not start lamotrigine within two weeks of a viral infection, skin rash or vaccination.

Side effects

Common side effects include headaches, dizziness and insomnia. Others include acne and skin irritation (as mentioned above), vivid dreams or nightmares, night sweats, body aches and cramps, muscle aches, dry mouth, mouth ulcers, damage to tooth enamel, fatigue, memory and cognitive problems, irritability, weight changes, hair loss, changes in libido, frequent urination, nausea, and appetite changes. In very rare cases, lamotrigine has been known to cause Stevens–Johnson syndrome (see page 214).

Special considerations

Unlike most other anticonvulsants, women are more likely than men to experience side effects with lamotrigine. This may be due to an interaction between lamotrigine and female hormones. It is of concern for women on oestrogen-containing hormonal contraceptives, which have been shown to decrease blood serum levels of lamotrigine by up to 66 per cent (Reimers, 2019). Women starting an oestrogen-based oral contraceptive may need to increase the dosage of lamotrigine to maintain its level of efficacy. Similarly, women may experience an increase in lamotrigine side effects upon discontinuation of a contraceptive. This may include the 'pill-free' week, where lamotrigine serum levels have been shown to increase twofold. There is a significant increase in **follicle-stimulating hormone (FSH)** and **luteinising hormone (LH)** in women taking lamotrigine with oral contraceptives when compared with women taking oral contraceptives alone.

The use of lamotrigine in pregnancy is normally restricted and should only be used if its potential benefits clearly outweigh the risks, as there is tentative evidence that it may cause cleft palates in babies. Lamotrigine is excreted in breast milk, and therefore breastfeeding is not normally recommended during treatment. Infant serum levels can be between 25 and 30 per cent of those of the mother, and this risks a life-threatening rash in the baby. Lamotrigine can inhibit sleep, so the medicine is best taken in the morning. Evidence from case studies and retrospective studies indicate that lamotrigine overdose is usually benign. However, there are reported cases of cardiac arrest and mortality following lamotrigine overdose. Most cases reporting lamotrigine exposures observed mild or no toxicity; however, large exposures were associated with severe CNS depression, seizures, cardiac conduction delays, wide complex tachycardia, and death. In adults with a serum concentration of greater than 25 mg/L, severe toxicity may occur. In children of less than 4 years of age, ingestions of greater than 525 mg may produce severe CNS depression and seizures (Alyahya et al., 2018). Before you read further, try Activity 7.4.

Activity 7.4   Critical thinking

You have just visited Charles, a patient in the community who suffers from bipolar disorder. He has recently had his mood stabiliser switched to lamotrigine. During the visit, you notice that Charles has developed a skin rash, skin lesions and bleeding.

- What action would you take?

An outline answer is provided at the end of the chapter.

For the management of common lamotrigine side effects, see those outlined above for carbamazepine, lithium and sodium valproic acid.

Atypical antipsychotics

In the past, typical as well as atypical antipsychotics have been used as adjunct treatments for bipolar disorder, but there is emerging evidence for the monotherapy use of these medicines as mood stabilisers. Olanzapine and quetiapine have been mostly used in the treatment of bipolar disorder, but other antipsychotics such as risperidone, zisprasidone, aripiprazole and clozapine have also been used, although evidence from meta-analysis is poor (Lindstrom et al., 2017). Usually, the severity of the symptoms, as well as the side effects profile of the antipsychotic, are determining factors in choosing the right antipsychotic. Where a patient is suffering from psychotic symptoms such as delusions and hallucinations, antipsychotics are recommended. Combination treatment with a second-generation agent and a mood stabiliser has a higher response rate in manic episodes than monotherapy with either medicine alone (Malhi et al., 2012a). For antipsychotic modes of action, as well as side effects and their management, see Chapter 8.

Common treatment errors to avoid

Because of its low therapeutic index, lithium is toxic, and as such requires careful monitoring for adverse effects, both in acute and long-term treatment. Lithium should not be administered to patients under the age of 12 years as no data on safety or on the efficacy are available in this age group, and the dose has yet to be established. Suicidal ideation should be monitored even in those suffering from the manic phase of the disorder. Dehydration can be a problem, particularly in manic patients who may be overactive, and therefore you should encourage adequate fluid intake. In general, people with bipolar illness require lifelong treatment. Discontinuation of mood stabilisers will often result in a relapse that is even more severe. If discontinuation must be undertaken, the medicine should be gradually withdrawn over a period of six weeks. Sustained-release medication should never be crushed as this will result in rapid absorption, causing toxic symptoms.

What the patient needs to know

- Lithium, valproic acid, carbamazepine, lamotrigine, and other medicines such as olanzapine and quetiapine are drugs that will treat mood or emotional problems. They also help with preventing relapse. It is important to take these medicines and follow instructions as prescribed.
- Mood stabilisers such as lithium, valproic acid, lamotrigine and carbamazepine are not addictive.
- Many side effects of mood stabilisers can be minimised by taking the medicines in divided doses.
- Because the therapeutic dosage and toxic dosage of lithium are so close to each other, regular blood tests should be performed to ensure that blood lithium levels are within the therapeutic range only.
- Bipolar disorder is biological, not a moral defect or character flaw. It is a treatable illness that runs in families. When severe, the patient may not always be able to control their behaviour.
- Patients taking lithium should be warned not to take over-the-counter non-steroidal anti-inflammatory drugs (NSAIDs) such as ibuprofen. Prescribing NSAIDs to such patients should be avoided if possible; and if they are prescribed, the patient should be closely monitored.
- Anticonvulsant mood stabilisers can cause birth defects; so if the patient is planning to have a family, she should contact the prescriber for more advice.
- Lifestyle changes that promote both physical and mental health should be discussed with the patient. These include the avoidance of sleep deprivation, even for one night, and avoidance of shift work, alcohol, illicit drugs, and other substances that interfere with sleep such as caffeine and decongestants.
- Decreased exposure to light in winter can trigger bipolar depression, and excessive exposure to sunlight, particularly in summer, can trigger mania.
- There are many self-help groups that provide support for bipolar patients and their families. You should provide information on these and other relevant organisations within the patient's area.

Chapter summary

Bipolar illness belongs to a group of mood disorders that are typically a mixture of depressive and manic phases. During the depressive phase of the illness, the patient may present with typical symptoms of major depressive disorder such as a low mood, apathy, poor concentration, poor appetite and sleep, cognitive changes, and suicidal ideation. In the manic phase of the illness, the patient typically presents with a euphoric mood that is not matched by their circumstances. Other symptoms may include irritability, grandiosity, racing thoughts, delusions, and hallucinations.

Subtle differences between unipolar and bipolar depression exist. Bipolar depression tends to occur at a younger age and is almost sudden in onset. Also, recovery from bipolar depression can be spontaneous, and patients can go into a manic phase after recovery from depression. Mood stabilisers are a group of medicines that prevent the patient from having extremes of mood (depressed or manic). The most used mood stabilisers are lithium, sodium valproic acid, carbamazepine, and lamotrigine.

Activities: brief outline answers

Activity 7.1 Critical thinking (page 207)

Slow-release medicine is designed so that a small amount of the medicine is released into the blood to avoid toxic levels. Therefore, if ordinary lithium tablets are administered in high doses, they will be absorbed very quickly into the bloodstream, thus elevating blood serum levels and risking lithium toxicity.

Activity 7.2 Evidence-based practice and research (page 208)

Medicines that reduce glomerular filtration rate (GFR):

- non-steroidal anti-inflammatory drugs (NSAIDS);
- renin-angiotensin system inhibitors.

Medicines that promote renal tubular reabsorption:

- thiazide diuretics;
- spironolactone.

Medicines that have uncertain mechanisms:

- calcium channel blockers (diltiazem, verapamil);
- nifedipine has been shown to reduce lithium clearance when administered chronically.

Activity 7.3 Critical thinking (page 209)

As Steven is going to Cyprus in August, the weather is likely to be hot and therefore he is likely to sweat a lot. In turn, this is likely to raise his blood lithium to toxic levels. He should be advised to drink lots of water. Alternatively, and more appropriately, you should ask the prescriber to review his lithium with a view to reducing the dose for the period that he is on holiday.

Activity 7.4 Critical thinking (page 218)

You should advise Charles not to take any more lamotrigine until it is confirmed that the skin rash and lesions are not due to lamotrigine side effects. You should contact the prescriber as well as his GP without delay.

Further reading

Preston, J.D., O'Neal, J.H. and Talaga, M.C. (2017) *A Handbook of Clinical Psychopharmacology,* 8th edition. Oakland, CA: New Harbinger.

This is a clearly written book that is particularly useful for those from a non-medical background. It explains non-pharmacological mental healthcare well.

Stahl, S.M. (2013) *Stahl's Essential Psychopharmacology: The Prescriber's Guide,* 4th edition. Cambridge: Cambridge University Press.

This is a comprehensive guide to psychopharmacology that is clearly written and has good illustrations.

Taylor, D.M., Barnes, T.R.E. and Young, A.H. (2018) *The Maudsley Prescribing Guidelines in Psychiatry,* 13th edition. London: Informa Healthcare.

This is a very useful, easy-to-understand, evidence-based prescribing and general medicines management manual. It is particularly useful for prescribers.

Useful websites

www.bmj.com/content/bmj/349/bmj.g5673.full.pdf

This is a very good article on how to manage people with bipolar disorder.

www.drugs.com

This website provides a lot of useful information that ranges from pill identification to different types of medicines and their interactions, as well as new medicines on the market.

www.medicines.org.uk/emc

This website explains all drug actions, side effects and interactions. It is a very good reference source, particularly for those who prescribe medicines.

www.mhf.org.uk/information/mental-health-a-z

The Mental Health Foundation (MHF) offers information and publications to download on research, good practice in services, mental health problems, and key issues. It provides a daily mental health news service, as well as directories of organisations, websites and events.

Chapter 8 Management and treatment of psychotic disorders

Chapter aims

By the end of this chapter, you will have an understanding of:

- the key aetiological factors of schizophrenia or psychosis, as well as the biological mechanisms involved in the treatment of psychosis;
- the therapeutic mechanism of different classes of antipsychotics and how these medications cause side effects;
- the treatment and management of special groups, as well as common errors to avoid and what to communicate to the patient.

Introduction

We can define schizophrenia as severe mental disorders that are characterised by abnormal thinking and distorted perceptions – schizophrenia is one such disorder. The term 'schizophrenia' is over 100 years old. Neurologist Emil Kraepelin first identified the disease as a separate mental illness in 1887. Written documents that identify schizophrenia can be traced back to ancient Egypt, as far back as the second millennium BC. Depression, dementia and thought disturbances that are typical of schizophrenia are described in detail in the *Ebers Papyrus*, or the *Book of Hearts*; the heart and the mind seem to have been synonymous in ancient Egypt (Joachim, 1890). The public health importance of schizophrenia is clear. Schizophrenia affects seven out of every 1,000 persons; males are twice as likely to suffer from schizophrenia as females, and it starts in adolescence or early adulthood. Studies have found an increase in the prevalence of schizophrenia in people living in countries at higher latitudes. As in psychosis in general, the symptoms of schizophrenia are many and diverse, but can be broadly divided into five syndromes: positive, negative, disorganisation, affective and cognitive. For a more comprehensive coverage of these syndromes, consult a specialist book on schizophrenia and its symptoms, but Figure 8.1 lists the common symptom domains of schizophrenia (we will use the terms 'schizophrenia' and 'psychosis' interchangeably).

Because schizophrenia is the most prevalent form of psychosis, this chapter provides an overview of the pharmacological treatment of schizophrenia. The chapter begins by outlining the physical illnesses and medicines that are associated with psychosis. This should encourage the perception of psychoses as illnesses that are a result of a complex interplay of social, psychological and biological factors. The chapter then explores the dopamine theory of schizophrenia as a way of providing the necessary background knowledge to understand the mechanism of action of antipsychotic medicines. The chapter explores the difference between first-generation (conventional) and second-generation (atypical) antipsychotics before discussing the common side effects of antipsychotics. The final sections of the chapter discuss advising patients on how to manage different types of side effects, errors to avoid during treatment, and what the patient needs to know.

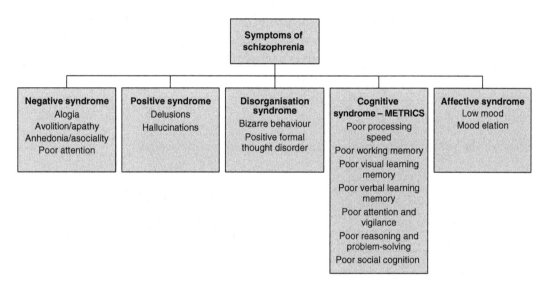

Figure 8.1   The common symptom domains of schizophrenia – cognitive symptoms have recently been added as part of the schizophrenia symptoms framework, and key cognitive symptoms should fit in with the Measurement and Treatment Research to Improve Cognition in Schizophrenia (METRICS)

Physical diseases that are associated with psychosis

Some physical illnesses can result in a person developing a type of schizophrenia that we call *secondary psychosis*. During consultation with a patient (see Chapter 4), it is important to be aware of their full medical history as this is a prerequisite to good clinical decision-making. If a patient's psychotic symptoms are secondary to a physical health disorder, it is essential and more effective to treat the underlying physical illness first.

Case study: Neil

A 45-year-old man with a history of alcohol dependence and sleeping rough was found wandering the streets in the early hours of the morning. He was not intoxicated but was confused and could not remember where he was. He gave his name as Neil but could not elaborate further. The police noticed that he was talking to himself a lot and trying to 'pick up things' from the floor that were not there. Also, he kept scratching his skin and complained of insects crawling all over his body. He was brought to hospital under the terms of the Mental Health Act 1983. He refused to go to bed for fear of ghosts and he could see spiders on the floor. As his condition was unknown, the team decided to monitor his condition without administering medication for at least a week. However, the team noticed that he was emaciated, which suggested that his dietary intake before admission to hospital was inadequate. He was prescribed vitamin supplements and part of the care plan was 'to encourage adequate fluid and dietary intake'. Neil's condition gradually improved, and he was able to give his full name and address, as well as naming the hospitals he had been admitted to for alcohol detoxification.

Some of the physical illnesses that can cause secondary psychosis are:

• Addison's disease	• Dementia with Lewy bodies (DLB)
• Cushing's syndrome	• Multiple sclerosis
• Brain injury	• Myxoedema
• Vitamin deficiency: folic acid (B_{12})	• Pancreatitis
• Vitamin D_3 deficiency	• Pellagra
• Toxic states (delirium)	• Pernicious anaemia
• Huntington's disease	• Porphyria
• Thyrotoxicosis	• Temporal lobe epilepsy

In summary, the physical conditions that may induce psychosis are many and diverse; therefore, it is important to be attentive to a patient's physical state as this can provide important information that can help to explain their mental state. The above case study of Neil is typical of how physical disorder can lead to the patient developing mental health symptoms. In his case, it is possible that alcohol withdrawal and poor diet may have precitpitated symptoms via various mechanisms, including an imbalance of inhibitory and excitatory mechanisms in the participating neurotransmitter systems. Therefore, thorough assessment of the patient's problems is the first important step towards correct treatment that leads to good recovery. Now that you understand how some physical illnesses can cause secondary psychosis, try Activity 8.1.

Activity 8.1   Critical thinking

You notice that a doctor has taken a blood sample for biochemistry analysis from a 68-year-old lady who lives alone. She has recently been admitted to your ward. She looks emaciated, disoriented and restless. The doctor has written in her notes 'For electrolyte test'.

- What might be the importance of testing for electrolytes in older people?

An outline answer is provided at the end of the chapter.

Medicines that are associated with psychosis

Ingesting some medicines, chemicals, toxins or substances may induce psychotic symptoms; therefore, it is important to have knowledge of medicines in clinical practice that may trigger psychosis. Table 8.1 lists some of these medicines and chemicals.

Table 8.1   Substances and medicines that can induce psychosis

Substance	Medicine
L-dopa	Fluoroquinolone
Hallucinogenic substances	Corticosteroids
Anticholinergic	Ketamine
Anti-inflammatory	Ecstasy (MDMA)
CNS stimulants (psychostimulants)	Barbiturates

Before you read further, complete Activity 8.2.

Activity 8.2   Decision-making

You have been asked to complete admission procedures for a 19-year-old man who has been brought to your ward suffering from a psychotic episode that seemed to have come on two days ago after his birthday party. He has no previous history of psychiatric illness. He has agreed to provide a urine sample for routine examination.

- What might you include in the screening process?

An outline answer is provided at the end of the chapter.

How psychotic symptoms arise

To be able to understand how antipsychotics work, it is important to begin by determining how psychotic symptoms arise in the first place. A comprehensive coverage of psychopathology is beyond the scope of this book, so do consult a specialist textbook on the subject. However, the following section discusses commonly accepted theories of the mechanism of psychosis.

Psychosis, like many mental health disorders, is thought to be the result of an interaction between a person's intrinsic biological factors and the stress they experience in life. The best articulation of this viewpoint comes from the *stress vulnerability model* (Zubin and Spring, 1977), which suggests that people become ill when the stress they face becomes more than they can cope with. Also, people's ability to deal with stress (i.e. their vulnerability) differs from person to person: a problem that one person may take in their stride might be enough to cause another person to become depressed or develop psychotic symptoms. A person's vulnerability has a close link with genetic factors.

In the case of schizophrenia, more than 100 candidate genes for condition have been identified with high levels of statistical significance. The most consistently identified genes include Neuregulin 1 (NRG1), disrupted in schizophrenia 1 (DISC1) and 22q11.2 deletion syndrome (22q11.2DS). Together with early environmental influences, these genes play an important role in the development of schizophrenia.

A range of structural and functional abnormalities of the brain usually accompany the development of schizophrenia. These include neuronal abnormalities in parts of the brain such as the parahippocampal pyramidal, insula and entorhinal cortex cells. Further, there is also a decrease in neuronal density in the superficial white matter and an increase in density in the deep white matter. Other structural abnormalities we see in schizophrenia include a reduction in overall grey and white matter volume, ventricular enlargement, a reduction in the volume of some limbic structures such as the hippocampus, parahippocampus, thalamus, amygdala and in entorhinal region volume and cingulate gyrus reduction. However, cortical brain abnormalities have been reported in people at ultra-high risk (UHR) for the development of schizophrenia, and specific abnormalities of the thalamocortical circuit may be biomarkers for the development of psychosis (Zhu et al., 2019). UHR refers to people with multiple risk factors, which leads to a high likelihood for the development of a psychotic disorder such as schizophrenia. In this regard, structural neurodevelopmental abnormalities are associated with a predisposition (vulnerability) for the development of a psychotic illness. Many imaging studies show that structural brain abnormalities often coexist with functional brain abnormalities. In psychosis, there is evidence from meta-analytic studies suggesting that a reduction of regional grey matter volume is associated with an impairment of brain function in a range of cognitive tasks, and this impairment includes regional brain hypoactivation (Radua et al., 2012). A functional abnormality that best links to the mechanism of action of antipsychotic medication is the dopamine theory, first proposed by Carlsson and Lindqvist (1963).

Early dopamine theory proposes that schizophrenia is due to excess dopamine activity or hyperdopaminergia of the mesolimbic pathway, but this conceptualisation has no direct empirical evidence base. However, recent positron emission tomography (PET) studies suggest that dopamine dysfunction is in fact greatest within the dorsal regions of the striatum (see Figure 8.2). Furthermore, we can see dopamine dysfunction in other subdivisions of the striatum such as the associative and sensorimotor regions, but dopamine dysfunction does not appear to be significant in the limbic subdivision of the striatum, as previously thought (McCutcheon et al., 2017). This provides direct evidence suggesting an elevation of presynaptic striatal dopamine in people with schizophrenia, and this elevation is also present before the development of symptoms in people at risk of developing psychosis (Egerton et al., 2013). This discovery stimulated the modification of the original dopamine theory.

The identified neurobiological abnormalities translate to diverse symptoms, and there are several mechanisms where presynaptic striatal dopamine dysfunction could contribute to the clinical manifestation of psychosis. The assigning of importance or salience stimuli involves excessive spontaneous dorsal striatal dopamine signalling. Thus, an increase in dopamine activity in the striatum results in an abherent (abnormal) motivational salience. Motivational salience is a form of cognitive activity that refers to the process of how reward-associated stimuli come to be *attention-grabbing* (salient) for the person and the focus of goal-directed behaviour (Kapur et al., 2005). In other words, a person experiencing schizophrenia shows an abnormally amplified response to neutral or irrelevant stimuli, and this in turn leads to the formation of positive symptoms of schizophrenia, such as paranoid delusions or ideas of reference where everyday occurrences may be layered with a heightened sense of bizarre significance. In recent years, neuroimaging techniques have been used to examine abherent motivational salience in people with schizophrenia, and they largely support this hypothesis (Wijayendran et al., 2018).

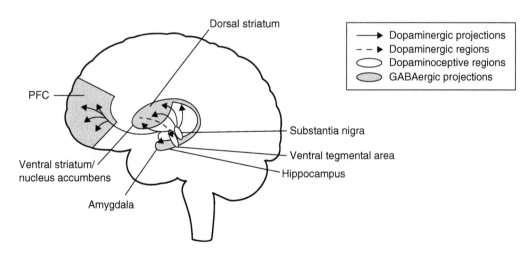

Figure 8.2 Four critical dopamine pathways: the mesocortical, mesolimbic, tuberoinfundibular and nigrostriatal pathways

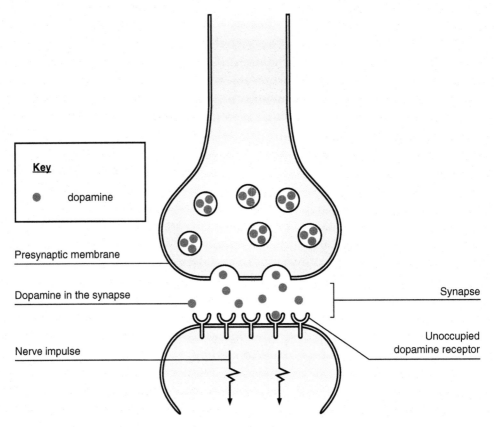

Figure 8.3 Normal dopamine release into the synaptic cleft

With regard to the negative and cognitive symptoms of schizophrenia, the first major reconceptualisation of the dopamine hypothesis was in the late 1980s. This originated from the recognition of enduring cognitive deficits in schizophrenia and the discovery of the critical role of prefrontal dopamine for cognitive functions (Davis et al., 1991). The current conceptualisation proposes that there might be a decrease in prefrontal dopamine function (hypodopaminergia) in schizophrenia, leading to cognitive and negative symptoms such as avolition and anhedonia. This view is supported by recent studies that provide *in vivo* evidence for a deficit in the capacity to release dopamine in the dorsolateral prefrontal cortex (DLPFC) in schizophrenia. Furthermore, there is an association between hypodopaminergia and cognitive symptoms such as poor working memory (Slifstein et al., 2015). However, much of the evidence has a limited empirical base at this stage. Furthermore, schizophrenia is a heterogeneous disorder, so no single brain region or neurotransmitter is likely to account for all symptoms in all patients.

Treatment of positive symptoms

The discovery of the medicines that can effectively treat psychoses (primarily schizophrenia) began in the 1940s. A French surgeon, Henri Laborit, convinced that many of

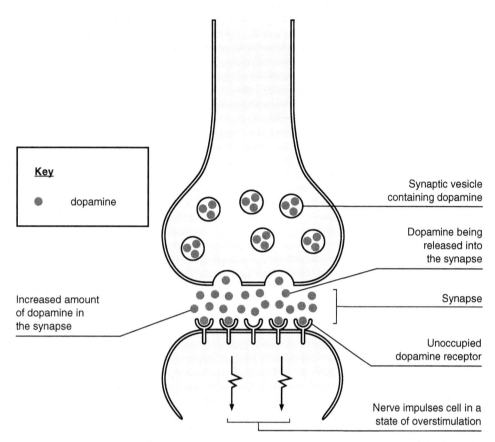

Figure 8.4 An elevated release of dopamine into the synaptic cleft, or hyperdopaminergia, resulting in positive symptoms of psychosis

the deaths associated with surgery could be attributed to patients' fears, discovered the sedatives promethazine and chlorpromazine, both of which proved to be dramatically effective. The use of chlorpromazine spread to the psychiatric clinic in the mid-1950s and was found to produce not only sedation, but also an equally dramatic reversal of the psychotic symptoms of schizophrenia. The discovery of chlorpromazine stimulated the discovery of several other antipsychotics that we now refer to as first-generation antipsychotics.

As previously discussed, schizophrenia results from an abnormal reward prediction and abnormal attribution of salience caused by disordered dopamine transmission. This results in positive symptoms of schizophrenia-like delusions, hallucinations and thought disorder. All antipsychotics work by blocking or antagonising dopamine. While several efforts have been made to develop antipsychotics that bypass the dopamine system, a blockade of the dopamine D_2 theory remains a necessary condition for antipsychotic activity to date. Previous and recent literature supports the effectiveness of D_2 antagonism compared to any alternative pharmacological intervention in psychosis (Amato et al., 2018; Pilowsky et al., 1993). By blocking striatal dopamine D_2

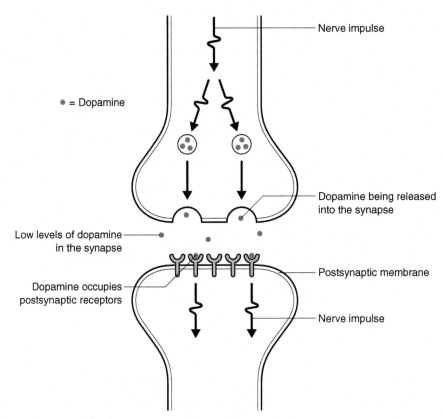

Figure 8.5 Low levels of dopamine release in the synapse, or hypodopaminergia, resulting in negative, cognitive and mood symptoms

transmission at postsynaptic receptors, this dampens or weakens motivational salience. Antipsychotics do not directly erase positive symptoms, but provide a neurochemical environment to block the effects of dopamine; therefore, new aberrant salience is less likely to form (see Figure 8.6). In the initial stage of an antipsychotic response, the patient experiences a detachment from symptoms, a downgrading of the delusions and hallucinations to the back of their minds, rather than a complete erasure of the symptoms. Only with time, and only in some patients, is there a complete resolution of symptoms. Contrary to popular belief, there is no delay in antipsychotic effect, and this effect can start within the first few days after treatment initiation. There is more improvement in the first two weeks than in any subsequent period thereafter (Kapur et al., 2006).

However, blocking dopamine receptors is not an effective therapeutic mechanism for all individuals with psychosis. For example, some patients with first-episode schizophrenia do not respond to antipsychotic treatment. A study that followed up 323 first-episode schizophrenia patients for ten years found that 74 patients did not respond to antipsychotics at the ten-year follow-up. Of these, 62 patients did not respond to antipsychotics from treatment initiation (Demjaha et al., 2017). This stimulated the view that current explanations of how antipsychotics work may be simplistic.

A more comprehensive understanding of the mechanisms underlying antipsychotic responsiveness should not simply describe the chemical interactions between antipsychotic medicines and their target receptors, but should consider modifications induced by antipsychotics at the cellular and circuit levels, and this view is supported by a growing body of literature (Amato et al., 2019). Further, explanations, should not only consider the action of antipsychotics on central D_2 receptors, but also interactions with other neurotransmitter receptors (i.e. adrenergic, serotoninergic, etc.).

Treatment of negative symptoms

A decrease in the white matter volume of the prefrontal (especially the orbitofrontal) region, volume loss in the anterior cingulate, the insular cortex and the left temporal cortex, and ventricular enlargement are associated with severity of negative symptoms. This loss is present even before the onset of symptoms, continues with the course of illness (Hovington and Lepage, 2012). Similarly, there is a reduction in cerebral blood perfusions in the frontal, prefrontal, posterior cingulate, thalamus, some parietal, and striatal regions in those with negative symptoms (Winograd-Gurvich et al., 2006). From a biochemical perspective, lower cortical dopamine transmission in the mesocortical

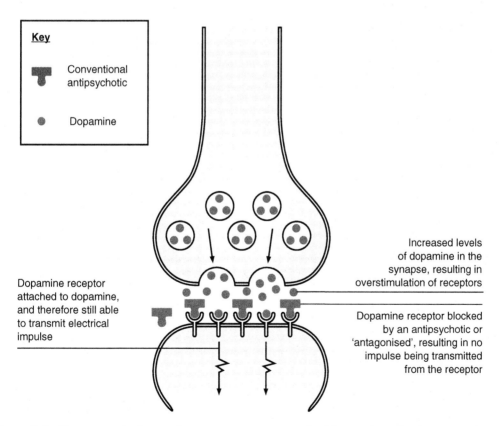

Key

Conventional antipsychotic

Dopamine

Increased levels of dopamine in the synapse, resulting in overstimulation of receptors

Dopamine receptor attached to dopamine, and therefore still able to transmit electrical impulse

Dopamine receptor blocked by an antipsychotic or 'antagonised', resulting in no impulse being transmitted from the receptor

Figure 8.6 Postsynaptic dopamine receptors antagonised by antipsychotics, reversing the effects of overstimulation by dopamine

pathway gives rise to negative symptoms. By antagonising dopamine receptors in an area with reduced dopamine activity (hypodopaminergia), antipsychotics are less effective in treating these symptoms. In fact, antipsychotic receptor antagonism in the mesocortical region may worsen negative, cognitive and mood symptoms. This is likely to be the case if first-generation antipsychotics are used, though the evidence is less clear-cut.

As many as 25–60 per cent of patients on first-generation antipsychotics are largely treatment-resistant or partially responsive to treatment. The challenge, therefore, is to find a medicine that can simultaneously reduce hyperactivity of dopamine in the mesolimbic region and improve hypoactivity in the mesocortical regions. In other words, we need to find an antipsychotic that can effectively treat positive as well as negative symptoms with minimal extrapyramidal symptoms. To some degree, the second-generation antipsychotics partially meet this challenge and will be discussed next. Before you read further, try Activity 8.3.

Activity 8.3   Critical thinking

A 46-year-old woman with a long history of being involved with mental health services was readmitted to your ward four days ago. She believes that her neighbours have been spying on her using CCTV cameras planted in her house. She spends most of the time sleeping in bed. She has been prescribed and is taking 20 mg of haloperidol per day.

- What concerns do you have about this woman taking haloperidol, particularly at such a high dose?
- How would you improve the situation?

An outline answer is provided at the end of the chapter.

Second-generation 'atypical' antipsychotics

As previously discussed, older first-generation antipsychotics such as haloperidol are effective in treating positive symptoms of psychosis, but they may cause other problems such as the worsening of negative symptoms, although recent evidence seems to suggest this may be overstated (Marques et al., 2014). In support of this view, a meta-analysis of 150 double-blind studies with an overall population of 21,533 participants comparing first-generation antipsychotics to second-generation antipsychotis found that some second-generation antipsychotics (quetiapine, sertindole, ziprasidone and zotepine) were only as efficacious as first-generation antipsychotics in treating negative symptoms. Most of these studies, however, only lasted for up to 12 weeks and were heterogeneous regarding the phase of the illness. Large scale pragmatic studies, such as the Cost Utility of the Latest Antipsychotic Drugs in Schizophrenia Study

(CUtLASS), did not demonstrate any significant difference between second- and first-generation antipsychotics in the treatment of negative symptoms (Jones et al., 2006). Despite this evidence from naturalistic studies, there is still a preference for second-generation antipsychotics for their purported superiority in improving functional outcomes and improving cognitive functioning, but the benefits are only modest. So, what is an atypical (second-generation) antipsychotic?

From a pharmacological point of view, an atypical antipsychotic may mean a medicine that is effective at treating symptoms of schizophrenia without inducing extrapyramidal side effects or prolactin. We will now turn to the mechanisms of action of these two distinguishing features of atypicality, and the first of these relates to the role of serotonin in defining atypicality.

The role of serotonin in defining atypicality

Apart from antagonising dopamine D_2 receptors, almost all second-generation antipsychotics block serotonin receptors as well (mainly $5HT_2$ and $5HT_1$). The blockade of serotonin serves two functions depending on the region of the brain. In the striatal region, the serotonin receptors blockade slows down dopamine release into the synapse, leading to a reduction of positive symptoms in the striatum (remember that positive symptoms are due to excess dopamine activity, particularly in the dorsal striatal region).

In the mesocortical region, blockade of serotonin receptors (presynaptic) by a second-generation antipsychotic such as olanzapine leads to the release of more dopamine into the synapse. As previously discussed, this theorectically improves negative, cognitive and mood symptoms (remember that negative, cognitive and mood symptoms are due to insufficient dopamine activity in the mesocortical region).

As we have previously discussed, one of the disadvantages of all antipsychotics is that they block dopamine receptors in non-therapeutic pathways such as the nigrostriatal. The *nigrostriatal pathway* is one of the four major dopamine pathways in the brain (see Figure 8.2 on page 227) and it is involved with the regulation of body movement. It is part of the **basal ganglia** (of which the striatum is part) motor loop system. Previously, we used to believe that dopamine output in the nigrostriatal pathway is normal in psychosis, but recent evidence points to the nigrostriatal pathway as the area of highest dopamine dysregulation, and it may potentially play an important role in the pathology of psychosis (Kuepper et al., 2012). Because of its importance in the regulation of body movement, the dopamine receptor blockade by antipsychotics causes extrapyramidal side effects, which are a variety of movement- and coordination-related side effects. This is particularly the case with the use of first-generation antipsychotics such as haloperidol. If we use a second-generation antipsychotic such as olanzapine, the situation is slightly different. The blockade of presynaptic serotonin receptors by second-generation antipsychotics results in the release of more dopamine in the synapse, therefore counteracting the effects of blocking postsynaptic dopamine receptors by the same agent.

Antipsychotics also act on a fourth dopamine pathway, the *tuberoinfundibular pathway* (see Figure 8.2 on page 227). In this pathway, dopamine levels are normal in people with psychosis. Therefore, the antipsychotic blockade in the tuberoinfundibular pathway has no therapeutic value. It only causes the stimulation of hormones, resulting in related side effects. These side effects include an increase in prolactin levels, disruptions to the menstrual cycle, visual problems, headaches, and sexual dysfunction. This is particularly so if we use first-generation antipsychotics such as haloperidol that have a strong and lasting blockade of dopamine D_2 receptors. The situation is slightly different if we use second-generation antipsychotics such as clozapine, olanzapine or quetiapine.

Keeping prolactin at normal levels

While the antagonism of dopamine D_2 receptors in the tuberoinfundibular pathway stimulates the release of prolactin, the antagonism of serotonin receptors in the same region inhibits the release of prolactin, thus counteracting the effect of dopamine antagonism. These opposing and simultaneous effect of dopamine and serotonin antagonism result in normal levels of prolactin being maintained when we use a second-generation antipsychotic. In theory, an antipsychotic's ability to keep prolactin at normal levels is another definition of a second-generation medicine (atypicality).

Loose blockage of dopamine D_2 receptors

The last definition of atypicality relates to the 'fast-off theory'. This theory proposes that atypical medicines bind loosely and are released rapidly from D_2 receptors in the synapse, and this may explain their lower tendency to induce extrapyramidal side effects and high prolactin levels (Bostoen et al., 2012). This contrasts with first-generation antipsychotics that block dopamine D_2 receptors firmly and in a more lasting way. According to some authorities, this may be the only necessary and sufficient criterion for atypicality (Kapur and Seeman, 2001). However, support for this hypothesis is limited to a relatively small number of studies made across several decades and under different experimental conditions; other investigations have questioned the utility of this theory (Meltzer, 2013). More studies are required to confirm the validity of this hypothesis. Before proceeding further, try Activity 8.4.

Activity 8.4   Critical thinking

Which of these medicines would you expect to cause the most sexual dysfunction in patients?

- haloperidol
- olanzapine
- quetiapine

An outline answer is provided at the end of the chapter.

Partial agonists and the treatment of psychosis

More recently, third-generation antipsychotics such as aripiprazole, with a unique mechanism of action and a more favourable side effects profile, are in use in practice. We refer to these medicines as partial agonists because of their dual mechanism of action. They have both agonist and antagonist properties; in other words, they can partly stimulate (act as a neurotransmitter) or partly block (act as an antipsychotic) depending on the situation. In an area of high synaptic dopamine activity such as the striatal region (involved in positive symptoms), the medicine's antagonist properties are more prominent, but only causing partial antagonism (i.e. it partially blocks the receptor), thus offering therapeutic benefit. In the mesocortical region, where dopamine activity is low, the medicine's agonistic properties are more prominent, causing partial agonism (i.e. partial activation of receptors), thus lessening negative, mood and cognitive symptoms. Several partial agonists are in clinical use, but the most widely used is aripiprazole.

Aripiprazole is effective at treating the positive and negative symptoms of schizophrenia with minimal extrapyramidal or metabolic side effects. An early systematic review of short- and long-term studies found that it is associated with improvements in the positive, negative, cognitive and affective symptoms of schizophrenia (Stip and Tourjman, 2010). This is supported by a relatively recent systematic review of 14 studies, which shows that aripiprazole has a similar efficacy to other antipsychotics but has a better safety profile (i.e. significantly fewer general extrapyramidal side effects, less use of anti-Parkinsonian drugs, akathisia). Moreover, aripiprazole causes significantly lower weight gain and alterations in glucose and cholesterol levels, compared to clozapine, risperidone and olanzapine (Ribeiro et al., 2018).

Common antipsychotic side effects

Although antipsychotics do not provide a permanent cure for psychosis, they are central to the treatment and recovery of persons with psychosis. Therefore, their beneficial effects have been established beyond doubt. Cunningham Owens (2014) has asserted that these medicines have played an important role in reversing centuries-old misconceptions of psychosis, both lay and professional; they have also played a part in making it possible to implement humane models of care for some of the most vulnerable and misunderstood people.

From an efficacy point of view, all classes of antipsychotics are equally effective, with only clozapine exerting a marginal superiority over the others. A relatively recent multi-treatment meta-analysis of 212 trials supports this view (Leucht et al., 2013).

Like all medicines, antipsychotics come as part of a package that includes therapeutic and non-therapeutic effects. The non-therapeutic effects are mainly side effects that we can broadly divide into two groups. The extrapyramidal side effects are due to antipsychotic action on the nigrostriatal pathway, and the non-extrapyramidal side effects are due to the effect of antipsychotics on other systems, such as their antagonism of the histamine, muscarinic and alpha-adrenergic receptors and the tuberoinfundibular pathway. The following sections will discuss the common side effects that patients experience in more detail.

Extrapyramidal side effects

PET studies of dopamine suggest that antipsychotic antagonism of nigrostriatal D_2 has a strong association with extrapyramidal side effects. The likelihood of the development of extrapyramidal side effects is highest when there is more than 80 per cent antagonism of D_2 receptors in the striatal part of the region by first-generation antipsychotics. Second-generation antipsychotics such as olanzapine achieve strong antipsychotic activity at a dopamine receptor antagonism of approximately 65 per cent, which may partly explain their clinical efficacy with minimal extrapyramidal side effects (Kapur and Seeman, 2001). Risk factors for extrapyramidal side effects are the choice of antipsychotic and a second-generation antipsychotic (with clozapine carrying the lowest risk and risperidone the highest), high doses, age, a history of previous extrapyramidal symptoms, and co-morbidity. Extrapyramidal side effects can take several forms, including dystonia, akathisia, pseudo-Parkinsonism and tardive dyskinesia, and we will look at these next.

Dystonia

Dystonia refers to an abnormality of voluntary muscle tone. Its characteristics are involuntary contraction or spasm of the muscles, most commonly affecting the head and neck, which can be painful and frightening. For example, the jaw may be forced to open, which can result in dislocation. The patient may suffer laryngeal spasms, which can be life-threatening. Acute dystonia is common with treatment using first-generation antipsychotics such as haloperidol, and 10 per cent of all patients taking first-generation antipsychotics experience dystonia as a side effect, typically within hours of initiating treatment. Dystonia is most common with intramuscular injections of high-potency antipsychotics and in young men below the age of 40. It is also common in those with a history of substance abuse and a family history of dystonia. Acute dystonia has been reported to be present in approximately 8.2 per cent of people taking long-acting injections of risperidone. For those who are at high risk of the condition, prophylactic treatment with anticholinergic medication such as procyclidine is generally recommended (see Chapter 12).

Activity 8.5   Critical thinking

Dave is a 23-year-old man who has been admitted to hospital following attempted suicide. He has been troubled for some time because he hears 'the voice of the devil' and bad people saying derogatory things about him. He was prescribed 15 mg of trifluperazine per day. After three days of taking trifluperazine, his condition deteriorated, and he became more restless and irritable, and at times aggressive.

- In your care plan review, what issues are you likely to consider?

An outline answer is provided at the end of the chapter.

Akathisia

Akathisia is a subjective feeling of muscular discomfort and inner restlessness; a compulsion to move the legs when sitting and an inability to stand still in one place are the most observed features. About 25 per cent of patients on first-generation treatment develop akathisia, and it occurs mostly within the first three months of treatment. It is also common in people taking second-generation antipsychotics, though at a much-reduced rate. Women are twice as likely to experience akathisia. There is ongoing debate about the propensity of different classes of antipsychotics in inducing akathisia. Some researchers suggest that rates of akathisia do not differ between first- and second-generation antipsychotics (Shirzadi and Ghaemi, 2006). For example, the Clinical Antipsychotic Trials of Intervention Effectiveness (CATIE) study found that both risperidone and perphenazine cause akathisia in 7 per cent of patients (Miller et al., 2008). The essential features of antipsychotic-induced acute akathisia are subjective complaints of restlessness and at least one of the following observed movements: (1) fidgety movements or swinging of the legs while seated; (2) rocking from foot to foot or 'walking on the spot' while standing; or (3) pacing to relieve restlessness or an inability to sit or stand still for several minutes. Akathisia is probably the most disabling and intolerable side effect that develops early during the treatment process. It can resemble psychotic agitation and is often associated with higher doses of medication, and may exist in tandem with other extrapyramidal side effects. One of the more effective ways to assess akathisia is the use of a rating scale such as the Barnes Akathisia Rating Scale (Barnes, 1989).

Pseudo-Parkinsonism

Symptoms of antipsychotic-induced Parkinsonism, or pseudo-Parkinsonism, include muscle stiffness, cogwheel rigidity, shuffling gait, stooped posture and drooling. Mask-like faces, abnormal slowness of movement (bradykinesia) and an indifference towards the environment (ataraxia), which are also part of the Parkinsonian syndrome, are often misdiagnosed as the negative symptoms of schizophrenia. Pseudo-Parkinsonism occurs in about 15 per cent of patients who are on antipsychotic treatment, usually developing within 5 to 90 days of starting treatment. The pathophysiological mechanism underlying pseudo-Parkinsonism involves a decrease in the activity of the nigrostriatal dopamine pathway due to the action of antipsychotic medicines. This decrease in activity causes a compensatory increase in the acetylcholine (cholinergic) activity, and this may account for some of the symptoms of drug-induced Parkinsonism.

Pseudo-Parkinsonism affects women twice as often as men, and the disorder can occur at all ages, although older persons are particularly at risk. It is important to note that in practice, Parkinsonian side effects can be difficult to diagnose in some patients because of an overlap of symptoms between this condition and negative and depressive symptoms. A failure to recognise and treat symptoms of pseudo-Parkinsonism can lead to increased morbidity and mortality in patients. We can use anticholinergic medication such as procylidine to treat pseudo-Parkinsonism (see Chapter 12), but it may be necessary to switch medication to an antipsychotic that has a low propensity for causing Parkinsonism.

Case study: Pete

Pete is a 34-year-old man who has suffered from schizophrenia for six years and takes a flupenthixol decanoate depot injection to control his symptoms. Initially, he was happy with his treatment, but after about six months he became increasingly unhappy with this medication, complaining that it was turning him into a zombie and that his neck and muscles ached. At a review meeting, it was agreed that the flupenthixol depot injection should be tapered off in favour of risperidone (Risperdal Consta). After three months, Pete's mental state improved and he was more socially active. He was making frequent bus journeys to visit his grandmother who lived nearby.

Pete was experiencing extrapyramidal side effects because of having the flupenthixol depot injection. Flupenthixol decanoate is a first-generation antipsychotic that blocks dopamine receptors in the therapeutic pathways (mesocortical and mesolimbic pathways) but also blocks dopamine D_2 receptors in the nigrostriatal and tubertoinfundibular pathways. It is this antagonising action of flupenthixol decanoate that is giving Pete pseudo-Parkinsonian side effects. Many patients who experience these types of side effects complain of muscle stiffness and painful muscles, particularly of the neck, jaw and limbs, as in Pete's case. After Pete's depot injection was switched to risperidone (a second-generation antipsychotic), he experienced fewer extrapyramidal symptoms, most likely because of its reduced propensity to cause extrapyramidal side effects.

Tardive dyskinesia

From a historical perspective, tardive dyskinesia (TD) is a term that is used to refer to delayed and persistent abnormal movements that are due to antipsychotic receptor antagonism of the nigrostriatal dopamine region. It rarely occurs until after six months of treatment. The disorder consists of endless involuntary movements of the tongue, jaw, trunk or extremities, and may be irregular (choreiform, athetoid) or stereotypic in nature. Most common are darting, twisting and protruding movements of the tongue, chewing and lateral jaw movements, lip puckering, and facial grimacing. Finger movements and hand clenching are also common. Overall, the prevalence of TD ranges from 20–50 per cent in outpatients treated with antipsychotics (Aquino and Lang, 2014). TD also occurs in patients with untreated schizophrenia. In 19 studies involving 11,000 untreated patients not exposed to antipsychotics, the prevalence of spontaneous dyskinesia was approximately 5 per cent. Moreover, siblings of patients with schizophrenia have higher prevalence rates of dyskinesia than matched controls (Tenback and van Harten, 2011), which suggests a genetic risk for the disorder in some patients. Other risk factors for TD are older age, female gender, history of brain damage or dementia, presence of a major affective disorder, and longer exposure to antipsychotics. The prevalence estimate of TD in older adults is a high as 57 per cent after three years' cumulative use of first-generation antipsychotics, according to a systematic review (O'Brien, 2016). TD can add to the subjective experience of disability and to the objective feelings of 'oddness', both of which affect rehabilitation and social inclusion.

Hormonal and sexual side effects

Earlier in the chapter, we explained that antipsychotics act in a non-therapeutic fourth dopamine pathway called the tuberoinfundibular pathway. Dopamine in this pathway is implicated in the production of the hormone prolactin, discovered more than 80 years ago. Prolactin is involved in more than 300 different functions. The main physiological functions include the stimulation and maintenance of milk production, breast enlargement during pregnancy, inhibition of the hypothalamic gonadotrophin-releasing hormone, and maintenance of proper ovarian function and progesterone-secreting structures (Peuskens et al., 2014). Antipsychotic antagonisim of the tuberoinfundibular dopamine pathway results in hormonal or endocrinological side effects, including irregular periods and excessive discharge of breast milk (galactorrhoea) and excessive development of the breasts (gynaecomastia), as well as sexual dysfunction due to **hyperprolactinaemia**. Sexual side effects are common with the use of all classes of antipsychotics and have an important quality of life dimension, but patients rarely report this side effect freely. Further, mental health professionals often fail to ask about sexual dysfunction. First-generation antipsychotic medicines are more likely to cause hyperprolactinemia than second-generation antipsychotics, and in particular haloperidol has an association with high prolactin levels of up to 60 per cent (Serretti and Chiesa, 2011). Up to 60 per cent of all men taking first-generation antipsychotics experience impotence and ejaculatory problems (Knegtering et al., 2006). All second-generation antipsychotics can induce hyperprolactinemia, especially at the beginning of treatment. The second-generation antipsychotics showing a consistent association with hyperprolactinemia are amisulpride, risperidone and paliperidone, while aripiprazole and quetiapine have the least association. The newer antipsychotics such as asenapine, iloperidone and lurasidone have a prolactin-elevating profile like that of clozapine and olanzapine. Prolactin elevations with antipsychotic medication are generally dose-dependant. By contrast, antipsychotics that have a minimal effect on prolactin, even at high doses, are quetiapine and aripiprazole. Apart from the effect of raised prolactin on sexual function, there are other explanatory mechanisms for antipsychotic-induced sexual dysfunction.

First, the elevation of prolactin gives rise to secondary effects such as a reduction in plasma levels of testosterone, oestrogen, luteinising hormone (LH) and follicle-stimulating hormone (FSH). A reduction of these hormones can cause sexual side effects. Second, dopamine plays a part in sexual arousal and orgasm; therefore, antagonising dopamine D_2 receptors contribute to loss of libido and orgasm disturbance. Third, the histamine-blocking effect of antipsychotics causes sedation, which leads to a diminishing of sexual performance. Moreover, many antipsychotics antagonise alpha-adrenergic receptors, and this may diminish erection, vaginal lubrication, and ejaculation. Women may experience orgasmic dysfunction and a rduction in libido, which is most likely to be due to alpha-adrenergic activity and calcium channel blockade.

A special problem in assessing sexual dysfunction in patients is that some patients with schizophrenia may experience alterations in sexual performance as a result of their primary illness and the social consequences of this illness (Dembler-Stamm et al., 2018). Sexual dysfunction can be as high as 25 per cent in medication-naive patients, according to a relatively recent study (Ravichandran et al., 2019). This makes it difficult to tease apart sexual dysfunction that is due to medication and that which is due to illness.

Case study: Jack

Jack, a 25-year-old man, was admitted to hospital after he was found in the early hours of the morning in the street, muttering and shouting to himself. As part of his treatment plan, he was prescribed 15 mg of haloperidol per day in divided doses. After a week of taking haloperidol, he complained of feeling unhappy about his medication because it was making his genitals melt away, and he felt his genitals had changed to a woman's genitals. He had never expressed this view before, and the doctor was made aware of Jack's deteriorating mental state. His medication was subsequently increased to 20 mg per day. Jack continued to repeat claims that his genitals had melted and morphed to a woman's. Because of the high dose of haloperidol that Jack was prescribed, as well as the nature of his complaint, the consultant psychiatrist ordered a prolactin levels test, which revealed that Jack had prolactin levels of 30 mcg/L, which is way above the normal threshold. Haloperidol was tapered off in favour of quetiapine, which was titrated up. After a month of taking quetiapine, Jack no longer complained about his genitals melting away.

Jack's case demonstrates the metaphorical way in which patients with schizophrenia can sometimes communicate. It also shows that it is important for you to recognise that first-generation antipsychotics can often cause sexual side effects. Jack's mental state may be deteriorating, but in many cases patients with schizophrenia may express themselves in metaphors (**secondary delusions**) to communicate an issue of importance to them. When Jack said that his medicine had made his genitals disappear, this was his own way of explaining the sexual side effects he was experiencing. For the management of sexual side effects, see Chapter 11.

Non-extrapyramidal side effects of antipsychotics

As has been discussed previously, antipsychotics in general also have affinity for other receptors, such as the muscarinic, histamine and alpha-adrenergic receptors. Each antipsychotic interacts with these non-dopamine receptors in a unique way, and this accounts for each medicine's unique side effects profile. This is a critical point to remember when choosing an antipsychotic. The following sections describe the action of antipsychotics on muscarinic, histamine and alpha-adrenergic receptors, as well as how this causes side effects.

Muscarinic receptors

Muscarinic receptors are in fact acetylcholine receptors that we find in the plasma membranes of some neurons. They have a widespread tissue distribution, particularly in the parasympathetic nervous system, where they exert both inhibitory and excitatory effects. They also play a role in the contraction of smooth muscle, particularly of the airway, ileum, iris and bladder. In addition, they play a role in the secretory glands.

The blockade of muscarinic receptors by antipsychotics causes adverse side effects such as dry mouth, blurry vision, constipation and cognitive blunting. In general, antipsychotics that cause the most extrapyramidal side effects are also known to exert a weak anticholinergic (muscarinic) action. An example of such medicines is the butyrophenones group, which includes haloperidol. However, haloperidol has little or no action on the muscarinic receptors, thus causing few or no cholinergic side effects. This makes butyrophenones such as haloperidol the medicine of choice for patients who are intolerant to muscarinic side effects. By contrast, medicines that cause fewer extrapyramidal side effects tend to cause pronounced cholinergic effects. The phenothiazine group of antipsychotics, such as chlorpromazine, and most second-generation antipsychotics, such as olanzapine, are good examples of these types of medicines.

Due to antipsychotics' antagonism of central and peripheral muscarinic receptors, we may observe antimuscarinic delirium in patients who have taken an overdose of antipsychotics, particularly second-generation antipsychotics. The most offending medications are clozapine, olanzapine and quetiapine, and to a lesser extent risperidone, ziprasidone and aripiprazole. Antimuscarinic toxicity includes hyperthermia, tachycardia, blurred vision, flushed dry skin, absent bowel sounds, urinary retention, agitation, hallucinations, lethargy, mumbling speech, undressing behaviour that is likely to be due to hyperthermia, and repetitive picking behaviour. Blurry vision and photophobia may be due to mydriasis (dilated pupils). Antimuscarinic effects slow down the rate at which food leaves the stomach, potentially prolonging toxicity. Patients may be amnesic to the events. We treat antimuscarinic delirium symptomatically.

Alpha-adrenergic receptors

The adrenergic receptors are a class of receptors that are targets for noradrenaline and adrenaline neurotransmitters. Many body cells possess these receptors, and the excitatory binding of noradrenaline or adrenaline generally causes the 'fight or flight' sympathetic response (see Chapter 4). There are two main groups of adrenergic receptors, alpha and beta, with several subtypes for each group. We are concerned only with the actions of the alpha receptors because of their relevance to antipsychotic treatment. When noradrenaline binds to both alpha-$_1$ and alpha-$_2$ adrenergic receptors, it causes vasoconstriction, leading to an increase in blood pressure and cognitive alertness. Antipsychotic antagonism of these receptors causes dizziness, drowsiness and decreased blood pressure. Low-potency antipsychotics and second-generation antipsychotics antagonise the alpha-$_1$ adrenergic receptors more than the alpha-$_2$ adrenergic receptors.

Histamine receptors

Histamine is a substance that plays a major role in many allergic reactions (see Chapter 4). When histamine reacts with receptors, it alters the body's neurochemistry to make a person more awake and alert. The antagonism of histamine receptors is associated with adverse side effects such as weight gain and drowsiness. In general, low-potency antipsychotics such as chlorpromazine and second-generation antipsychotics such as olanzapine tend to antagonise histamine H$_1$ subtype. Long-term use of many second-generation antipsychotics, particularly clozapine or olanzapine, has an association with weight gain and metabolic syndrome. A putative mechanism is through the antagonising effect of these antipsychotics on H$_1$ receptors in the hypothalamus. During short-term treatment with low-potency or second-generation antipsychotics, antagonising histamine receptors in the hypothalamus rapidly increase calorie intake, resulting in weight gain. In long-term treatment with second-generation antipsychotics, antagonising H$_1$ receptors in the hypothalamus reduce the production of heat in the body (thermogenesis reduction). Additionally, antagonising these receptors may contribute to fat accumulation through simultaneously decreasing the breakdown of fat (lipolysis) and increasing the formation of fat (lipogenesis) in white adipose tissue (He et al., 2013). Recent evidence also points to the role of second-generation antipsychotics in altering the gut microbiome. The suggestion is that second-generation antipsychotic-induced weight gain may be due to their microbiome environment altering effect, though an explanatory mechanism is unclear at this stage (Bretler et al., 2019).

As previously mentioned, excessive weight gain in patients on antipsychotics renders them vulnerable to obesity-related illnesses such as cardiovascular diseases and non-insulin-dependent diabetes. The term *metabolic syndrome* has been used to describe this group of cardio-metabolic risk factors, and a recent meta-analysis found that second-generation antipsychotics such as olanzapine and clozapine were associated with a higher incidence of diabetes in patients (Holt, 2019). In contrast, risperidone and quetiapine were not associated with a higher incidence of developing diabetes. Clearly, metabolic syndrome presents a considerable health risk to patients, and its prevention – or management once it has occurred – is very important (for management, see Chapter 12). Now, before we turn to haematological side effects, test your understanding of antipsychotics by completing Activity 8.6.

Activity 8.6   Critical thinking

Why is olanzapine medication administered mostly before bedtime?

An outline answer is provided at the end of the chapter.

Haematological effects

Case study: Millie

Millie, a 44-year-old Caucasian woman with a history of depression with psychotic symptoms, was admitted to hospital for treatment following a relapse of symptoms. After two weeks in hospital, she was discharged home on lamotrigine, mirtazapine, olanzapine and venlafaxine. Four months later, Millie developed severe ocular cellulitis, severe oral thrush and febrile neutropenia, which necessitated an urgent admission to hospital. On admission, her white blood cell count was 600 cells/mm^3, her absolute neutrophil count was 18 cells/mm^3, and microbial pathogens were isolated in peripheral blood and tracheal aspirate cultures. Despite treatment with antibiotics and filgrastim, Millie developed multiple organ dysfunction and died five days later from septic shock.

Antipsychotic side effects acting on the blood system include an increase or decrease in the number of white blood cells (leucocytosis or leucopenia), which usually occurs between six and eight weeks after antipsychotic initiation, as in the above case study of Millie. This decrease in white blood cells is due to the suppressive effect that some antipsychotics have on the bone marrow. In most cases, this condition is not permanent with most antipsychotic medications, except for clozapine. A life-threatening form of leucopenia is *agranulocytosis*, a condition where the granulocyte-producing ability of the bone marrow is severely diminished. Millie was taking olanzapine, which suppresses the bone marrow's ability to produce granulocytes. Agranulocytosis usually appears within three to four weeks after initiation of antipsychotic medication. It affects people in a dose-dependent manner and affects the elderly and females more severely, as with Millie in the above case study. Its mortality rate can be as high as 30 per cent, with clozapine being the most offending medicine, though olanzapine and phenothiazines such as chlorpromazine pose a significant risk of both neutropenia and agranulocytosis.

Cardiovascular effects

Cardiovascular effects can be a direct result of hypotension and anticholinergic-induced tachycardia, and there is a current concern and a focus on the prevalence of cardiovascular disease (CVD) in people with mental health problems. Although this high prevalence is due to a combination of factors, both lifestyle and biological, it has been known for a long time that antipsychotics have an association with cardiovascular disorders. In general, antipsychotic medicines that have an affinity for the acetylcholine receptors (antimuscarinic or anticholinergic) can cause cardiovascular complications. These include low-potency first-generation medicines, such as chlorpromazine, as well as second-generation antipsychotics. Specifically, second-generation antipsychotic medicines such as olanzapine, risperidone and quetiapine are a chemically diverse group that vary in their effect on the cardiovascular system in both type and degree.

One cardiovascular risk that is common to most antipsychotics is sudden unexpected death. Reports of sudden unexpected death due to antipsychotics began in the early 1960s. There are several mechanisms whereby antipsychotics can cause sudden death. One common mechanism is that antipsychotics cause QT_c elongation, which can lead to *torsade de pointes*. The main feature of *torsade de pointes* is ventricular tachycardia that has distinct characteristics on the electrocardiogram (ECG). Ventricular tachycardia can develop into ventricular arrhythmia, which ultimately leads to ventricular fibrillation and sudden death.

Other cardiovascular effects of all antipsychotics, including second-generation antipsychotics, are low blood pressure, and in rare cases they can cause congestive heart failure and myocarditis. In addition, all second-generation antipsychotics, except for ziprasidone and aripiprazole, increase serum triglycerides to an extent. Specifically, severe high levels of triglycerides (hypertriglyceridemia) occur predominantly with clozapine and olanzapine.

Risk factors for adverse cardiovascular effects that have an association with the use of second-generation antipsychotic medicines include advanced age, autonomic nervous system dysfunction, pre-existing CVD, female gender, electrolyte imbalances (particularly low calcium and magnesium), elevated serum antipsychotic drug concentrations, genetic characteristics, and the psychiatric illness itself (Mutsatsa, 2015) (see Chapter 1).

Neuroleptic malignant syndrome

Case study: Rajiv

Rajiv, a 25-year-old man with paranoid schizophrenia, presented at hospital with an acute psychotic episode after having stopped taking his medication. He reported auditory hallucinations and appeared aggressive and dishevelled, and had loud, pressured speech, disorganisation of thought processes and he believed MI5 had planted listening devices in his bedroom. Because of his condition, he was administered a total of 10 mg of intramuscular haloperidol (5 mg each) injections, as well as requiring physical restraint after he attempted to strike another patient. The following morning, Rajiv was noted to be sweating profusely. His pulse was 140 bpm, blood pressure 145/96 mmHg, respiratory rate 26 breaths per minute and temperature 40°C. Physical examination demonstrated generalised rigidity and trembling in all extremities, and his mental status was consistent with delirium. Levels of serum transaminases (creatine phosphokinase) were elevated, but levels of electrolytes, blood urea nitrogen and creatinine were all within normal limits, and a urine toxicology screen was negative. He was diagnosed with neuroleptic malignant syndrome and all of his medication was discontinued.

Neuroleptic malignant syndrome (NMS), like agranulocytosis, is a potentially fatal side effect of many psychotropic and antipsychotic medications. It can occur any time during treatment, as in the above case study of Rajiv. It has a prevalence of 0.02–3 per cent in patients taking antipsychotics. The main symptoms of NMS are hyperthermia, muscle rigidity, mental status changes, slow movements (bradykinesia) and muscle rigidity, blood pressure instability, profuse perspiration (diaphoresis), tachycardia, and altered consciousness. Rajiv showed most of these symptoms. There are several biochemical abnormalities that accompany NMS, such as high serum levels of the enzyme **creatine phosphokinase (CPK)**, as in Rajiv's case. Other biochemical abnormalities include an increase in **aldolase**, **transaminases** and lactic acid dehydrogenase, a reduction in serum iron concentrations, and the presence of metabolic acidosis and **leucocytosis**. Although there is ongoing debate regarding the diagnosis of NMS, there is general agreement that a patient must show at least four of the following symptoms for a diagnosis of NMS: fever, rigidity, CPK elevation, increased white blood count, altered consciousness, and urinary incontinence. Of these, fever and rigidity must be present, and Rajiv had both.

Although high-potency antipsychotics such as haloperidol have a strong relationship with NMS, all antipsychotics, including first- and second-generation antipsychotics, may precipitate the syndrome. The symptoms of NMS usually evolve over 72 hours, and if there is no treatment they can last 10 to 14 days. Quite often this diagnosis is missed during the early stages as the symptoms are frequently mistake for agitation due to NMS as a worsening of psychosis. NMS affects men more frequently, especially those who are agitated and have received intramuscular injections of antipsychotic medication in high and rapidly escalating doses, as in the case of Rajiv. It especially affects younger men, and the mortality rate can reach 30 per cent or higher with the use of conventional antipsychotics.

The pathophysiology of this serious condition is currently not clear. Multiple factors probably contribute to NMS, including dehydration, co-morbid medical conditions and agitation. Other clinical, systemic and metabolic factors that have an association with NMS aetiology include agitation, poor oral intake, being physically restrained,

Table 8.2 The adverse effect of different antipsychotics on various risk measures (adapted from forest plots by Huhn et al., 2014)

Positive symptoms	Negative symptoms	Weight gain	Akathisia	Prolactin levels	QTC elongation	Sedation	Use of anti-Parkinsonian medication effects	Best choice
AMISULPIRIDE	CLOZAPINE	ZIPRASIDONE	CLOZAPINE	CLOZAPINE	LURASIDONE	PLACEBO	CLOZAPINE	↓ (Best choice at top)
RISPERIDONE	ZOTEPINE	PLACEBO	PERAZINE	ZOTEPINE	BREXPIPRAZOLE	PIMOZIDE	PERAZINE	
CLOZAPINE	AMISULPIRIDE	LURASIDONE	SERTINDOLE	ARIPIPRAZOLE	CARIPRAZINE	PERPHENAZINE.	SERTINDOLE	
OLANZAPINE	OLANZAPINE	ARIPIPRAZOLE	ILOPERIDONE	FLUPENTIXOL	ARIPIPRAZOLE	FLUPHENAZINE	PLACEBO	
PALIPERIDONE	ASENAPINE	HALOPERIDOL	OLANZAPINE	PERAZINE	PLACEBO	CARIPRAZINE	OLANZAPINE	
CHLORPROMAZINE	PERPHENAZINE.	BREXPIPRAZOLE	PLACEBO	CARIPRAZINE	PALIPERIDONE	LEVOMEPROMAZINE	QUETIAPINE	
HALOPERIDOL	RISPERIDONE	CARIPRAZINE	QUETIAPINE	QUETIAPINE	HALOPERIDOL	PENFLURIDOL	ASENAPINE	
ASENAPINE	PALIPERIDONE	CLOPENTHIXOL	BREXPIPRAZOLE	PLACEBO	QUETIAPINE	PALIPERIDONE	LEVOMEPROMAZINE	
PERPHENAZINE	SERTINDOLE	AMISULPIRIDE	ZOTEPINE	BREXPIPRAZOLE	OLANZAPINE	ILOPERIDONE	ARIPIPRAZOLE	
ZUCLOPENTHIXOL	CHLORPROMAZINE	ZUCLOPENTHIXOL.	PALIPERIDONE	PIMOZIDE	RISPERIDONE	MOLINDONE	THIORIDAZINE	
ZIPRASIDONE	ZIPRASIDONE	FLUPENTIXOL	ARIPIPRAZOLE	ZIPRASIDONE	ASENAPINE	SERTINDOLE	AMISULPIRIDE	
SERTINDOLE	ARIPIPRAZOLE	PERAZINE	ZIPRASIDONE	OLANZAPINE	ILOPERIDONE	ARIPIPRAZOLE	ILOPERIDONE	
QUETIAPINE	CARIPRAZINE	MOLINDONE	THIORIDAZINE	ILOPERIDONE	ZIPRASIDONE	AMISULPIRIDE	BREXPIPRAZOLE	
FLUPENTIXOL	QUETIAPINE	LOXAPINE	ASENAPINE	ASENAPINE	AMISULPIRIDE	TRIFLUPERAZINE	PALIPERIDONE	
ARIPIPRAZOLE	LURASIDONE	ASENAPINE	AMISULPIRIDE	CHLORPROMAZINE	SERTINDOLE	BREXPIPRAZOLE	ZIPRASIDONE	
LURASIDONE	HALOPERIDOL	SULPIRIDE	CHLORPROMAZINE	LURASIDONE		LURASIDONE	RISPERIDONE	
CARIPRAZINE	ZUCLOPENTHIXOL.	LEVOMEPROMAZINE	RISPERIDONE	SERTINDOLE		RISPERIDONE	LURASIDONE	
ZOTEPINE	BREXPIPRAZOLE	RISPERIDONE	THIOTIXENE	HALOPERIDOL		FLUPENTIXOL	ZOTEPINE	
ILOPERIDONE	LEVOMEPROMAZINE	TRIFLUPERAZINE	CARIPRAZINE	AMISULPIRIDE		HALOPERIDOL	CARIPRAZINE	
LEVOMEPROMAZINE	ILOPERIDONE	PALIPERIDONE	PERPHENAZINE.	RISPERIDONE		THIORIDAZINE	CHLORPROMAZINE	
BREXPIPRAZOLE	FLUPENTIXOL	CLOZAPINE	LOXAPINE	PALIPERIDONE		ASENAPINE	SULPIRIDE	
PLACEBO	PLACEBO	QUETIAPINE	HALOPERIDOL			LOXAPINE	PERPHENAZINE.	
		ILOPERIDONE	LURASIDONE			OLANZAPINE	MOLINDONE	
		CHLORPROMAZINE	TRIFLUPERAZINE			THIOTIXENE	ZUCLOPENTHIXOL.	
		SERTINDOLE	SULPIRIDE			ZIPRASIDONE	TRIFLUPERAZINE	
		OLANZAPINE	MOLINDONE			QUETIAPINE	FLUPENTIXOL	
		ZOTEPINE	PENFLURIDOL			PERAZINE	PENFLURIDOL	
			PIMOZIDE			CHLORPROMAZINE	LOXAPINE	
			FLUPHENAZINE			SULPIRIDE	FLUPHENAZINE	
			ZUCLOPENTHIXOL.			ZOTEPINE	HALOPERIDOL	
						CLOPENTHIXOL	THIOTIXENE	
						CLOZAPINE	CLOPENTHIXOL	
			FLUPHENAZINE			ZUCLOPENTHIXOL.	PIMOZIDE	Worst choice (at bottom)

pre-existing abnormalities of CNS dopamine activity or receptor function, iron deficiency, traumatic brain injury, sudden stopping of muscle relaxant (dantrolene), and the psychological stress of physical disease.

Seizures

All antipsychotics reduce the seizure threshold to some degree, and therefore seizures are a potential early complication of antipsychotic treatment. Among the first-generation antipsychotics, chlorpromazine appears to have the greatest association with seizure risks; and among the second-generation antipsychotics, clozapine is the most likely to cause seizures. Risperidone, fluphenazine, pimozide, haloperidol and trifluoperazine seem to be the least likely antipsychotics to induce seizures. However, the use of antipsychotics in people with epilepsy does not seem to increase seizure frequencies, according to a case-controlled study of 450 patients (Okazaki et al., 2014).

However, the practical risk of seizures is low, being 0.5–0.9 per cent of all patients taking antipsychotic treatment. Rapid increase of dosage (upward titration) is a risk factor, and others include CNS disease and electroencephalogram (EEG) abnormalities. Low starting doses, use of minimum effective doses, and avoidance of unnecessary antipsychotic polypharmacy are strategies that may lower the risk of seizure provocation associated with these medicines.

Long-term depot medication

Soon after the introduction of antipsychotics in the 1950s, poor adherence to oral medication was found to be a critical issue. This led to the development of long-acting injectables, or 'depot injections'; the first depot injections were fluphenazine enanthate and fluphenazine deconoate. Clinical trial results showed a dramatic reduction in the morbidity of schizophrenia. However, initially, the idea of depot injections for schizophrenia was not received enthusiastically by the mental health profession because of worries about an increase in side effects and a lack of efficacy. Also, this was perceived as an attempt to impose treatment upon patients without due respect for their feelings or human rights. In addition, there were concerns about the potential for medico-legal problems. However, subsequent surveys and trials provided evidence of their benefits (Schooler et al., 1980). Several studies have reported advantages of long-acting depot injections over oral medication in terms of relapse prevention and adherence. A meta-analysis of ten randomised trials showed a significant reduction in relapse rates with the use of depot as opposed to oral medication (Leucht et al., 2011), and a smaller systematic review found that long-acting depot formulations outperformed oral antipsychotics in terms of discontinuation due to inefficacy and non-adherence (Kishi et al., 2016). Medication discontinuation rates with oral antipsychotics can reach 74 per cent in comparison with 33 per cent for second-generation depot injection (Marcus et al., 2015). A further study found that risk of rehospitalisation for patients receiving long-acting depot injections was about one-third of that for patients receiving equivalent oral medications (Tiihonen et al., 2011). Table 8.3 provides some of the advantages and disadvantages of using long-term depot injections.

Despite the advantages that depot injections offer, a negative attitude among clinicians towards these formulations is common, particularly in the prescribing for those with first-episode psychosis. A survey of 891 European psychiatrists and nurses revealed that 96 per cent preferred depot injection to oral treatment for patients with chronic schizophrenia, whereas only 40 per cent preferred them for first-episode patients (Geerts et al., 2013). In respect to patients, a systematic review of 12 studies found that the most positive attitudes were seen in those already prescribed long-term depot injection, and patients said that they 'feel better', have a more 'normal life' and find injections 'easier to remember' (Waddell and Taylor, 2009). The positive attitude of staff correlated closely with the extent of their knowledge of long-term depot antipsychotics (Waddell and Taylor, 2009). However, evidence suggests that staff do not fully inform patients about long-term depot injections and tend to make treatment decisions without consulting patients or caregivers (Potkin et al., 2013).

Among pharmacological interventions that aim to enhance adherence, recent guidelines propose a switch to long-term depot injection if the patient lacks insight, has co-morbid substance use, has persistent symptoms, logistic problems, lack of routines or of family/social support that makes adherence to oral antipsychotics problematic (Kane and Garcia-Ribera, 2009). Table 8.3 shows the pharmacokinetic and clinical features of common depot injections in clinical use.

Table 8.3 A summary of potential advantages and disadvantages of long-acting injectable antipsychotics as compared with oral antipsychotics (adapted from Brissos et al., 2014)

Advantages of depot injection	Disadvantages of depot injection
1. No need for daily administration.	1. Low dose titration.
2. Guaranteed administration and transparency of adherence.	2. Longer time to achieve steady-state levels.
3. Allows healthcare professionals to be alerted and to intervene appropriately if patients fail to take their medication.	3. Less flexibility of dose adjustment.
4. Less probability of rebound symptoms and rapidly occurring/abrupt relapses.	4. Delayed disappearance of distressing and/or severe side effects.
5. Overcomes partial adherence or overt non-adherence.	5. Pain at the injection site can occur and leakage into the subcutaneous tissue and/or the skin may cause irritation and lesions (especially for oily long-acting injectables).
6. If a relapse occurs, it is due to other reasons beyond non-compliance.	
7. Reduced risk of unintentional or deliberate overdose.	
8. Minimal gastrointestinal absorption problems, circumventing first-pass metabolism.	6. Burden of frequent travel to outpatient clinics or home visits by community nurses for their administration.
9. More consistent bioavailability.	
10. More predictable correlation between dosage and plasma levels.	7. Risperidone long-acting injectable needs refrigeration, which may be cumbersome in some latitudes.
11. Reduced peak-trough plasma levels.	
12. Improved patient outcomes.	
13. Improved patient satisfaction.	8. Perception of stigma.
14. Regular contact between the patient and the mental healthcare team.	

Special considerations

Clozapine

Clozapine is one of the original second-generation antipsychotics, but it was withdrawn from the market in 1975 because of haematological safety concerns, particularly agranulocytosis. This was partly due to the release of alarming reports of agranulocytosis in Finnish patients that created panic among prescribers. A total of 17 patients had agranulocytosis and eight of these died. Clozapine was immediately withdrawn. However, since 1989, it has enjoyed a renaissance for the management of treatment-resistant schizophrenia under strict blood monitoring systems. In a multicentre double-blind study of patients who were not responsive to antipsychotics, Kane et al. (1988) found that at least 30 per cent of patients prescribed clozapine improved in comparison to only 4 per cent who were treated with chlorpromazine. This superiority was subsequently reported in later studies, including in patients who had failed to improve on two or more antipsychotics (Lewis et al., 2006), as well as its superiority over quetiapine and risperidone (Stroup et al., 2009). Other purported advantages of clozapine over other antipsychotics include a reduction in suicide (Kasckow et al., 2011) and a reduction in aggression and violence (Frogley et al., 2012).

As a second-generation antipsychotic, clozapine antagonises serotonin ($5HT_{2A}$) receptors and weakly antagonises dopamine D_2 receptors, but interestingly it has a higher affinity for non-dopamine receptors such as alpha-adrenergic, histamine and muscarinic, in comparison with its affinity for dopamine D_2 receptors. This may partly explain clozapine's tendency to be effective with minimal extrapyramidal side effects.

The risk of agranulocytosis (1–2 per cent) that clozapine poses is managed by a mandatory monitoring of blood to assure that patients undergo routine blood testing before each dispensation. National Institute for Health and Care Excellence (NICE) guidelines mandate that service providers such as GPs, community health services, mental health services and hospitals ensure that there are procedures and protocols in place to monitor the prescribing of clozapine for adults with schizophrenia (NICE, 2015c).

We initiate clozapine therapy gradually (usually 12.5 mg per day); monitoring of vital signs is essential and should be at least hourly for the first six hours because of clozapine's hypotensive effects. However, this monitoring is not necessary if we give the first dose at night. It is important to inform the prescriber if the patient experiences the following: body temperature rises above 38°C, pulse of over 100 bpm (a sign of myocarditis), postural blood pressure drop of 30 mmHg (a sign that the patient is clearly sedated), or any other intolerable side effect. If the patient is tolerant of clozapine, increase the dose gradually until you reach a dose of 300 mg per day. Where sedation is an issue, slower titration is necessary. Because around 2 per cent of patients on clozapine treatment develop **neutropenia**, it is important to maintain a normal white blood cell count (WBC) and an absolute neutrophil count (ANC) at safe levels (WBC should be greater than 3,500 per mm³ and ANC should be greater than 2,000 per mm³) throughout treatment. This allows the identification of patients at risk of developing

Table 8.4 Pharmacokinetic and clinical features of the most commonly used depot antipsychotics injection (adapted from Brissos et al., 2014)

Name	Vehicle	Dose range (mg)	Administration interval (weeks)	Time to achieve peak plasma concentration (days)	Half-life (days) (multiple dose)	Time to steady state (weeks)	Injection site	Storage
Fluphenazine decanoate	Sesame oil	12.5–100	1–4	0.3–1.5	14	3	Gluteal muscle	15–30°C
Flupenthixol decanoate	Viscoleo	10–50	2–4	7	17		Gluteal muscle	15–30°C
Zuclopenthixol decanoate	Viscoleo	200–400	2–4	4–7	7–19	8	Gluteal muscle	15–30°C
Haloperidol decanoate	Sesame oil	50–400	4	3–9	21	8–12	Gluteal muscle	15–30°C
Risperidone long-acting	Water (microsphere polymers suspension)	25–50	2	28	4–6	8	Gluteal or deltoid muscle	2–8°C (up to 25°C for one week)
Paliperidone palmitate	Water (suspension of nanoparticles)	25–150	4–12		25–49		Gluteal or deltoid muscle	15–30°C
Olanzapine pamoate	Water (microcrystalline suspension)	150–300	2 or 4	2–4	14–30	8–12	Gluteal muscle	15–30°C
Aripiprazole long-acting	Water (microparticles)	300–400	4	5–7	29–46	12	Gluteal muscle	

agranulocytosis and neutropenia before the conditions become life-threatening. In fact, the implementation of registries for the monitoring of haematological toxicity has significantly contributed to a reduction in mortality and morbidity in patients on clozapine treatment.

Asenapine

Asenapine is one of the newer second-generation antipsychotics, and it has a chemical structure like that of mirtazapine. Like mirtazapine, it antagonises a range of serotonin receptor subtypes, including $5HT_{2A}$, $5HT_{2C}$, $5HT_7$ and $5HT_5$. Theoretically, this suggests that asenapine may have some antidepressant properties and may be suitable for psychotic patients with concomitant depression.

Additionally, indirect evidence, mainly from animal studies, suggests that asenapine has a high affinity (antagonistic property) for a range of alpha-adrenergic (α), histamine (H) and dopamine receptor subtypes. It antagonises dopamine D_4 more than D_2 receptors. It has a low antagonistic action on the muscarinic–cholinergic receptors, suggesting that it is less likely to cause side effects such as constipation, dry mouth and urinary retention. Further studies on asenapine receptor activity suggest that it has an upregulating effect on dopamine D_1-like receptors (Tarazi et al., 2008). This finding is important because some evidence suggests that the upregulation of dopamine D_1 and D_2 receptors has links with a reduction in the likelihood of extrapyramidal symptoms (Tarazi et al., 2008). This is a unique property of asenapine as no other antipsychotic significantly upregulates dopamine receptors. However, a systematic review of eight randomised clinical trials, including 3,765 patients, that compared asenapine with placebo or olanzapine found asenapine to be of similar or superior efficacy to placebo. Further, asenapine was similar or inferior to olanzapine on most efficacy outcomes. It demonstrated fewer adverse metabolic outcomes than olanzapine, though rates of extrapyramidal symptom-related adverse effects were higher with asenapine (Orr et al., 2017). Overall, we require more naturalistic studies to determine the effectiveness of asenapine in relation to other antipsychotics.

We normally administer asenapine sublingually, because if we give it orally the stomach extensively metabolises it before absorbing it into the bloodstream, so its bioavailability via the oral route is negligible. Because of its rapid absorption when we give it sublingually, there is the suggestion that it is possible to use it as an oral rapid tranquillisation medicine without resorting to an injection. However, one potential adverse effect of sublingual administration of asenapine is a reduction in oral sensitivity (hypoesthesia). It is important to advise the patient not to eat or drink for ten minutes following sublingual administration of asenapine, to avoid the medicine being washed out of the sublingual absorption sites into the stomach where extensive first-pass metabolism of the medicine takes place.

As with most antipsychotics, asenapine has a black box warning that it may increase mortality in older adults with dementia-related psychosis. In long-term treatment with asenapine, common adverse side effects are weight gain, insomnia, sedation, somnolence, gastrointestinal symptoms and akathisia. These side effects are usually mild to moderate.

Olanzapine pamoate

Olanzapine long-acting injection, or olanzapine pamoate, is one of three second-generation antipsychotics now available. It is a microcrystalline salt of pamoic acid and olanzapine suspended in an aqueous solution that slowly dissociates into the separate components after intramuscular injection into gluteal muscle. Olanzapine depot injection can achieve efficacy in the short term, and for maintenance treatment of people with schizophrenia at doses of 150–300 mg every two weeks or 405 mg every four weeks. The overall side effects profile of the depot formulation is like that of oral olanzapine. Injection site complications are mild. However, there is a 0.07 per cent chance of developing post-injection delirium/sedation syndrome (PDSS) after injection. The symptoms of PDSS evolve over a period of hours, during which the olanzapine plasma concentrations rise. The symptoms are very similar to an oral olanzapine overdose; we can categorise them into delirium (which manifests as disorientation), confusion, ataxia, difficulty in articulating words (dysarthria), irritability, anxiety and aggression. The other part of PDSS symptoms is sedation-related adverse effects such as sleepiness (somnolence), sedation, or other changes in the level of consciousness. The presence of PDSS symptoms has led to a PDSS event that requires a 'risk management plan'. There are several safety measures that can help reduce the risk of PDSS events. The most obvious precaution is using the proper injection technique to prevent olanzapine pamoate monohydrate from contacting the blood system. For gluteal injections, the needle of choice is a 35 mm 19G needle (1{1/2} inches), or a 50 mm needle (2 inches) for obese patients, allowing an application deep into the muscle. During the procedure, the nurse should place emphasis on the proper aspiration to allow removal of the syringe when blood is visible. If a blood vessel is punctured, it is important to withdraw the syringe and repeat the injection technique into an alternate injection site.

Since the time of onset of symptoms associated with PDSS varies individually, the current recommendation is that an appropriate healthcare professional (nurse) should observe the patient for a three-hour period after administration. The nurse should monitor vital signs during this period and report any signs of PDSS symptoms. Furthermore, the nurse should ask the patient not to drive or operate machinery for that day, and the patient should be advised to be attentive for potential symptoms and call for assistance if needed.

Common treatment errors to avoid

The long-term use of antipsychotics, and second-generation antipsychotics specifically, has a strong link with weight gain and CVD. The nurse should screen patients for a familial history of metabolic and cardiovascular disorders. Weigh the patient before they start antipsychotics to find out if they are already overweight or obese. A body mass index (BMI) of greater than 25 indicates that the person is overweight. If a patient gains more than 5 per cent of their initial weight, discuss switching to another second-generation antipsychotic such as aripiprazole or lurasidone (see Table 8.2).

Most antipsychotics can cause hypotension, so it is important to check blood pressure before commencing antipsychotics and regularly for a few weeks afterwards. Also, patients can suffer hypotension after the administration of intramuscular short-acting low-potency antipsychotics. To avoid such an occurrence, advise the patient to lie on their back (supine position) for 30 minutes after administration. Take the patient's blood pressure before and after each intramuscular dose. Patients on olanzapine pamoate depot injection can suffer PDSS, and it is important to observe and record their vital signs for the first three hours after injection.

Akathisia is an extremely uncomfortable side effect, frequently misdiagnosed as psychotic agitation. It is important to routinely assess for the presence of akathisia, particularly in those prescribed high-potency antipsychotics. Patients taking antipsychotics and experiencing emotional blunting can be misconstrued as having negative symptoms or as being depressed. We should use anticholinergic medication only to alleviate extrapyramidal side effects; excessive use or abuse can cause toxic psychosis. Monitor patients' fluid intake and be particularly vigilant for urinary retention in older patients. Abrupt discontinuation of an antipsychotic is only necessary in situations that have the potential to cause sudden death or severe adverse reactions. The nurse should advise patients that sudden withdrawal of medication can cause discontinuation syndrome, which involves several symptoms, including nausea, vomiting, diarrhoea, cold sweats, and muscle aches and pains. Movement disorder (withdrawal dyskinesia) can appear within the first two to three weeks after discontinuation. Withdrawal dystonia, Parkinsonism and akathisia are known to occur within days of discontinuation.

What the patient needs to know

- You should explain to patients that most psychotic illness and schizophrenia are relapsing conditions, and taking medication regularly is important to prevent relapse. Even if someone is in remission, it is necessary to emphasise the importance of continual medication-taking to act as an insurance against relapse.
- It is important that you tell the patient the name of the medication, the dosage, and the number of times the medicine is to be taken. You should emphasise the importance of taking medication with food or soon after mealtimes to avoid gastrointestinal irritation. Patients prescribed lurasidone should take their medicine with at least 500 calories of food for the medicine to be effective.
- Antipsychotic medications are not addictive, but coming off them should be done slowly to avoid unpleasant complications such as antipsychotic rebound syndrome. You should encourage the patient to speak to the prescriber if they wish to stop taking antipsychotics.

- You should explain in simple terms, depending on the level of the patient's understanding, the likely side effects that the patient may suffer. You should explain extrapyramidal side effects such as akathisia, tardive dyskinesia, dystonia and Parkinsonism, particularly for those prescribed first-generation antipsychotics.
- You should inform patients in their first episode of illness that treatment is likely to be for a year, but treatment for those who have had two or more episodes is likely to be indefinite, as stated by the NICE guidelines (NICE, 2014).
- You should explain to the patient the role of psychostimulants, such as cocaine, amphetamines and cannabis, in triggering or worsening psychosis.
- If medication to alleviate extrapyramidal side effects is prescribed, it should be continued for a few weeks after antipsychotics have been discontinued.
- You should inform the patient that because antipsychotics can cause cardiac arrhythmia, they can be fatal if taken in overdose.
- Most antipsychotics can cause drowsiness due to their effect on histamine receptors. You should warn the patient not to drive a car or operate machinery while taking antipsychotic medication.

Chapter summary

Schizophrenia is the most common of all psychotic disorders and perhaps the most widely investigated. It affects 0.1 per cent of the population. The most common types of symptoms for schizophrenia are hallucinations, delusions, thought disorder, bizarre behaviour, negative cognitive deficits, and affective symptoms.

Some medicines and many physical illnesses can cause psychotic symptoms. Positive symptoms of schizophrenia are due to an increase in dopamine activity in the synapse in the striatal region of the brain. This is corrected by antagonising postsynaptic dopamine D_2 receptors with antipsychotics. Apart from antagonising postsynaptic receptors, dopamine also blocks other regions and receptors in the brain, giving rise to adverse side effects. The older first-generation antipsychotics cause more extrapyramidal side effects by antagonising dopamine D_2 receptors in the nigrostriatal pathway. The newer second-generation antipsychotics have a better, more tolerable side effects profile than conventional forms, but they still have worrying side effects such as sedation and weight gain. Antipsychotic medications are generally started at low doses and titrated up to minimise side effects. The multiple receptor binding profile of second-generation antipsychotics has been linked to these medicines causing cardio-metabolic problems. Clozapine is effective for people who have responded poorly to other antipsychotics. Blood should be taken regularly to monitor for neutropenia. The medicines to prescribe should be driven by the patient's preference and lifestyle.

Activities: brief outline answers

Activity 8.1 Critical thinking (page 225)

Electrolyte imbalance will generally cause toxic confusional states, particularly in the elderly.

Activity 8.2 Decision-making (page 225)

You should recommend a thyroid function test. She is restless and thought disordered, which are common signs of psychosis due to excess thyroxine. Thyrotoxicosis is a genetically inheritable disease.

Activity 8.3 Critical thinking (page 232)

She is on a high dose of haloperidol, which is likely to induce extrapyramidal symptoms such as akathisia, Parkinsonism, dystonia and tardive dyskinesia. More importantly, haloperidol has a very strong affinity for dopamine D_2 receptors and will block a considerable amount of these receptors in the mesocortical region, therefore worsening her negative symptoms. To improve the situation, suggest an alternative such as a second-generation antipsychotic or a third-generation partial agonist such as aripiprazole.

Activity 8.4 Critical thinking (page 234)

Out of the three, the medication you would expect to cause sexual dysfunction is haloperidol because it is a potent dopamine receptor antagonist in the tuberoinfundibular pathway.

Activity 8.5 Critical thinking (page 236)

Dave is most likely experiencing akathisia: he is young, taking a conventional antipsychotic, and his restlessness coincided with the initiation of trifluperazine. In this case, a change of antipsychotic may be the best course of action. If this is not possible, Dave can be given beta blockers or benzodiazepines in the short term.

Activity 8.6 Critical thinking (page 243)

Apart from its antipsychotic effect due to its antagonism of D_2 receptors, olanzapine blocks histamine and alpha-adrenergic receptors, giving rise to drowsiness. If given at night, it can have the dual role of relieving psychotic symptoms and helping a person to sleep. By contrast, if olanzapine is given during the daytime, its sedative effects can interfere with normal social functioning.

Further reading

Stahl, S.M. (2013) *Stahl's Essential Psychopharmacology: The Prescriber's Guide*, 4th edition. Cambridge: Cambridge University Press.

This is a comprehensive guide to psychopharmacology that is clearly written and has good illustrations.

Taylor, D.M., Barnes, T.R.E. and Young, A.H. (2018) *The Maudsley Prescribing Guidelines in Psychiatry*, 13th edition. London: Informa Healthcare.

This is a very useful, easy-to-understand, evidence-based prescribing and general medicines management manual. It is particularly useful for prescribers.

Useful websites

www.bnf.org

The *British National Formulary* (BNF) is very useful for finding out about drug information, including normal dosages, interactions and side effects.

www.medicines.org.uk/emc

This website supplies very detailed information on medicine side effects and interactions.

www.rethink.org

This very useful website publishes material on service users and carers of people with serious mental illness.

Chapter 9 Management and treatment of dementias

Chapter aims

By the end of this chapter, you should be able to:

- outline the main clinical features of dementia;
- describe anti-dementia medication and its mechanism of action, as well as recognising its side effects;
- describe common mistakes to avoid and communicate necessary information to patients in the treatment of dementia.

Introduction

Case study: Marjorie

Marjorie is 68 years old and retired from her job as a personal secretary after 45 years. She noticed that driving long distances confused her; she frequently forgot how to get to her destination, and because of this she stopped driving altogether. Her troubles with memory deteriorated so much that coping with the activities of daily living (ADLs) became progressively more difficult. Her short-term memory had deteriorated significantly, though her long-term memory was still intact. She suffered gastrointestinal problems that led to dramatic weight loss, causing her to be depressed. Recently, she was rushed to hospital after she found it difficult to walk or talk; she was weak and unable to absorb food properly.

After several investigations, doctors could not find the cause of Marjorie's gastrointestinal problems but took a particular interest in the results of an MRI scan. This

(Continued)

257

(Continued)

and her non-existent short-term memory led the doctor to conclude that Marjorie was suffering from Alzheimer's disease. Because of her deteriorating physical and mental health, her only daughter moved in with her to look after her full-time. Her daughter was able to slow down Marjorie's deterioration by monitoring what she ate and how often. The good care provided by her daughter was essential for her survival. However, Marjorie's condition continued to deteriorate, though gradually, which had a hugely stressful effect on her daughter. Because of this, Marjorie was admitted to a nursing home where her daughter now regularly visits her.

Dementia is any decline in cognition that is significant enough to interfere with independent, daily functioning, and it is best characterised as a syndrome rather than one disease. Although dementia is far more common in the older population, it may occur at any stage of adulthood. It is a non-specific illness that affects areas of cognition, memory, attention, language or problem-solving, as in the above case study of Marjorie. A useful way to classify different types of dementia is into one of three categories: reversible, non-progressive or progressive (Rabins et al., 2008). To diagnose dementia, symptoms should normally be present for at least six months; but if cognitive dysfunction has been present for only a short time, especially less than a week, we must call this delirium. Further, research suggests that dementia may develop in individuals over the course of decades. If this view is correct, then dementia is a disease that most people are in the process of developing throughout adulthood. There are several types of dementia, including Alzheimer's disease, Pick's disease, Lewy body dementia (LBD), vascular dementia, Huntington's disease, Parkinson's disease, and trauma- and HIV-induced dementia. Of these, Alzheimer's disease is the most prevalent form of dementia, constituting over 70 per cent of all cases, and for this reason this chapter mainly focuses on Alzheimer's disease.

The chapter briefly reviews the mechanisms underlying Alzheimer's disease, first describing the common clinical features of the condition, before discussing the treatment and care of people with dementia. The final section covers treatment errors to avoid, as well as what you as a nurse need to discuss with patients who have dementia and their carers.

Alzheimer's disease

In 1907, Alois Alzheimer first described the illness that later assumed his name. According to experts, without the introduction of disease-modifying treatments, Alzheimer's disease is poised to increase rapidly throughout the world; current estimates are that it will quadruple over the next 40 years to affect one in every 85 people.

Alzheimer's disease is a devastating neurodegenerative disease and the predominant form of dementia, accounting for 50–75 per cent of all types of dementia. In 2015, approximately 44 million people worldwide were estimated to have Alzheimer's disease or a related dementia. Each year, 4.6 million new cases are predicted, with numbers expected to almost double by 2030 and to reach 131 million by 2050 (Lilford and Hughes, 2018). There are over 800,000 people with Alzheimer's dementia currently living in the UK, with an estimated cost of £23 billion to the NHS and associated care agencies.

Although the cause of Alzheimer's disease is currently uncertain, genetic factors play an important part, and in this regard it is possible that Marjorie's condition has a genetic basis. Approximately 40 per cent of people with Alzheimer's disease have a family history of dementia. Also, the concordance rate for illness in monozygotic (identical) twins is high (43 per cent), compared with that of dizygotic twins (8 per cent).

The role of molecular genetics in Alzheimer's disease has been confirmed with the discovery of fully penetrant mutations of the *amyloid precursor protein (APP)*, *presenilin-1 (PSEN1)* and *presenilin-2 (PSEN2)* genes explaining 5–10 per cent of the occurrence of early-onset alzheimer's disease. This supports the earlier discovery of the gene variant *ε4 of apolipoprotein E (APOE)* a quarter of a century ago as a strong genetic risk factor for Alzheimer's disease. More recently, the identification of at least 21 additional genetic risk loci for the more genetically complex form of Alzheimer's disease re-emphasised the multifactorial nature of Alzheimer's disease (Carmona et al., 2018).

Other risk factors of developing Alzheimer's disease include being female, having a first-degree relative who has the disorder, and having a history of head injury. The brain of an individual with Alzheimer's disease is characterised by shrinkage (atrophy) and an enlargement of cerebral ventricles. The current thinking is that the neurotransmitters acetylcholine and noradrenaline are underactive in people with Alzheimer's disease. Cholinergic antagonists (e.g. atropine) impair, whereas cholinergic agonists (e.g. physostigmine) enhance cognitive abilities.

The cognitive dysfunctions in dementia include general intelligence, learning, memory, language, problem-solving, orientation, perception, attention, concentration, judgement, and social ability, as in the above case study of Marjorie. Alzheimer's disease can also affect an individual's personality, and it is mostly progressive and permanent.

Amyloid cascade and neurofibrillary theory

This theory originated from early findings of profound acetylcholine neural loss in people with Alzheimer's dementia. The death of these acetylcholine neurons is brought about by *amyloid plaques*. Amyloids are an aggregation of low molecular weight proteins that form plaques outside neurons (see Figure 9.1). These plaques interfere with the normal biochemical function of the neurons, causing conditions such as inflammation of the neuron and the release of toxic chemicals, including cytokines and free radicals. Further, these amyloid plaques induce the conversion of cell microtubules into tangles, which will result in neuronal cell dysfunction that ultimately leads to neuronal cell death. Other changes include synaptic degeneration, hippocampal neuronal loss, and an abnormal number of chromosomes in a cell.

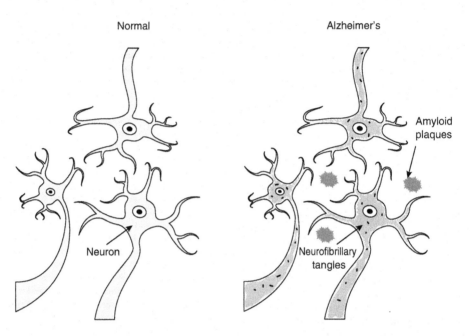

Normal vs. Alzheimer's Diseased Brain

Figure 9.1 Normal neurons and Alzheimer's neurons with amyloid plaques and neurofibrillary tangles

Much investigation has focused on neurofibrillary tangles (see Figure 9.1). These are intracellular masses containing abnormally formed and excessively **phosphorylated** tau protein. We see tau protein mainly in the central nervous system and neurons, and its function is to stabilise cell microtubules. In phosphorylated tau protein, there is alteration to the tau's normal function due to gene mutation. This is associated with frontotemporal dementia (FTD), especially in cases with coexistent Parkinsonism. FTD is an uncommon type of dementia that starts early in an individual's life (from 45 years upwards) and causes problems with behaviour and language. Despite the genetic and cell-biological evidence that supports the amyloid hypothesis, it is becoming increasingly clear that Alzheimer's disease aetiology is complex, and that the amyloid plaque theory alone is unable to account for all aspects of Alzheimer's disease.

Clinical features of Alzheimer dementia

Case study: David

David is a 58-year-old man who worked as a painter and decorator for most of his life. He is married with three grown-up children and five grandchildren. Recently, his wife noticed that David was doing 'silly things' without realising it. On several occasions, he had been paid cash for his work, and when his wife asked him about the money he would have no idea what she was talking about. Sometimes David would leave the money in the car or lose it completely. He would often get irritable for no reason. Lately, he has had problems remembering the names of his children. It was at this point that David saw his GP and was referred to a specialist who diagnosed Alzheimer's disease.

Alzheimer's disease pathology accumulates years before the onset of clinical symptoms and has been termed 'preclinical dementia'. Thus, the onset of the disease is insidious and symptoms manifest themselves slowly over a period of years, as is apparent in the above case study of David. In the initial stages of the illness, patients show fatigue, difficulty in sustaining mental performance, and a tendency to fail when a task is new, complex or requires a shift in problem-solving strategy. One of the early prominent and classical signs in people with Alzheimer's disease is memory impairment. The case of David's forgetfulness is typical of someone showing early signs of Alzheimer's disease. The individual loses the ability to perform ADLs, such as shopping, managing finances or using the telephone, early in the course of the illness, while they lose abilities such as eating and grooming at later stages. Patients in residential care with dementia can forget how to get back to their rooms after going to the toilet. Also, those with Alzheimer's and vascular dementia can suffer difficulties in language processing, which can be characterised by vague, imprecise or **circumstantial speech**. They may have difficulties in naming objects and may also undergo personality changes that can be profoundly disturbing for the patient's family. The patient may become quite introverted and show no concern for their relatives, or they may become very hostile towards them. Patients with frontal and temporal lobe dementia may experience marked changes in their personality, which include being explosive and irritable. It is estimated that up to 30 per cent of patients with Alzheimer's disease experience hallucinations, and up to 40 per cent have paranoid delusions and are generally hostile to their families. In the end, people with dementia will need supervision and assistance with ADLs, which may be particularly distressing. Therefore, identification of ADLs that are important to the patient and their family is paramount in order to tailor treatment and management to target these activities. More importantly, in collaboration with the patient and their carers, it is crucial to periodically revisit the issue of which activities are most important, as priorities may change over the course of treatment. People with dementia face a gradual but downward progression of disease symptoms, with an average timescale from onset of illness to death of between eight and ten years.

Care and management of people with dementia

Many of the effective treatments for dementia focus on increasing the availability of the neurotransmitter acetylcholine in the brain synapses. Acetylcholine is broken down by two enzymes – acetylcholinesterase and butylcholinesterase – into the inactive compounds choline and acetate. Inhibiting (disabling) these enzymes will result in the accumulation of acetylcholine in the cholinergic system, rendering more acetylcholine available for neurotransmission. An increase in the levels of acetylcholine in the cholinergic system improves memory and cognitive ability. It therefore follows that substances which block (antagonise) acetylcholine receptors in normal humans produce memory disturbances such as those seen in Alzheimer's disease. An example of such a substance is scolopamine. Overall, an important approach to nursing intervention is to tailor interventions around the recovery approach.

At first glance, we may think that the current emphasis on promoting 'recovery' has little relevance to people with dementia. However, there are striking similarities between the values and aspirations of the recovery model and the principles of person-centred care that guide dementia care in the NHS. In this regard, we aim to promote people's capacity to care for themselves for as long as they can do so. One way that we can achieve this is by combining pharmacological with non-pharmacological approaches, which is what we will look at next.

Non-pharmacological approaches to the care of people with dementia

There is considerable debate about the quality of nursing home care for people with dementia. The care at traditional nursing homes often focuses on physical care, keeping residents safe, and preventing healthcare problems (Foebel et al., 2016). However, in recent years, there has been more emphasis on a psychosocial and more home-like care concept, with increasing interest in values such as quality of life, autonomy, and striving to allow residents of nursing homes to continue the life they had before admission as much as possible (Tolson et al., 2011). Policies, strategies or frameworks launched in many countries aiming at improving the quality of care and quality of life for people with dementia now reflect this change. Caring for a person with dementia is a complex task that requires paying attention to a variety of physical, psychological, emotional, social and informational needs of the person, as well as those of their formal and informal caregivers.

Life expectancy is more emphatically curtailed by dementia than it is by other mental health syndromes, yet the evidence for suboptimal care persists, especially in the later stages of the illness. In an early retrospective survey of carers in England, McCarthy et al. (1997) reported a host of common signs and symptoms experienced by people with dementia in the last year of life: confusion, urinary incontinence, pain, low mood, constipation and loss of appetite. The study found similar frequencies of such symptoms in cancer patients, but people with dementia experienced the symptoms for longer.

People with dementia tend to have difficulties with nutritional intake, and these can be present even during the early stages of the illness. The impact of poor nutrition is profound, and this may be due to an inability to request food or drink, feed themselves, and recognise food, due to refusing to eat or having significant problems with swallowing food. While it is difficult to reverse the problem of malnutrition in people with late-stage dementia, treating malnutrition to maintain or slow down deterioration that may be due to poor nutrition is critical. It is important to bear in mind that older people with dementia generally have a lower body mass index (BMI), and this is usually associated with higher frequency and severity of behavioural problems.

Bladder and bowel function are compromised, and incontinence of urine is common, which itself can threaten skin integrity, causing discomfort. Seek advice from a continence specialist as this can often be helpful. Constipation, which can sometimes lead to faecal impaction or overflow incontinence, can occur when the diet or fluid intake is poor, or when medication slows bowel transit times. Immobility and a reduction of awareness of the call to stool make matters worse. Constipation itself impedes bladder function, and discomfort, pain or toxicity can follow. The person may become more confused or more agitated. A common sign of constipation is the tendency to lean to one side. Therefore, it is important to incorporate strategies that reduce the risk of constipation, such as adequate fluid intake, encouraging a high-fibre diet and promoting exercise.

General levels of functioning need attention, and providing the right amount of support is necessary to allow as much independence as possible while still maintaining the person's dignity. In addition to physical care, non-pharmacological care of people with Alzheimer's disease includes techniques that help to compensate for cognitive losses, such as employing the use of memory books, which contain important pieces of information that may be forgotten by the affected patient, as well as environmental modifications that promote intellectual functioning (e.g. improvements in lighting, the establishment of a quiet environment). Individualising the non-pharmacological care of people with Alzheimer's disease according to the stage of deterioration the patient is at is important. Paying attention to the patient's safety, even in the early stages, and the use of technology can be particularly useful, as illustrated in the following case study.

Case study: Peter

Peter is a 76-year-old man who was diagnosed with Alzheimer's disease soon after his wife died a year ago. It was reported on several occasions that Peter was found outside during the day wearing pyjamas, appearing disorientated and in need of reassurance. After the diagnosis, his only daughter, who lived about 80 miles away, visited him frequently but found it increasingly difficult and was becoming distressed. Because of the safety risk Peter presented, an electronic device with a recording of his daughter's voice was installed at his front door. This voice device was activated every time he approached the front door, telling him not to go out and to wait for the home care staff to arrive. There were no reports of Peter wandering outside the house distressed after the device was installed. His daughter reported reduced levels of stress and distress.

As the above case study shows, we can usefully employ technology to assist people with dementia. Helpful equipment is available that may support the independence of people with dementia (see the useful websites at the end of the chapter). Assistive technology not only allows people with dementia to live more independently; it may also help to support and reassure their carers, as in the above case of Peter's daughter. As much as assistive care is helpful, it is not the answer for every patient with dementia. In the main, it can be useful for those patients who are still in the early stages of the illness. Patients in the early stages of the disease may also benefit from being discouraged from performing certain ADLs in which they have shown impairment (e.g. lighting a gas cooker, using a telephone).

However, as patients progressively deteriorate to the later stages of Alzheimer's disease, deficits in cognition and functioning become more profound. At this stage, it may be appropriate to introduce pharmacological interventions to focus on behavioural disturbances. Before you proceed further, try Activity 9.1.

Activity 9.1   Critical thinking

Good physical healthcare is very important in people with dementia.

*   What are the key physical healthcare interventions required to optimise patient well-being?

An outline answer is provided at the end of the chapter.

Pharmacological approaches to dementia

Cholinesterase inhibitors have a useful place in arresting the rate of memory and cognitive decline in patients. The only cholinesterase inhibitors approved for the treatment of Alzheimer's disease are donepezil, galantamine and rivastigmine. The N-methyl-D-aspartate (NMDA) receptor antagonist memantine is the only non-cholinesterase inhibitor approved for the treatment of Alzheimer's disease.

Cholinesterase inhibitors

Randomised placebo-controlled clinical trials of cholinesterase inhibitors have included patients with mainly mild to moderate Alzheimer's disease, and have shown significant benefits with respect to cognition, daily function and behaviour. The condition of patients who are taking these medicines can remain stable for a year or more, and then it may decline, though at a rate that is slower than that of untreated patients. In other words, although these medicines may not be able to arrest intellectual decline in patients, they are able to slow down the rate at which deterioration takes place.

The European Federation of Neurological Societies (EFNS) has published recommendations for the diagnosis and management of Alzheimer's disease. Based on available research evidence, treatment with cholinesterase inhibitors is recommended even for mild or early disease; no specific cholinesterase inhibitor is recommended over another (Hort et al., 2010). In 2006, the American Association for Geriatric Psychiatry (AAGP) published practice recommendations that also emphasised treatment with approved medications for cognitive symptoms, as well as symptomatic treatment for neuropsychiatric manifestations, such as depression and psychosis, and issues related to safety, such as driving, living alone and medication administration (Lyketsos et al., 2006). In the UK, National Institute for Health and Care Excellence (NICE) guidelines recommend that the three acetylcholinesterase inhibitors – donepezil, galantamine and rivastigmine – are options in the management of patients with Alzheimer's disease of mild to moderate severity only (NICE, 2018a). Before you proceed to the next section, try Activity 9.2.

Activity 9.2 Critical thinking

Albert is a 72-year-old man with Alzheimer's disease who is known to have enjoyed music and dancing in his youth. He is currently quite restless and agitated for no obvious reason.

* How might you get Albert to be settled and less agitated?

An outline answer is provided at the end of the chapter.

All currently available cholinesterase inhibitors (donepezil, galantamine and rivastigmine) show some evidence of a beneficial effect on patients with respect to ADLs. *Donepezil* is mainly used to increase levels of acetylcholine in the cortical region of the brain and therefore improve a patient's cognition. Furthermore, donepezil may improve a patient's behavioural disturbances, such as apathy, depression, anxiety and disinhibition. It is recommended as a treatment option for people with mild to moderately severe Alzheimer's disease only, and it has no effect on people suffering from vascular dementia. It can take up to six weeks before any improvements in the patient's memory can be noticed. In many cases, the degenerative process of Alzheimer's disease can take several months to arrest. NICE guidelines recommend that only specialists in dementia should prescribe and review these medicines (NICE, 2011). The prescriber should carry out a review of the patient's treatment every six months. Also, it is important to always seek the views of the carer. The normal doses for this medicine are 5 mg per day, and this can be increased to 10 mg per day.

Galantamine has been used for decades in Eastern Europe and the Soviet Union for various indications, such as the treatment of sensorimotor dysfunction associated with disorders of the CNS. It is a selective, competitive and reversible inhibitor of acetylcholineesterase and is suitable for the symptomatic treatment of people with mild to moderately severe Alzheimer's disease. It has been found to be effective in vascular dementia as well (Chen et al., 2016). In addition, galantamine enhances the action of acetylcholine on nicotinic receptors, thereby improving cognition in people with dementia. The maintenance dosage is 16–24 mg per day.

Rivastigmine is an acetylcholinesterase and butyrylcholinesterase inhibitor, licensed in the UK. It was developed by Marta Weinstock-Rosin in Israel and is useful in the symptomatic treatment of people with mild to moderately severe Alzheimer's disease. Rivastigmine has been shown to provide meaningful symptomatic effects that may allow patients to remain independent and 'be themselves' for longer. In particular, rivastigmine appears to show marked positive treatment effects in patients showing a more aggressive form of Alzheimer's disease, such as those with a younger age of onset or a poor nutritional status, or those experiencing symptoms such as delusions or hallucinations (Gauthier et al., 2006). For example, the presence of hallucinations appears to be a predictor of especially strong treatment response to rivastigmine, both in Alzheimer's disease and other illnesses such as Parkinson's disease (Kandiah et al., 2017). These effects might reflect the additional inhibition of butyrylcholinesterase, which is implicated in symptom progression and may provide added benefits over medicines that selectively inhibit acetylcholinesterase. The usual maintenance dosage is 3–6 mg twice per day, taken with food to minimise incidences of nausea.

All cholinesterase inhibitors can cause similar side effects; the most common are nausea, vomiting, appetite loss, increased gastric acid secretion, weight loss, insomnia and dizziness. These side effects tend to occur early during the treatment process and most are transient. For general side effects management, see Chapter 12. This medicine can exacerbate asthma or other pulmonary diseases. Donepezil can be lethal in overdose and can cause a cholinergic crisis, which is characterised by nausea, vomiting, salivation, sweating, bradycardia and hypotension, followed by increased muscle weakness, respiratory depression and convulsions. If there is the suspicion that someone has taken an overdose of donepezil, it is important to notify the prescriber without delay. The most likely treatment for donepezil toxicity is 1–2 mg of atropine intravenously, and this dose can be increased depending on the condition of the patient.

Non-cholinesterase inhibitor memantine

Memantine is an NMDA receptor antagonist that blocks the effects of unusually elevated levels of glutamate which may lead to neuronal dysfunction. Its use is in the treatment of people with moderate to severe dementia. For example, a 28-week double-blind study involving patients with moderate to severe Alzheimer's disease found that patients receiving 20 mg of memantine per day experience substantially slower functional deterioration than patients treated with a placebo, as measured by changes in ADLs (Reisberg et al., 2003). Significantly, a Cochrane systematic review concludes that memantine has a beneficial effect on CNS activity and is a potential treatment for Alzheimer's disease, as well as for vascular and mixed dementia (McShane et al., 2019). It is also purported to have a beneficial effect on cognitive function in patients with moderate to severe Alzheimer's disease and those with vascular dementia. More notably, its adverse effects profile and tolerability are good, and agitation is less common with memantine. Therefore, glutamate antagonist treatment with memantine can reduce clinical deterioration in people with moderate to severe Alzheimer's disease. However, memantine's effect on people with mild to moderate Alzheimer's disease is unclear. The recommended maintenance dosage is 10 mg twice per day.

Much debate surrounds the use of combination therapy of cholinesterase inhibitors with memantine. An industry-sponsored systematic review suggests that combination therapy of memantine and donepezil is effective, safe and well tolerated, and may represent a gold standard for the treatment of moderate to severe Alzheimer's disease (Patel and Grossberg, 2011), as well as improving patient adherence to medication and reducing caregiver burden (Calhoun et al., 2018). However, NICE guidelines do not recommend combination treatment with memantine and AChE inhibitors because of a lack of evidence of additional clinical efficacy over and beyond that with memantine monotherapy (NICE, 2018b). Overall, there seems to be a lack of robust evidence for the use of combination therapy despite its use in clinical practice. This rather unclear situation may be because the clinical heterogeneity that is present in Alzheimer's disease makes it unlikely that any single drug will have a large effect size. This means that optimal drug treatment may involve multiple drugs, each having an effect size that may be less than the minimum clinically important difference (McShane et al., 2019).

Because of the limited efficacy of current medicines for dementia, the development of novel medicines with strong disease-modifying properties represents one of the greatest challenges in modern medicine. Ongoing preclinical studies in academic as well as industrial settings focus on many potential molecular targets involving the pathogenesis of Alzheimer's disease.

Unfortunately, behavioural and psychiatric symptoms typically increase with disease progression in people with Alzheimer's disease. The most experienced symptoms tend to be anxiety, depression and psychotic symptoms. As such, it is important to take account of the presence of these symptoms in the care of people with Alzheimer's disease, and we will look at this next.

Management of the psychiatric symptoms of dementia

Not surprisingly, available evidence suggests that depression is very common in people with Alzheimer's disease. At least 25 per cent of patients are likely to experience depression at the time of, or just before, the onset of the illness. In patients for whom medication is appropriate, selective serotonin reuptake inhibitors (SSRIs) are the medication of choice in order to avoid prescribing tricyclic antidepressants (TCAs), because their anticholinergic effects can cause or worsen confusion (see Chapter 6). Also, TCAs' cardiotoxic profile makes them unsuitable for use in older people. Before continuing, try Activity 9.3.

Activity 9.3   Critical thinking

Jan is an 86-year-old lady with Alzheimer's disease. You notice that her dietary intake has been poor lately and that she is restless. Also, you notice that her stomach is slightly distended and that she has been refusing to take medication.

- How might you encourage her to take medication and food?

An outline answer is provided at the end of the chapter.

According to the Alzheimer's Society (2018), at least 90 per cent of people with dementia also experience behavioural and psychological symptoms, such as aggression, loss of inhibitions, agitation, delusions, hallucinations and irritability. But the occurrence of these behavioural and psychological symptoms early in the course of illness also raises the possibility of an alternative diagnosis, such as dementia with Lewy bodies (DLB). These symptoms can be distressing for the person and their carers, as well as putting the person at risk. To overcome the problem, *cautious* treatment with antipsychotics can be helpful because they are associated with serious side effects (see Chapter 8). A systematic review of 47 studies found that the use of antipsychotics in this population is disproportionately associated with cerebrovascular events, hip fracture, pneumonia and death (Pratt et al., 2012). In this regard, the prescribing of antipsychotics in this population should be accompanied by a plan to aggressively manage side effects in the event of their occurrence (for side effects management, see Chapter 12). The next section deals with the importance of providing support to caregivers; but before you move on, try Activity 9.4.

Activity 9.4   Decision-making

Ahmed, a third-year student nurse, was on practice learning experience in a nursing home. One day, at lunchtime, he noticed Jeff, a resident, using his hands instead of cutlery to eat with. Ahmed rightly thought that Jeff was having problems using cutlery, so he assisted him with his meal. However, he was stopped from assisting Jeff by the staff nurse, who insisted, 'Jeff is doing all right'.

- Do you agree with the staff nurse's view? If so, why?

An outline answer is provided at the end of the chapter.

Caregiver support

The Alzheimer's Society estimates that there are about 850,000 people in the UK acting as primary carers for people with dementia (**www.alzheimers.org.uk**). Evidence suggests that carers of people with dementia experience greater stress than carers of other older people (Anand et al., 2016). This comes as no surprise, as caring for an individual with Alzheimer's disease can be a physically and emotionally draining experience that can bring irreversible changes to people's lives and relationships. Depression, emotional and physical exhaustion, and general poor health are common in carers. Many carers of people with dementia are old themselves, with physical frailty and health conditions of their own. Routinely offering support assistance with day-to-day caring and access to respite and short breaks, support groups, online groups, as well as assistance with financial benefits such as the carer's allowance, is important.

Important points to consider

Prior to commencing medication, you should ensure that the patient has undergone a full physical check-up, which may include full blood count, liver function test, electrolytes and kidney function. Ensure that medication is taken with food to avoid gastrointestinal irritation. Good fluid intake is also very important and should be encouraged. If possible, the use of TCAs should be avoided in older people because of their tendency to cause drowsiness and constipation. If they are to be prescribed, they should be administered at night to minimise the incidence of daytime sedation. If antipsychotics are prescribed, this should only be for a short duration; you need to be particularly vigilant for the occurrence of adverse side effects and manage these aggressively. Older people are particularly sensitive to the disabling effects of extrapyramidal side effects (see Chapter 7).

What the patient and carers need to know

- Alzheimer's dementia is a progressively deteriorating illness that affects a person's memory and cognitive abilities.
- There is currently no cure for Alzheimer's disease and other related dementias, but there are some treatments that can temporarily help with some of the symptoms.
- It is common for people with dementia to have poor dietary intake; therefore, patients should be encouraged to eat more and to follow a good diet to help with general well-being.
- Poor physical health is very common in people suffering from dementia. Patients may be taking medication for physical health conditions in addition to medicines to relieve symptoms of dementia. Check for medicine interactions and inform relatives where appropriate.

Chapter summary

Dementia is a condition that is characterised by gradual memory and cognitive impairment, mostly in elderly people. There are many forms of dementia but the most common is Alzheimer's disease, and the prevalence of this illness is set to increase fourfold in the next 40 years. Alzheimer's disease is thought to be caused by a reduction in acetylcholine in the brain. Therefore, the treatment of Alzheimer's disease symptoms aims to correct acetylcholine deficiency, and this is achieved by using cholinesterase inhibitors. Donepezil, galantamine and rivastigmine are the main cholinesterase inhibitors used in the treatment of Alzheimer's disease. In addition to patients suffering symptoms of dementia, they may also experience depression and other mental health problems. Therefore, it is important for you to be vigilant for the presence of these problems. You should also use non-pharmacological approaches to supplement the use of medicines and involve carers in the treatment of people with dementia.

Activities: brief outline answers

Activity 9.1 Critical thinking (page 264)

You should ensure a good diet and sufficient fluid intake, adequate sleep, adequate exercise during the day that involves adequate mental stimulation, and good oral hygiene. Always promote good bowel movements (e.g. high-fibre diet, fluids, exercise) to limit the chances of constipation.

Activity 9.2 Critical thinking (page 265)

It is quite possible that Albert is bored. The use of multidimensional activities can be very useful in this situation. He is known to be interested in music, so activities along these lines might be helpful.

Activity 9.3 Critical thinking (page 268)

It is important to assess whether Jan is constipated or not. Constipation is relatively common in the elderly. Jan has a distended stomach, restlessness and a poor appetite; all of these can be signs of constipation. Initially, you should promote good bowel movements by encouraging exercise, a high-fibre diet and plenty of fluids.

Activity 9.4 Decision-making (page 269)

The staff nurse is correct. It is important for dementia patients to retain their independence as much as possible. Although Jeff has lost the skill to use cutlery, at least he has not lost the skill to feed himself using his hands without assistance. The aim is to promote independence as much as possible.

Further reading

Martin, G. and Sabbagh, M. (2010) *Palliative Care for Advanced Alzheimer's and Dementia: Guidelines and Standards for Evidence-Based Care.* New York: Springer.

This is a very good book that offers practical advice for those looking after people with advanced dementia.

Mittelman, M. (2003) *Counseling the Alzheimer's Care Giver: A Resource for Healthcare Professionals.* Chicago, IL: American Medical Association Press.

This book is useful for those who intend to give carers support, advice and information.

Useful websites

www.alzheimers.org.uk

This is a very useful website that provides information about dementia in general, and particularly Alzheimer's disease, including care and treatment and current research breakthroughs.

www.atdementia.org.uk

This website brings together information about assistive technology that has the potential to support the independence and leisure opportunities of people with dementia.

www.carersuk.org

This website provides a forum for carers in the UK. Carers can share their experiences with other carers and professionals alike.

Chapter 10 Management and treatment of anxiety disorders

Chapter aims

By the end of this chapter, you should have knowledge and understanding of:

- the pathophysiological mechanisms underpinning anxiety disorders and the mechanisms of action underpinning anti-anxiety medicines;
- how to manage the side effects of anti-anxiety medication and of common errors to avoid in the treatment of anxiety disorders;
- what information to communicate to patients and carers.

Introduction

Case study: Amy

Just before she sat her A levels, Amy experienced a state of uneasiness and worry because she feared failing. In addition to worry and fear, she experienced poor concentration and poor appetite. Her experiences impacted on her studies in several ways. She was continually in a state of anxiety and sometimes had panic attacks. She found it difficult to leave her house as she was worried about having a panic attack on the journey to school. In addition, Amy encountered difficulties with concentration on her work in class. She felt too embarrassed to tell her teachers about the problem, and as a result she did not do well in her exams. After the exams, however, she continued to worry, even about things she considered minor, and she was unable to stop herself from worrying. Much later, she sought help from her GP and was diagnosed with anxiety and referred for counselling.

In common parlance, 'anxiety' is an unpleasant state of mental uneasiness or concern about some uncertain event, or a state of restlessness and agitation like that experienced by Amy in the above case study. A distressing sense of oppression or tightness in the stomach may accompany anxiety. The disorder of anxiety probably existed long before recorded history and is not unique to human beings, although human anxiety appears to be the most complex. The earliest interpretations of anxiety disorders appear to be mostly spiritual; early spiritual treatments of the disorder somewhat resemble modern psychotherapies. It is also interesting that ancient and traditional natural remedies for anxiety have some surprising similarities to modern medicines.

Anxiety and anxiety disorders have played substantial roles in human history, most prominently in times of hardship, war or social change. However, in more pleasant times, societies tend to embrace the illusion that anxiety is a minor issue that deserves little attention or respect, and ignore it easily. Lack of interest in the fundamental nature of anxiety has often left societies ill-prepared for unforeseen challenges.

Anxiety disorders are common worldwide, affecting one in every 14 people at any point in their lives. The prevalence rates are significantly higher in populations exposed to conflict than in non-conflict situations. An anxiety disorder generally starts early in life and follows a repetitive, intermittent course, causing substantial disability in terms of health loss, role impairment, and disadvantage across the lifespan in areas such as income, education and interpersonal relationships. In fact, anxiety is the sixth leading cause of disability, in terms of Years Lived with Disability (YLDs) in all countries (Baxter et al., 2014). In addition, 7 per cent of all suicide mortality was estimated to be attributable to anxiety disorders (Baxter et al., 2013). Women are more likely than men to develop an anxiety disorder throughout their lifespan; they have a lifetime prevalence rate of 40 per cent in comparison with men, who have a lifetime prevalence rate of 26 per cent (Kessler et al., 2012). Genetic factors seem to play a part in the aetiology of the disorder, with epidemiological studies reporting heritability estimates of between 30 and 50 per cent. At a molecular genetic level, a meta-analysis of studies across different ethnic populations identifies three genes (MFAP3L on 4q32.3, NDUFAB1, and PALB2 on 16p12) implicated in anxiety disorders (Otowa et al., 2014). There is good evidence suggesting that there are significant anatomical changes in the brain related to anxiety neurocircuitry in those suffering from the condition. For example, there is an increase in grey matter volume in the amygdala, especially the right amygdala volume, in females with generalised anxiety disorders (Maron and Nutt, 2017). In addition, living in an urban environment, marital status, socio-economic disadvantage, relationship difficulties, and exposure to violence, trauma and conflict are associated with a higher incidence of anxiety.

Anxiety is a normal emotion under threatening circumstances, and we believe it to be part of the evolutionary 'fight or flight' reaction to aid survival. Not only is it normal to be anxious; it is also adaptive. From a biological perspective, a balance normally exists between the pathophysiological mechanisms that produce neural excitation and those that produce neural inhibition. In such cases, anxiety levels remain within normal limits. If this balance is lost, as in Amy's case, anxiety becomes problematic and psychiatric symptoms develop. This chapter initially provides an overview of anxiety symptoms and how they arise before discussing in more depth the medicines we use to treat anxiety and their management. The final sections discuss common treatment errors to avoid, and what patients and carers need to know.

Symptoms of anxiety

Freud's fundamental notions of the psychological origin of anxiety dominated aetiological explanations of the disorder in the early part of the twentieth century. In his theory, Freud suggests that anxiety disorders are a result of an unconscious perception of danger. Such unconscious judgements involving potential danger provoke 'signal anxiety' and trigger defensive operations. When these defensive operations fail, the patient experiences symptoms of anxiety. One other dominant psychological explanation of anxiety originates from Beck (1976), who suggests that anxiety is generated when people overestimate danger or underestimate their coping ability. Although these psychological theories were developed before biological explanations were formulated, the two have converged to form the behavioural neuroscience of anxiety. The core symptoms of anxiety are excessive fear and worry, which is the next point of discussion.

Within the systems of humans exists a complex network of nerve pathways and endocrine glands that are responsible for initiating the fight or flight response in a dangerous situation. When a person perceives a threat, the body shuts down non-essential physiological processes (e.g. digestion, reproduction) and directs energy to a variety of essential bodily functions in preparation for fast action. The nervous system goes into a state of hyper-stimulation and alertness. All of these changes happen very quickly and automatically, and these actions are an adaptive evolutionary response to ensure our survival. Anxiety involves several neurotransmitters in different parts of the brain.

The neurotransmitters involved in anxiety

To understand how medicines for anxiety work, an appreciation of the involment of neurotransmitters is important in this condition. A revision of the anatomy involved is necessary, and you may wish to revisit Chapter 3.

The three main neurotransmitters involved in anxiety are gamma-aminobutyric acid (GABA), serotonin and noradrenaline. As discussed in Chapter 3, GABA is the key inhibitory neurotransmitter and it plays a role in the reduction of activity of many neurons in the brain, including those that we find in the amygdala. There are three major types of GABA receptors and numerous subtypes. The major types are $GABA_A$, $GABA_B$ and $GABA_C$ receptors. When neurons are in an excited state and fire rapidly, GABA slows down this excitation to 'normal' by binding to its own receptors (see Figure 10.1b). In other words, GABA works as the body's own natural anti-anxiety medicine.

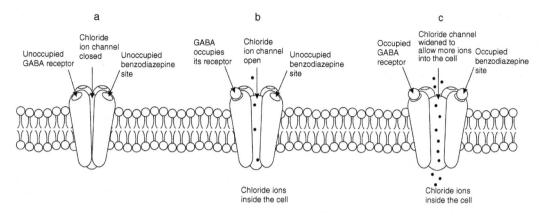

Figure 10.1 Chloride ion channels at different levels of opening

The anti-anxiety effect of GABA increases when a benzodiazepine medicine binds to the $GABA_A$ receptor (see Figure 10.1c). Thus, benzodiazepines only exert their therapeutic effect in the presence of the GABA neurotransmitter. If the GABA neurotransmitter is absent, benzodiazepines alone have no effect on neurons. Furthermore, benzodiazepines only exert a therapeutic effect on synaptic $GABA_A$ receptors and have no effect on the $GABA_B$ or $GABA_C$ receptors. In summary, benzodiazepines enhance the inhibitory action of postsynaptic $GABA_A$ receptors. This theoretically reduces amygdala and cortico-striatal-thalamo-cortical (CSTC) loop hyperactivity, resulting in blunting fear and worry associated outputs.

The role of serotonin

Earlier in this chapter, we looked at the overlap in symptoms of depression and anxiety; not surprisingly, the neural circuitry of these two disorders also overlap. It is also not surprising that the neurotransmitter serotonin links both depression and anxiety symptoms. Serotonin is involved in the regulation of mood, impulse control, sleep, vigilance, eating, libido, and cognitive functions such as memory and learning. Serotonin is present in the amygdala neurons as well as all the elements of CSTC circuits, namely the prefrontal cortex, the striatum and the thalamus. In other words, we find serotonin in both the fear and worry circuits. It is the shortage of a serotonin subtype ($5HT_1$) in key areas of the brain, such as the hippocampus, the amygdala, and the anterior cingulate cortex and raphe nuclei, that contributes to these anxiety symptoms. This partly explains why selective serotonin reuptake inhibitors (SSRIs) have become the first-line treatment for people with anxiety (see Chapter 6).

The role of noradrenaline

The third neurotransmitter involved in anxiety is the excitatory neurotransmitter noradrenaline. Excessive output of noradrenaline in the *locus coeruleus* part of the brainstem (see the next section on the amygdala and the generation of fear) can result in symptoms of anxiety such as fear, flashbacks, panic attacks, sweating and night-mares. Currently, the hypothesis is that alpha$_1$ and beta$_1$ adrenergic receptors may have specific involvement in these reactions. Studies of fear conditioning consistently demonstrate that the amygdala has a critical involvement in the formation, consolidation and recovery of associative fear memory.

The amygdala and the generation of fear

Neuroimaging studies in humans confirms the central role of the amygdala in fear, though other brain networks, such as the anterior cingulate cortex, the hippocampus, the insula and the ventral medial prefrontal cortex (vmPFC), are also involved. The amygdala integrates emotional and cognitive information from the environment and then determines whether to evoke a fear response. In the presence of a threat, the amygdala activates the hypothalamus and the sympathetic nervous system. It also triggers a variety of biological processes, including the production of cortisol, thyroxine and adrenaline. Further, the activation of the amygdala also triggers a burst of neural stimulation in the locus coeruleus part of the brainstem with connections to the limbic system. Neurons that control fear are mediated by various neurotransmitters and hormones, including serotonin (5HT$_1$), glutamate, GABA, noradrenaline and corticotrophin-releasing hormone (CRH).

The cortico-striatal-thalamo-cortical loop and the generation of worry

The second core symptom of anxiety is worry, which involves feelings of anxiousness, misery, apprehension, catastrophic thinking and obsession. The CSTC feedback loop, which originates in the frontal cortex, mediates the symptom of worry. Several neurotransmitters and regulators, including serotonin, GABA, dopamine, noradrenaline, glutamate and voltage-gated ion channels, modulate this loop. In a normal person, the excitatory neurotransmitter glutamate transmits impulses from the frontal cortex, which leads to neural excitation in the striatum. Striatal activation triggers the inhibitory neurotransmitter GABA to transmit impulses to the **globus pallidus interna** (GPi) and the substantia nigra (SNr) (see Figure 10.2). This decreases GABA output from the GPi and the SNr to the thalamus, resulting in the triggering of excitatory glutamate output from the thalamus to the frontal cortex. This direct pathway is a positive feedback loop.

In an indirect external loop, the GABA from the striatum inhibits the **globus pallidus externa** (GPe). In turn, the inhibition of the GPe lessens the production of GABA in the subthalamic nucleus (STN). The decreased production of GABA frees the excitatory glutamate from the STN to excite the GPi and SNr. Exciting the GPi and SNr promotes the production of GABA, which will then inhibit the thalamus (see Figure 10.2). In patients with obsessive-compulsive disorder (OCD), the direct pathway is more hyperactive than the indirect pathway. The hyperactivity in the frontal cortex increases with symptom severity but decreases following successful treatment.

In addition to these functional abnormalities seen in people with anxiety, structural volumetric and grey matter density abnormalities are present in the aforementioned structures. In summary, symptoms of worry are therefore associated with malfunctioning of the CSTC loops that are regulated mainly by glutamate and GABA. Serotonin, dopamine, noradrenaline and voltage-gated ion channels are also involved in their regulation.

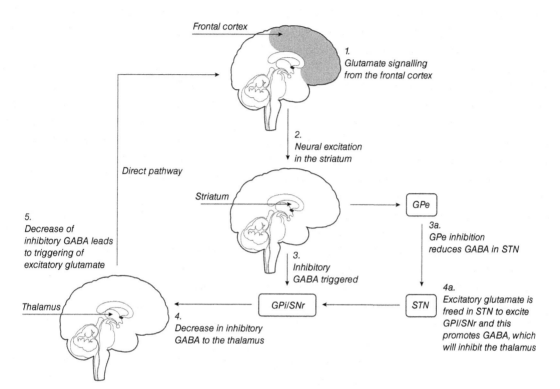

Figure 10.2 The CSTC loop in anxiety

In general, patients with anxiety experience some of the following symptoms: trembling, feeling shaky, restlessness, muscle tension, shortness of breath, smothering sensation, rapid heartbeat (tachycardia), sweating and cold hands and feet, lightheadedness, dizziness, tingling of the skin, frequent urination, diarrhoea, feelings of unreality, difficulty in falling asleep, impaired attention and concentration, and nervousness. Some of these symptoms are present in one type of anxiety but may not be present in another – a complex situation that we will now turn to.

The overlapping symptoms of anxiety

Anxiety disorders encompass a broad group of psychiatric problems and – like depression – have many underlying causes. This results in different types of anxiety disorders, and they all have a great deal of symptom overlap. Some forms of anxiety appear to have a clear relationship to biochemical abnormalities, while others seem to have a mainly psychological or emotional origin. Also, anxiety disorders tend to occur in tandem with other psychiatric disorders, such as depression, schizophrenia, and substance use and bipolar disorders. There are at least six different types of anxiety disorder, as listed below:

- generalised anxiety disorder (GAD);
- phobias;
- panic disorders;
- obsessive-compulsive disorder (OCD);
- post-traumatic stress disorder (PTSD);
- social anxiety/phobia.

Although there are different diagnostic criteria for different anxiety disorders, these diagnostic criteria are constantly changing, and many authorities no longer consider OCD to be an anxiety disorder. However, as previously mentioned, all anxiety disorders have the overlapping symptoms of fear and worry. What differentiates one anxiety subtype from another may not be the anatomical localisation of the neurotransmitter regulating fear and worry in each of the anxiety subtypes, but the specific nature of the malfunctioning within these similar circuits.

For example, in GAD, the malfunctioning of the loops in the amygdala and the CSTC may be persistent but not severe. In panic disorder, the malfunction may be intermittent, unexpected and catastrophic. In PTSD, the malfunction may be traumatic in origin, or the circuits may be trapped in a redundant repetitive loop such as in OCD.

In addition to fear and worry, each anxiety subtype has its own specific symptoms. For example, people suffering from GAD may also experience irritability, muscle tension, arousal, fatigue, poor concentration and sleep disturbance. Those suffering from panic disorder normally experience unexpected panic attacks and phobia or behavioural change, in addition to the core symptoms of fear and worry. Symptoms of social anxiety disorder (also called social phobia) normally include the expectation of panic attacks and phobic avoidance of the anxiety-provoking situations. In PTSD, the characteristic symptoms in addition to the core symptoms include the traumatic experience being relived, as well as worry about having other symptoms such as an increase in arousal, sleep difficulties such as nightmares, and avoidance behaviours. Obsessive-compulsive disorders include the core symptoms of fear and worry, which tend to trigger obsessions and compulsions to reduce the worry and the obsessions themselves.

Nurses will not only come across people with these different kinds of anxiety, but also people with different physical illnesses that have given rise to anxiety. It is to these illnesses that we now turn.

Physical illnesses associated with anxiety

It is important to be aware of the possibility that patients with the following conditions will also experience anxiety at some level:

- angina pectoris;
- cardiac arrhythmias;
- CNS degenerative disease;
- Cushing's syndrome;
- delirium;
- hyperthyroidism;
- hypoglycaemia;
- Ménière's disease.

Before you read any further, try Activities 10.1 and 10.2.

Activity 10.1 Critical thinking

The experience of anxiety is common to most people and it can be beneficial.

- At what point does anxiety become a problematic emotion?
- Name the two symptoms that are common to all anxiety disorders.

An outline answer is provided at the end of the chapter.

Activity 10.2 Critical thinking

Chris is a 26-year-old man who has an excessive fear of vomiting in public places. He is aware that his fear is irrational; nevertheless, he cannot stop himself worrying about vomiting in public places. Lately, his mood has been low because he is now socially restricted. He is not sure what medication he can benefit from and asks your advice.

- What is your advice to Chris?

An outline answer is provided at the end of the chapter.

Modern treatment of anxiety

Working in partnership and taking a shared decision-making approach is very important when working with people with anxiety disorders. While medication is helpful, it is not the only treatment option, as demonstrated later in this chapter, but information on medication must include potential side effects. It is important to provide patients, families and carers with information on self-help and support groups where appropriate. Before reading on, try Activity 10.3.

Activity 10.3 Communication

Use the internet to search for self-help groups and organisations in your area that help people suffering from anxiety. Make a list of the services they provide.

- If you were a patient who does not have internet access, how would this information be available to you?

An outline answer is provided at the end of the chapter.

For many common mental health disorders, the National Institute for Health and Care Excellence (NICE) advocates a stepwise approach to their management, offering – or referring people for – the least intrusive and most effective intervention first (NICE, 2016). Many patients with anxiety will choose psychological treatments. These include stress management, cognitive behavioural therapy (CBT), relaxation training, meditation, psychotherapy, and eye movement, desensitisation and reprocessing (EMDR) therapy. Where there is a need for medication, there are four main types of medicines available. Before we discuss these treatment options in more detail, read the following case study.

Antidepressants

Case study: Greg

Greg is a 40-year-old married artist with three children. He was diagnosed with pneumonia after a spell of feeling unwell. The doctor told him that he was lucky to be alive, and this made Greg very anxious that he had an illness which could have killed him. Although he recovered well from the pneumonia, he started experiencing dizzy spells – at times vertigo – and weakness, and he was sure his heart was weakening. Before long, his wife was rushing him to A&E because he was sure he was having a heart attack. The doctor examined him but pronounced him fit and healthy. Despite the doctor's pronouncement, he deprived himself of sleep, because he feared that if he slept he would have a heart attack and never wake up. This went on for so long that his behaviour was affecting his relationship with his family. He could not go too far away from home, where he felt safer. Greg continued to believe that there was something wrong with his heart, despite continual reassurance from a specialist doctor who carried out thorough investigations. Greg was finally referred to a psychiatrist who diagnosed Greg with GAD and prescribed 50 mg of sertraline per day. His psychiatrist referred him to a clinical psychologist where he had eight sessions of CBT. Towards the end of the sessions, Greg's condition improved so that he was able to go back to work part-time.

There is a growing body of evidence that antidepressants are effective in the treatment of primary anxiety disorders, as demonstrated in the above case study of Greg. They tend to work on the fear network by slowing down the action of the neurons. They have been extensively researched, and SSRIs such as sertraline are commonly considered the first-line treatment, particularly for GAD (NICE, 2011). Sertraline is the best medicine in limiting discontinuation due to side effects and the second-best medicine in achieving response in patients not discontinuing treatment due to side effects (Mavranezouli et al., 2013).

A systematic review and meta-analysis of 27 trials found several antidepressants, including fluoxetine, duloxetine, sertraline and escitolapram, to be effective in the treatment of GAD in terms of tolerability, response and remission (Baldwin et al., 2011). Another meta-analytic study of 57 trials ($n = 16,056$) also concluded that SSRIs and selective noradrenaline reuptake inhibitors (SNRIs) offer the the greatest incremental improvement from baseline. We see the greatest treatment benefits for both SSRIs and SNRIs in social anxiety disorder. Higher doses of SSRIs, but not SNRIs, are associated with significantly greater symptom improvement and likelihood of treatment response (Jakubovski et al., 2019).

Second in line in terms of effectiveness are the SNRI antidepressants mirtazapine and SNRIs. If treatment is unsuccessful with these medications, we can use tricyclic antidepressants (TCAs). Antidepressants seem to be effective in reducing the symptoms of GAD in the medium to long term.

When to consider antidepressants for anxiety disorders

Clinical situations in which antidepressants are more likely to be considered as the initial treatment for anxiety disorders include:

- post-traumatic stress disorder, obsessive-compulsive disorder;
- generalised anxiety disorder, social anxiety disorder (possibly in combination with a benzodiazepine);
- presence of a co-occurring depressive disorder or a history of depression;
- predominance of cognitive aspects of pathological anxiety (e.g. pathological worry);
- current or past alcohol or other substance misuse/dependence, concern about benzodiazepine dependence and misuse.

Before we discuss the next group of medicines used to treat anxiety, try Activity 10.4.

Activity 10.4 Critical thinking

A patient on your ward is suffering from GAD and the doctor has prescribed 40 mg of fluoxetine to be taken at night. A staff nurse later approaches the doctor and asks them to correct the mistake.

- What do you think the error could be?

An outline answer is provided at the end of the chapter.

Case study: Mavis

Mavis is 28 years old and recently gave birth to a baby girl by caesarean section after developing birth complications. After the birth of her child, she felt a little run-down, but she put this down to tiredness and the difficult time she experienced giving birth. Gradually, she began to worry about the health and safety of her newborn baby and the frequent trips she was making to the hospital. One day when she was shopping for groceries in her local supermarket, she began to feel a little unwell but pushed on with her shopping. By the time she got to the checkout, she was feeling uncomfortably stressed. She felt a tremendous sense of impending dread. Putting it down to tiredness, she continued unpacking her items from the trolley. That was when the first attack hit her. She could not breathe; her heart raced and felt like it would explode. Her legs almost crumpled under her, and she desperately wanted to run out of the shop, scream or grab somebody to help her. She did not know what was happening to her. All she knew was that she felt like she was going to die. She grabbed the items she needed, threw them into a bag, somehow managed to toss some cash at the operator, and fled from the shop. Back in the car, she settled down a little, but she still felt terrible. She slowly drove home, but by the time she pulled into her driveway she felt almost her old self again. She promptly forgot about the ordeal after a day or so. Unfortunately, this pattern of events repeated itself several times until she sought medical help. She was diagnosed with panic disorder and was initially prescribed 2 mg of clonazepam twice per day and 10 mg of fluoxetine once per day in the morning. Mavis experienced relief from her symptoms within three days; however, she still worried excessively about the welfare of her child. The clonazepam was slowly tapered off after two weeks, while the fluoxetine was titrated up to a maintenance dose of 40 mg per day. After about nine weeks of treatment with fluoxetine, she felt well enough to be able to attend the local anxiety management clinic.

Benzodiazepines

One of the medicines that Mavis was given in the above case study, clonazepam, is a benzodiazepine, usually prescribed for epileptic seizures but also useful in treating anxiety in the short term. Benzodiazepines were discovered in the late 1950s by Leo Sternbach. The first benzodiazepine, chlordiazepoxide, was followed by several others, which rapidly constituted one of the largest and most widely prescribed classes of psychotropic compounds. After more than 50 years, benzodiazepines are still routinely utilised not only in psychiatry, but more generally in the whole of medicine. Despite their wide therapeutic index, which makes benzodiazepines safer than other medicines such as barbiturates, there has been controversy over their wide use due to their addictive potential in the long term. However, they appear to be the most effective medicines available, and they are generally at least as effective as psychological treatments. It used to be believed that once treatment continues beyond two weeks, both psychological and other medication treatments, particularly antidepressants, become more effective than benzodiazepines (Tyrer et al., 1988), but this view is now under challenge.

Some recent studies have demonstrated that long-term use of benzodiazepines for anxiety disorders can be effective as well as safe. Additionally, in combination with psychological therapy and antidepressants, they can produce optimal outcomes (Starcevic, 2014). This is not only because other forms of treatment have a delayed onset of action, but also because they fail to convincingly show superiority to benzodiazepines even in the long term, as suggested by at least one meta-analysis of 22 studies (Offidani et al., 2013). A meta-analysis of 56 studies with 12,655 participants treated with either placebo, antidepressants or benzodiazepines further supports the efficacy of benzodiazepines over other agents. Overall, benzodiazepines show superiority over antidepressants or placebo in controlling symptoms of anxiety (Gomez et al., 2018).

Accumulating evidence seems to support the view that the risk of addiction to benzodiazepines during long-term treatment of anxiety and related disorders may be exaggerated. This may be partly due to the observation that when we use benzodiazepines in the long term, an all-encompassing preoccupation with, craving, compulsive or uncontrollable benzodiazepines-seeking behaviour seems to be less evident (Tyrer, 2012). However, what may not be in dispute is that the use of benzodiazepines is effective for the emergency short-term management of anxiety, such as the immediate relief of Mavis's panic attacks in the above case study, as well as for insomnia. In spite of the favourable review of benzodiazepines, NICE guidelines only recommend their use as a short-term measure (NICE, 2016).

From a risk perspective, benzodiazepines are remarkably safe when taken singly, have few adverse effects in normal circumstances, and patients prefer them, although they have additive effects when used with alcohol and other depressant medicines, particularly of the sedative-hypnotic type such as barbiturates. Benzodiazepines have no antidepressant action, which is a major disadvantage as co-morbidity between anxiety and depressive disorders is the rule rather than the exception.

In general, we should prescribe benzodiazepines in as low doses as possible to afford adequate symptom relief. Those benzodiazepines with higher potency and shorter half-life, such as lorazepam, are associated with a greater likelihood of developing dependence.

Generally, we should encourage a patient to withdraw benzodiazepine use gradually after long-term use unless there is a clear risk of more severe problems if the patient stops a benzodiazepine. Many patients previously on benzodiazepine treatment over long periods successfully withdraw, but dependence on these medicines is not waning because prescription of these medicines is not declining. Despite accumulating evidence in support of their relative safety in the long term, some patients on long-term benzodiazepine treatment are likely to have trouble discontinuing them unless we expertly manage the situation, including offering psychological and alternative therapies.

Side effects of benzodiazepines

All benzodiazepines can induce psychomotor impairments, including drowsiness, sedation, dizziness and ataxia. This particularly affects tasks that need coordination and vigilance, so it is important to warn patients of the risks of driving and operating machinery while on these medicines. According to many pharmacoepidemiological studies, the use of benzodiazepine has a link with an increased risk of road traffic accidents, over and above that which we see with untreated mental health disorders (Smink et al., 2010).

Because of serum drug accumulation, the use of benzodiazepines with a longer half-life (e.g. diazepam) may be more hazardous than the use of those with a shorter half-life (e.g. triazolam, midazolam). Older patients are more vulnerable to the cognitive and psychomotor adverse effects of benzodiazepines and eliminate long-acting medicines more slowly than younger patients. We should consider this as a potential risk for falls when we are deciding to prescribe benzodiazepines in this population.

Irrespective of the long-term therapeutic benefits of benzodiazepines, the risks increase when they are taken for four weeks or longer. This is mainly because of the risk of withdrawal symptoms, which is why Mavis in the above case study was weaned off clonazepam after two weeks. People who become 'dependent' on benzodiazepines may be suffering from discontinuation syndrome after reducing or stopping the medicine. Symptoms of withdrawal normally start within 24 hours of stopping a short-acting benzodiazepine and up to six days after stopping a long-acting one. We sometimes use the terms 'rebound insomnia' and 'rebound anxiety' in the context of withdrawal reactions. However, there is no fundamental difference between the symptoms of rebound and those of withdrawal; it is just more common to use the term 'withdrawal' when anti-anxiety medicines have been taken for a longer period. Withdrawal symptoms can be physical (e.g. flu-like complaints, muscle cramps) or psychological (e.g. irritability, insomnia, nightmares, perceptual changes, depersonalisation or derealisation). There may be a prolongation of symptoms that are sometimes hard to distinguish from those of underlying anxiety disorders, although perceptual disturbances are relatively infrequent in untreated patients with anxiety disorders. These withdrawal reactions generally do not last long; typically, they last less than one month, though the pharmacokinetic profile of the individual may influence the duration.

The other major features of drug dependence (i.e. craving, medicine-seeking behaviour, escalation of dosage, marked tolerance) are not nearly so prevalent with benzodiazepines, although tolerance is now seen as a much greater problem than in the past. There is also some evidence that the more potent benzodiazepines, particularly those with a short elimination half-life, such as triazolam or midazolam, may carry greater risks of inducing tolerance than others, such as diazepam and clonazepam. It is for this reason that Mavis in the above case study was prescribed clonazepam, a medicine with a relatively longer half-life and less 'dependence' potential. Though tolerance is less common and develops more slowly with benzodiazepines, it tends to be observed more in those who have been prescribed these medicines as a hypnotic or an anticonvulsant. It is unusual for patients to steadily increase their dosage, but this can occur in some patients, particularly those with a history of alcohol dependence or other substance misuse.

Management of benzodiazepine overdose

Overdose from oral ingestion of benzodiazepines alone is generally not fatal. Most fatalities reported with this class of medicines tend to involve multiple medications, especially those that depress the CNS, such as opiates, barbiturates and alcohol. Symptoms of benzodiazepine overdose include drowsiness, confusion, somnolence, tiredness, impaired coordination, clumsiness in walking (ataxia) and slow reflexes. When multiple medications are implicated in benzodiazepine overdose, severe symptoms include difficulty breathing, slowed heart rate, low blood pressure, loss of coordination, and loss of consciousness, leading to coma and potentially death. Respiratory depression is a potential complication, particularly if the patient has ingested opioids, ethanol (alcohol) and other CNS depressants. The management of overdose may require special attention if the patient has pre-existing chronic obstructive pulmonary disease (COPD).

If there is a suspicion that a person has taken a benzodiazepine overdose, treat it as an emergency. Take the person to A&E for observation and treatment and bring the prescription bottle of medication and any other medication suspected in the overdose to the hospital, because the information on the prescription label can be helpful to the treating doctor.

Generally, the only management required is careful nursing and supportive care, paying attention to a clear airway. The use of a specific benzodiazepine antagonist (flumazenil) is indicated in carefully selected patients. The efficacy of flumazenil can be determined by the level of clinical improvement in consciousness and respiration in the patient. Its use is reserved for patients in a coma, those with hypotension or respiratory depression, and those who have a history of epilepsy; they should not have ingested pro-convulsants (e.g. cocaine, amphetamines) recently. Caution should be exercised if the patient is a habitual benzodiazepine user to avoid acute withdrawal symptoms. Flumazenil has been known to precipitate convulsions and cardiac arrhythmias when TCAs have been taken; therefore, an electrocardiogram (ECG) should be taken before administration. Flumazenil has a short half-life (about one hour); therefore, patients in whom it is indicated may need a repeat dose (0.5 mg intravenously over one minute – the same dose should be repeated if there is no response or only a partial response). In addition to benzodiazepines, the use of antidepressants is also a popular option in the treatment of anxiety.

Azaspirones

Azaspirones are a group of medicines that work at the serotonin 5-HT$_{1A}$ receptor and are used to treat patients suffering from GAD. One of the medicines, buspirone, was initially thought to possess antipsychotic properties, but this later proved to be incorrect. Further pharmacological and clinical evaluation of buspirone showed marked anxiolytic effects similar to those of diazepam (Goldberg, 1979). Since then, extensive neuropharmacological and clinical studies in animals and humans have demonstrated a unique anxiolytic profile for buspirone. In a systematic review of 36 studies, Chessick et al. (2006) found that in general, azaspirones – and buspirone in particular – appear to be useful in the treatment of GAD, especially for those participants who had not been on a benzodiazepine. This medication offers the benefit of a reduction in rumination and worry without the problems of sedation and potential medicine dependence ostensibly seen with benzodiazepines. It is not addictive and thus provides a treatment option for patients with GAD who are at risk of substance abuse. Recently, however, the use of certain anticonvulsants in the treatment of anxiety disorders has been increasing.

Anticonvulsants

Based on the hypothesis that anxiety results from excessive activation of the fear and worry circuits, it has been theorised that anticonvulsant medication can reduce this excitation in similar ways to which they reduce epileptic bursts. Researchers have investigated the use of various atypical anticonvulsants in the treatment of anxiety, and so far the results for gabapentin, tiagabine, vigabatrin and levetiracetam have been modest (Ravindran and Stein, 2010). However, the use of pregabalin in the management of GAD has been widely investigated, and it has been found to be effective. A systematic review of 13 trials found pregabalin to be consistently efficacious across the licensed dose range of 150–600 mg per day. Its effectiveness as a monotherapy has been shown in older patients with GAD and patients with severe anxiety, as well as for adjunctive therapy when added to an SSRI or an SNRI in patients who fail to respond to an initial course of antidepressant therapy. More support for the utility of pregabalin in anxiety disorders comes from a more recent systemetic review and meta-analysis of eight randomised controlled trials ($n = 2{,}299$) comparing the use of pregabalin at different dosages and placebo. Pregabalin is superior to placebo in alleviating anxiety and is comparable to benzodiazepines in response rate (Generoso et al., 2017). Further, the efficacy and tolerability of pregabalin compared to sertraline is high according to a head-to-head study that also shows pregabalin to have a more rapid onset than sertraline, but with equal efficacy (Cvjetkovic-Bosnjak et al., 2015). An earlier study that compared pregabalin and venlafaxine also supports this finding (Montgomery et al., 2006).

Despite the clinical efficacy of pregabalin, there is concern over its addictive potential, and in the UK the medicine is now reclassified as a scheduled drug. However, a systematic review of 106 studies did not find convincing evidence of the vigorous addictive power of gabapentinoids, especially in those with no prior history of substance related dependence (Bonnet and Scherbaum, 2017). Overall, the use of gabapentinoids such as pregabalin seem effective in the treatment of anxiety but we should avoid their use in those with a history of substance use disorder. When discontinuing long-term pregabalin therapy, tapering over the course of at least one week is recommended (Baldwin et al., 2015).

Side effects of anticonvulsants

Common side effects of atypical anticonvulsants used for anxiety disorders include sedation, dizziness, ataxia, memory impairment, confusion, blurred vision and abnormal coordination. In overdose, atypical anticonvulsants frequently cause altered mental status. Seizures may be more common with tiagabine, lamotrigine and oxcarbazepine. With reference to pregabalin, the most frequent adverse side effects are mild central nervous system depression, tachycardia, tremor/muscular twitching, seizures and unconsciousness. The most severe symptoms are seizures and central nervous system depression (for the management of these side effects, see Chapter 12). Next is an overview of some anxiety subtypes, as well as their treatment and management.

Treatment and management of anxiety subtypes
Generalised anxiety disorder

Anxiety is often co-morbid with other illnesses such as depression or substance abuse. Psychotherapeutic strategies are recommended as the treatment of choice for those with GAD (NICE, 2011). In the event that the individual does not respond to psychotherapeutic strategies, we can prescribe SSRIs, particularly sertraline, or SNRIs such as venlafaxine. We should monitor blood pressure in patients taking venlafaxine due to its tendency to cause hypertension in those taking doses of above 300 mg per day. Mirtazapine is another effective anti-anxiety medicine.

Where this is not appropriate, we can use benzodiazepines (e.g. diazepam, clonazepam, alprazolam). Benzodiazepines have the advantage of providing rapid physical symptom relief, but unfortunately have no effect on the core symptom of worry. Older people have difficulties in tolerating the adverse effects of benzodiazepine, such as sedation and impaired physical coordination, therefore risking falls. For this reason, we should avoid their use in older people. Most patients with GAD respond well to 1–3 mg of alprazolam per day or 1–2 mg of clonazepam per day. Buspirone, an azaspirone partial agonist, is effective in treating GAD without sedating the patient, nor does it cause dependence problems, but it does not relieve the physical symptoms of GAD. In some cases, we can use second-generation antipsychotics as an adjunct treatment.

Obsessive-compulsive disorder

CBT can be effective and is a preferred psychotherapeutic option for OCD, providing a more lasting benefit than medicines. Other psychotherapeutic approaches are also effective. In any event, it is important to combine psychotherapeutic and psychopharmacological strategies to optimise treatment outcomes. SSRIs are the first-line treatment, and a Cochrane systematic review of 17 studies (3,097 participants) showed that all types of SSRIs are effective in reducing the symptoms of OCD (Soomro et al., 2008). In OCD, we usually initiate SSRIs at low doses, at approximately half the initiation dose for depression treatment, but the final therapeutic dose is usually higher than for other indications. Another meta-analytic study including 17 trials of SSRIs (3,276 subjects) concluded that the greatest incremental treatment gains in OCD are seen during the first two weeks of treatment (Issari et al., 2016). When effective, long-term treatment with an SSRI is a reasonable option to prevent relapse. If treatment is not effective, other options include switching to another SSRI or to venlafaxine, duloxetine or clomipramine. However, only 40–70 per cent of patients respond to first-line treatment with SSRIs. It may be possible in some instances to augment antidepressant treatment with low-dose antipsychotics for a period not exceeding three months in those who do not respond to antidepressant monotherapy. Recent evidence suggests that one in three SSRI non-responders improve with antipsychotic augmentation. Among antipsychotics, risperidone and aripiprazole have the best evidence, with haloperidol being considered second in line owing to its unfavourable side effects profile (Thamby and Jaisoorya, 2019).

Social phobia

The mainstay treatment for social phobia is exposure-based therapy. In this regard, CBT is the therapy of choice, and it is best augmented with SSRIs such as sertraline or escitoloapram. A meta-analytic study with a total of 1,598 patients from three randomised studies supports this view. The study found escitolapram to be superior to placebo in the treatment of those with social anxiety (Baldwin et al., 2016). As with OCD, SNRIs such as venlafaxine or duloxetine are effective in the treatment of social phobia. A meta-analysis of eight randomised controlled trials found that duloxetine results in a greater improvement in symptoms of anxiety in comparison to placebo during short-term treatment in adults with social anxiety, and its tolerability is acceptable (Li et al., 2018). Dose initiation is like that of OCD, and many patients do not respond to treatment until they are receiving higher doses. If a patient fails to respond to treatment, consider switching to another SSRI. If this fails, then consider augmenting the SSRI with a benzodiazepine; clonazepam is a popular choice in this respect. If this also fails, then the prescriber can augment treatment with newer anticonvulsants such as pregabalin or gabapentin. Treatment can be continued for up to a year and medication can slowly be tapered off. The non-reversible monoamine oxidase inhibitor (MAOI) phenelzine (see Chapter 6) may be more potent than other classes of antidepressants; but because of its food and medicine interaction liabilities, you should restrict its use to patients not responding to SSRIs or SNRIs.

Post-traumatic stress disorder

As in other anxiety subtypes, the augmentation of psychopharmacological treatment with psychotherapeutic approaches (especially EMDR) produces the best results. During the acute stages of PTSD, the combination of CBT and SSRIs is effective. Patients suffering from PTSD often experience depression and therefore the use of SSRIs is timely. SSRIs can make pre-existing anxiety worse, but this is only temporary. To counter this, starting doses should be very low and the patient should be warned that response time can be up to 12 weeks or longer. A systematic review and meta-analysis of 51 studies that found SSRIs to be superior to placebo in reducing PTSD symptoms supports the use of SSRIs (Hoskins et al., 2015). Many people with PTSD will still experience some symptoms despite treatment. For this reason, augmenting treatment is very common. For example, patients who continue to show impulsivity or lability of mood can be augmented with antipsychotics or mood stabilisers. In some situations, buspirone, mirtazapine or anticonvulsants can be effective augmentation, though benzodiazepines are not particularly effective for the treatment of PTSD and may worsen the condition (Guina et al., 2015).

Panic disorder

In acute situations, the priority is to control the frequency and intensity of symptoms. Benzodiazepines are particularly useful for people whose symptoms are so severe that they are unable to wait longer for antidepressants to take effect. An increasingly popular approach in the treatment of panic disorder is to concomitantly treat with benzodiazepines and antidepressants. We gradually taper off the benzodiazepine as we titrate the antidepressant up and the patient uses it long term. However, in older persons, we may prefer to use antidepressants over benzodiazepines because of the difficulty that older people have in tolerating the adverse effects of benzodiazepines. In the medium term, a combination of CBT and antidepressants is a better preference. Also, we may prefer the use of antidepressants if a patient is unsure about CBT or cannot invest enough time in therapy. A Cochrane systematic review of 21 randomised trials, with 1,709 participants undergoing combination treatment of CBT and antidepressants for panic disorder, concludes that combined therapy is superior to antidepressant pharmacotherapy in the medium term (Furukawa et al., 2007). Specific antidepressants are effective either in combination or as monotherapy in the treatment of panic disorder. A meta-analysis of 50 studies with 5,236 participants found that the following antidepressants are significantly superior to placebo in the treatment of panic disorder: citalopram, sertraline, paroxetine, fluoxetine and venlafaxine (Andrisano et al., 2013). Because panic disorders are typically chronic illnesses, treatment is usually for up to nine months after symptoms have remitted.

Common management errors to avoid

When a patient presents with anxiety, it is important to ask them for their full medical history as anxiety could be secondary to a pre-existing physical illness. In such cases, it is important to treat the underlying physical condition. Also, always take note of any current medication the patient may be taking as some medications may induce anxiety symptoms. Avoid using TCAs, especially in older people, because of their adverse effects (especially antimuscarinic effects). Also, avoid using benzodiazepines in this population as these medicines can cause confusion and coordination impairment. Some SSRIs such as fluoxetine are associated with sleep disturbance and are therefore best administered in the morning. Avoid prescribing benzodiazepines in patients who have a concurrent substance abuse problem. Psychotherapeutic approaches are quite effective in the treatment of anxiety, so it is important to offer these therapies in tandem with medication for maximum effect.

What the patient and carers need to know

- Normally, both fear and anxiety can be helpful, helping us to avoid dangerous situations, making us alert and giving us the motivation to deal with problems. However, if the feelings become too strong or go on for too long, they can stop us from doing the things we want to and can make our lives miserable.
- Talking about the problem to friends or family can be beneficial and finding ways of learning to relax can help to control anxiety and tension. Everything from books and video tapes to seeking professional advice can offer an insight on how to relax. Self-help groups and psychotherapy are other options that may help patients to come to terms with the reasons for their anxiety.
- Medication can play a role if the other options are not appropriate. The most common medications are benzodiazepines, antidepressants, buspirone and atypical anticonvulsants.
- Patients prescribed benzodiazepines should not drive or operate machinery.
- Patients prescribed SSRIs should not stop the medication abruptly as this will cause discontinuation syndrome. They should be informed that antidepressants can in some cases take up to six weeks or longer to have a significant effect. Also, if a patient misses an antidepressant dose, they should be advised to take it as soon as possible within two to three hours of the scheduled dose. If it is close to the next scheduled dose, they should skip the missed dose and continue the regular dosing schedule. Patients should not take double doses. Most antidepressants can be taken with or without food.

Chapter summary

Anxiety as a disorder has existed for a long time, and people who suffer from this condition typically experience feelings of apprehension, fear, physical tension, irritation and worry. There are several subtypes of anxiety, namely GAD, phobias, OCD, panic disorder and PTSD. Each subtype has its own characteristics and symptoms that require different treatment. Psychotherapeutic approaches to treatment are preferred for anxiety disorders, so it is important to offer these therapies in tandem with medication for maximum effect. SSRIs are the first medicine of choice, and other classic antidepressants are also effective. Benzodiazepines are also useful, particularly for GAD and during the acute stages of panic disorder. Their use in older people, however, should be restricted because of adverse side effects.

Activities: brief outline answers

Activity 10.1 Critical thinking (page 279)

Anxiety is normal, and in normal cases it allows us to overcome obstacles by preparing ourselves. However, it becomes a clinical problem when the individual cannot function normally as a result. Fear and worry are common to all anxiety disorders.

Activity 10.2 Critical thinking (page 279)

Chris is showing symptoms of fear, anxiety and depression. SSRIs are probably a good option because they act on the fear and worry loop. SSRIs will be able to relieve the symptoms of depression that Chris is experiencing.

Activity 10.3 Communication (page 280)

If patients and relatives have no internet access at home, you could advise them to use the internet in libraries or internet cafés. Alternatively, you could advise patients to seek information about local self-help groups from their GPs.

Activity 10.4 Critical thinking (page 281)

Fluoxetine, an SSRI, has an energising effect and can cause sleep disturbance. Increased electromyographic (EMG) tone and eye movements during non-REM sleep have been observed during sleep in fluoxetine-treated depressed patients. It is best taken in the morning rather than at night. By contrast, TCAs such as amitriptyline cause sedation, and are therefore best taken at night rather than in the morning.

Further reading

Clark, D.A. and Beck, A. (2011) *Cognitive Therapy for Anxiety Disorders: Science and Practice.* London: Guilford Press.

This is a useful book that deals with practical aspects of CBT for anxiety.

Wells, A. (1997) *Cognitive Therapy of Anxiety Disorders: A Practice Manual and Conceptual Guide.* Chichester: Wiley.

This is a good guide for those practising CBT for anxiety.

Useful websites

www.anxietyuk.org.uk

Anxiety UK is a national registered charity for agoraphobia and those affected by other anxiety disorders. It is run by sufferers and ex-sufferers, supported by a high-profile medical advisory panel, and provides information, support and understanding via an extensive range of services, including one-to-one therapy.

www.social-anxiety.org.uk

This website aims to provide information for people with social anxiety and related issues. It has links to further information and acts as a central hub for those with social anxiety problems in the UK.

Chapter 11 Management and treatment of substance use disorders

Chapter aims

By the end of this chapter, you should have an understanding of:

- the biological mechanisms that underpin the reward system in substance misuse;
- the mode of action of various medicines used in the treatment of substance misuse conditions and their side effects;
- what to communicate to patients and the common errors to avoid.

Introduction

Case study: Darren

Darren has just been released from prison where he was serving a five-year sentence for armed robbery. He uses cocaine, cannabis and heroin. Before Darren became a poly-drug user, he was employed as a physical fitness instructor in the army. He started using drugs after the death of his wife in a car crash in which he was the driver. His first experience of smoking cannabis was a feeling of extreme euphoria and pleasure, which contrasted greatly with the low mood he was then experiencing. However, the feeling of euphoria and pleasure did not last long, and soon he was looking for cocaine to gratify his need. In a very short period, Darren was addicted to drugs, and this had a dramatic effect on his life. He lost his job and many of his friends deserted him. He turned to crime to finance his habit and therefore came into conflict with the law. He has served prison sentences several times for offences related to drug use. He has tried to give up drugs several times but has not succeeded. While in prison, he made several attempts on his life. His probation officer has recommended that he attends a drug treatment centre as a condition of release, which he has gratefully accepted.

Substance use disorder is defined as the harmful use of substances such as drugs and alcohol for non-medical purposes. It is the sole pursuit of substance use despite the individual experiencing serious harm to themselves or others. The term 'substance misuse' often refers to illegal drugs, but can also include legal substances such as alcohol, prescription medications, caffeine, nicotine and volatile substances. 'Habitual use' of these substances can cause physical or mental health problems, while 'substance dependence' is diagnosed when the use of substances becomes compulsive, uncontrollable and associated with physiological withdrawal symptoms. Millions of people worldwide misuse substances each year, which has profound consequences for their health, as in the above case study of Darren. It is estimated that globally, around 164 million people had an alcohol or drug use disorder in 2016. Around 318,000 people died in 2016 as a direct result of a substance use disorder, and this number is likely to be an undestimate (Ritchie and Roser, 2019). Approximately 40 per cent of patients with mental health problems also use substances such as alcohol, illicit drugs or nicotine (Munro and Edward, 2008), and this figure is likely to be higher. The use of alcohol is the most common; it is estimated that in the UK, 24 per cent of adult men and 13 per cent of adult women drink in a hazardous or harmful way. The prevalence of drug use and dependence ranges from 0.4 to 4 per cent, and this includes heroin and cocaine use disorders (0.25 per cent). Overall, the highest rates of substance misuse occur during late adolescence and early adulthood. In those who will eventually have a substance use disorder, the pattern of use rapidly evolves from 'experimentation' to overt substance abuse.

Like Darren in the above case study, people with mental health problems may misuse more than one substance. Several studies have found a link between the use of substances and mental health (Mutsatsa, 2015). Critically, there is a clear association between the misuse of cannabis and psychosis, especially in those who present with an early onset of psychosis. In other words, the misuse of substances, especially cannabis, can expose an individual to psychotic illness at an earlier age. The misuse can occur at any phase of the person's illness and this usually includes multiple patterns of use.

Because of the complex nature of substance misuse and its accompanying social and health consequences, it is difficult to offer a single causal explanation that applies to all individuals in all cultures. However, popular theories suggest that the use of substances is a form of self-medication, a genetic vulnerability, or the result of environment and/ or lifestyle factors. In this regard, it is possible that Darren first used drugs as a form of self-medication after the death of his wife, or he is simply genetically vulnerable. At one end of the spectrum, it is possible to view substance misuse as criminal conduct, a moral failing, or evidence of the individual's social incompatibility. On the other end of the spectrum, you could consider the problematic use of substances as a biobehavioural act driven by an individual's genetic make-up. For example, some investigators estimate that up to 70 per cent of the **variance** associated with drug use disorders or dependence is genetically heritable (Kendler et al., 2007), though subsequent findings are inconsistent despite scientific interest in the area (Kotyuk et al., 2019). Apart from these two polar views, there is a general acceptance that environmental factors play an enormously powerful role in the development and continuation of problematic substance use, especially as they interact with individual characteristics (Sloboda et al., 2012). Irrespective of the aetiology of substance misuse, there is a clear neurobiological pathway responsible for the behaviour seen in many people with such problems.

While the use of substances arguably contributes to the propensity for aggression and recklessness, there is evidence that these traits in substance abusers date back to childhood and therefore predate the onset of substance abuse. It is also argued that the substance abuse by itself may be an attempt to self-medicate for these behavioural traits or other psychiatric disorders. This is a good reason to ask patients with any psychological disorder, such as depression or anxiety, whether they have found anything that seems to help their condition.

To better understand treatments for substance use disorders, it is necessary for us to understand the mechanism underlying addictive behaviour; the dopamine theory of reward offers a plausible explanation.

The dopamine theory of reward

There is a general acceptance that the reward circuit, or the dopamine mesolimbic system, is the common pathway of reward and reinforcement in people with substance use disorder. We refer to this pathway as the 'pleasure centre', and within it dopamine is the 'pleasure neurotransmitter'. It is a very old pathway from an evolutionary point of view, and the use of dopamine neurons to control behavioural responses to natural rewards is present even in worms and flies that evolved between 1 billion and 2 billion years ago. An increase in dopamine levels in the mesolimbic (reward) system produces a pleasurable feeling, and there are many natural ways to trigger the release of dopamine in the mesolimbic system. The mesolimbic system includes the dopamine-containing neurons of the ventral tegmental area (VTA), the nucleus accumbens and part of the prefrontal cortex. The pleasure experienced when passing an examination, listening to music we enjoy, watching a funny movie, eating food, drinking, sex, and so on are a result of dopamine release in these regions. To be able to produce these feelings of joy or 'natural highs', there are an array of chemicals that regulate dopamine in the mesolimbic pathway, and these include the brain's own natural drugs such as endorphins (opiates), anadamide (cannabis) and acetylcholine. Nearly all abusive substances directly or indirectly target the brain's reward system by flooding the circuit with dopamine.

When an individual takes abusive substances such as drugs, the release of dopamine in the reward system can be up to ten times the amount that natural rewards produce, thus dwarfing natural rewards production. In some cases, this release occurs almost immediately as in the intravenous injection or smoking of drugs. Further, the effects can last for much longer than those of natural rewards. Such a powerful reward strongly motivates people to take drugs repeatedly; therefore, this reaction sets in motion a pattern that 'teaches' people to repeat the behaviour of abusing these substances. By contrast, there is a depression of dopamine neurons when an individual is not using abusive substances, and this creates an omission of the expected reward. In other words, there is no release of dopamine in the reward pathway and this creates a 'need' in the individual. In nature, we learn to repeat behaviours that lead to maximising rewards; thus, we learn to repeat behaviours that lead to an increase in dopamine in the reward system.

Tolerance and addiction

Case study: Kevin

Kevin is a 24-year-old man who is currently living alone in rented accommodation. He has a history of committing crime, including multiple counts of burglary, usually to finance drug-taking behaviour. Kevin started smoking cannabis when he was 15 years old and he very quickly moved on to taking crack cocaine. He soon discovered that he had to increase his intake of cocaine to get the same level of satisfaction as before. For Kevin, this meant that he had to steal from houses to finance his drug habit.

As a person continues to abuse substances, the brain responds by adapting to the overwhelming surges in dopamine by producing less dopamine or by reducing the number of dopamine receptors in the reward circuit. This reduces the impact of dopamine on the reward circuit, therefore reducing the drug abuser's ability to enjoy the substances, and this may be why Kevin had to increase his cocaine intake in the above case study. The person may now require larger amounts of the drug than initially to achieve the original dopamine high; we call this effect *tolerance*.

Abusive substances facilitate non-conscious (conditioned) learning, which leads to the user experiencing uncontrollable cravings when they see a place or person that they associate with the drug experience, even when the drug itself is not available. The person may then be caught up in a cycle progressing through three stages: binge/intoxication, withdrawal/negative affect, and preoccupation/anticipation of substances. This becomes worse over time and ultimately leads to a severe neurobiological disorder, which may be the case with Kevin in the above case study. Brain imaging studies of drug-addicted individuals show changes in areas of the brain that are critical to judgement, decision-making, learning and memory, and behaviour control (Cosgrove, 2010).

In addition to the reward pathway, scientific evidence implicates the role of corticotropin-releasing factor (CRF) in driving addiction via actions in the central extended amygdala, producing anxiety-like behaviour, reward deficits, excessive compulsive drug self-administration and stress-induced reinstatement of drug-seeking behaviour.

Neuron activation by CRF in the medial prefrontal cortex may also contribute to the loss of control (Zorrilla et al., 2014). Together, these changes can drive an abuser to seek out and take substances compulsively despite adverse consequences. In other words, they become addicted to drugs. The addicted person may resort to committing crime to finance a substance abuse habit and this brings them into conflict with law enforcement agencies, as seen in the above case study of Kevin.

The treatment of substance use disorders

We use a wide variety of medications for the treatment of substance use disorder; these vary according to the type of substance the patient uses, as well as patient choice and motivation. Despite this variety, their use has a common theoretical base that will be briefly reviewed.

Care and management approaches

The core value or guiding principle for the treatment and management of those who misuse substances is that such persons have the same entitlement to health and social care as other patients. It is therefore the duty of all other healthcare professionals involved to provide for their general health and social needs in addition to their drug-related problems. We can divide the care and management of people with substance use disorders into two stages: detoxification and recovery. The key to a successful detoxification regime is good preparation. Before you read further, try Activity 11.1.

Activity 11.1   Critical thinking

You receive a phone call from one of your patients who drinks heavily, informing you that he wants to 'end it all'. He says that he has not been drinking for a day and feels irritable and sweaty. He is not sure whether he should continue to drink alcohol and he needs help to 'sort his life out'.

- How would you respond to this call?

An outline answer is provided at the end of the chapter.

The first responsibility for a nurse is to bring the patient to a point of readiness to change their substance misuse behaviour by applying the popular stages of change model (Prochaska and Diclemente, 1984) (see Chapter 2). This means that the patient must reach at least the contemplation stage. At this stage, the patient is likely to have enough motivation to make a sustained effort to change. In other words, the patient will have reached a good-quality decision to change because they feel physically unwell, are under pressure from family or work, or simply feel the need for a temporary break from their substance misuse.

Patients need to be given accurate information about what to expect during detoxification as this information is likely to reduce the severity of the withdrawal and increase adherence. In the course of discussion with the patient, it is often useful to map out a timetable for the week in which detoxification will take place, as well as for the following week, as this will bring up a number of important issues, such as work commitments, childcare arrangements, transport difficulties and personal support.

It is important to understand the cause of the problem and to assess its consequences in order to establish the patient's strengths and weaknesses. If the nurse carries out a good assessment, it is then possible to formulate a good overall care and medicines management plan. The nurse should provide care that is evidence-based, including harm reduction approaches (DoH, 1999). Another aspect that promotes good care is effective key working.

Effective key working

National Institute for Health and Care Excellence (NICE) guidelines stipulate that to ensure a person gets full benefit from care, it is important to adopt effective key working strategies because this helps to deliver high-quality outcomes for people who misuse substances (NICE, 2017). Key workers have a have a central role in coordinating a care plan and building a therapeutic alliance with the patient, as the benefits of any treatment approach in substance misuse can only be realised within the context of properly coordinated care. Also, it is important to take account of the patient's needs and preferences. People who misuse substances should have the opportunity to make informed decisions about their care and treatment, in partnership with the healthcare professional. If a patient does not have the capacity to make decisions, the Mental Capacity Act 2005 should guide professionals in the decision-making process (see Chapter 1). Good communication between the patient and the nurse is always important. We should support any information we give to the patient regarding their treatment with evidence, and the support should be culturally appropriate and tailored to the patient's needs, ensuring that any information the nurse gives to the patient is is accessible to people with additional needs, such as sensory or learning disabilities, as well as to people who do not speak or read English. If the patient agrees, families and carers should have the opportunity to be involved in the decision-making about care and management, and they will also need information and support. Because alcohol is the most widely used substance, we will now discuss this in more detail.

Alcohol

The production and use of alcoholic beverages is common in many cultures and may go as far back as the Egyptian and Mesopotamian civilisations. In many parts of the world, drinking alcoholic beverages is a common feature of social gatherings. Because alcohol is legal and is integral to the socialisation process in many cultures, it is not seen as a drug or as harmful to our health. Nevertheless, alcohol is intoxicating, toxic and dependence-producing, and its consumption carries a risk of adverse health and social consequences. The harmful use of alcohol is a global problem that compromises both individual and social development. It results in 3 million deaths per year (WHO, 2018). Alcohol is the world's third-largest risk factor for premature mortality, disability and loss of health; it is the leading risk factor in the Western world. The use of alcohol has a link with many serious social and developmental issues, including violence, child abuse, and absenteeism in the workplace. It also causes harm far beyond the physical and psychological health of the drinker; it harms the well-being and health of people around the drinker. An intoxicated person can harm others or put them at risk of traffic accidents and violent behaviour; they can negatively affect co-workers, relatives, friends or strangers. Thus, the impact of the harmful use of alcohol reaches deep into society.

In the UK, about 23 per cent of the adult population drink alcohol in a hazardous or harmful way (Drummond, 2004). Estimates are that 38 per cent of men and 16 per cent of women aged 16–64 in the UK consume more alcohol than the recommended sensible limit. The annual cost of alcohol-related crime and public disorder in the UK approximates £7.3 billion, workplace costs at up to £6.4 billion and healthcare costs at £1.4–1.7 billion per year. As well as this very significant public cost, there are direct effects on the individual, with alcohol causing around 60 different types of disease and medical conditions (Anderson and Baumberg, 2006). Alcohol is a CNS depressant that shares many pharmacological properties with the non-benzodiazepine sedative-hypnotics and barbiturates. It affects the CNS in a dose-dependent fashion (the larger the quantity, the more the effect), producing sedation that progresses to sleep, unconsciousness, coma, surgical anaesthesia, and finally fatal respiratory depression and cardiovascular collapse. Alcohol intake increases the body's own naturally occurring opiates, and this may be responsible for the euphoria experienced.

Alcohol is probably the most studied substance, mainly because it is the most abused. It is associated with dependence, abuse, withdrawal, intoxication, delirium, dementia, amnesia, delusions, hallucinations, mood disorder, anxiety disorder and sexual dysfunction. Psychiatric symptoms are very common in people who misuse alcohol, but most of these symptoms subside within weeks of stopping alcohol. From a co-morbidity perspective, schizophrenia, depression, bipolar disorder and personality disorder are the most common disorders associated with alcohol misuse. Since alcohol is a depressant, it tends to produce symptoms of depression during intoxication and anxiety symptoms during withdrawal and abstinence.

Some key changes that alcohol causes involve a decrease in both brain gamma-amino butyric acid (GABA) neurotransmitter levels and GABA receptor sensitivity. It also activates the glutamate systems, which leads to the hyperactivation of the nervous system in the absence of alcohol. With chronic alcohol exposure, GABA receptors become less sensitive and therefore require higher alcohol concentrations to achieve the same level of suppression (termed 'tolerance'). Even when the patient no longer uses alcohol in this altered nervous system, the GABA receptors remain less responsive, leading to an imbalance that favours excitatory neurotransmission. We observe this CNS excitation as clinically observed symptoms of alcohol withdrawal in the form of tachycardia, tremors, sweating, and neuropsychiatric complications such as delirium and seizures.

Alcohol also acts on N-methyl-D-aspartate (NMDA) glutamate receptors as an antagonist, thereby decreasing the CNS excitatory tone. This leads to an upregulation (sensitisation) of NMDA receptors (glutamate receptors) to maintain CNS balance.

The goals of treatment should normally include the suppression of symptoms and the prevention of complications that arise from abstinence. In general, less than half of patients who abuse report withdrawal symptoms. In most cases, these symptoms do not require intervention, often disappearing within two to seven days of the last drink. Patients should be considered for psychiatric inpatient detoxification if they:

- are severely dependent on alcohol;
- have a history of delirium tremens and alcohol withdrawal seizures;
- have a poor social support network;
- have poor physical health that includes cardiac, pulmonary, hepatic, kidney or cardiovascular diseases;
- have cognitive and memory impairment;
- have psychiatric co-morbidity (e.g. depression, psychosis, personality disorder).

It is important to be aware that the manifestation of alcohol withdrawal tends to differ from person to person but usually occurs within six to 24 hours after the last drink. Symptoms can include mild insomnia, increases in blood pressure and pulse rate, tremors, hyperreflexia, irritability, anxiety, and depression. Alcohol withdrawal syndrome (AWS) can be a life-threatening condition affecting some alcohol-dependent patients who discontinue or decrease their alcohol consumption too suddenly. Most cases of AWS are relatively mild (e.g. mild anxiety, agitation, tremors, nervousness, irritability, insomnia, gastrointestinal symptoms) and require only symptomatic management. In most cases, the symptoms of mild alcohol withdrawal do not require medical intervention and usually disappear within two to seven days of the last drink (see Table 11.1). However, the symptoms of severe AWS may progress to more complicated forms, characterised by *delirium tremens*, seizures and coma. Cardiac arrest and death may occur in 5–10 per cent of patients.

Table 11.1   The variation of signs and symptoms of AWS over time

Time of appearance after stopping alcohol use	Symptoms
6 to 12 hours	Minor withdrawal symptoms: insomnia, tremor, anxiety, gastrointestinal upset, headache, diaphoresis, palpitations, anorexia, nausea, tachycardia, hypertension
12 to 24 hours	Alcoholic hallucinosis: visual, auditory or tactile hallucinations
24 to 48 hours	Withdrawal seizures, generalised tonic clonic seizures
48 to 72 hours	Alcoholic withdrawal delirium: hallucinations

Moreover, research shows that alcohol withdrawal is detrimental to the CNS because it can cause neuronal degeneration and death. It can also increase the loss of hippocampal and cerebellar neurons and cause poor memory performance. For these reasons, it is important for nurses to systematically assess the level or severity of dependency in an individual, preferably using a clinical rating scale.

Table 11.2   The CIWA-Ar scale

Symptom severity	0	1	2	3	4	5	6	7
Agitation								
Anxiety								
Auditory disturbances								
Clouding of sensorium								
Headache								
Nausea/vomiting								
Paroxysmal sweats								
Tactile disturbances								
Tremor								
Visual disturbances								

There are many rating scales for the assessment of alcohol withdrawal but the best known and most extensively studied is the Clinical Institute Withdrawal Assessment for Alcohol (CIWA-A). A short version, the Clinical Institute Withdrawal Assessment for Alcohol revised (CIWA-Ar), is a carefully refined list of ten signs and symptoms (Wiehl et al., 1994); each item scores a minimum of 0 and maximum of 7 (see Table 11.2). The CIWA-Ar has added usefulness because high scores, in addition to indicating severe withdrawal, are also predictive of the development of seizures and delirium.

Total scores on the CIWA-Ar of less than 8 to 10 indicate minimal to mild withdrawal, scores of 8 to 15 indicate moderate withdrawal (marked autonomic arousal), and scores of 15 or more indicate severe withdrawal. A study of the CIWA-Ar predicted that those with a score of over 15 were at increased risk of severe alcohol withdrawal; the higher the score, the greater the risk. However, it is important to be aware that some patients, if left untreated, can suffer complications despite low scores. It is also essential to always explain procedures fully to the patient and answer any questions. As usual, always seek and document consent before carrying out procedures. A detoxification regime always follows an assessment, and we will now turn to this.

Alcohol detoxification

The process of alcohol detoxification requires the elimination of alcohol from the body, and any withdrawal or other symptoms that are bound to occur are treated medically, psychologically or both. As mentioned previously, it is important to be aware that

AWS can be quite distressing and can even become fatal if the addiction to alcohol is very severe. The patient needs to be an inpatient for at least a week to remain under constant supervision, as the sudden cessation of alcohol consumption can lead to other symptoms that require medical intervention. Some patients who undergo the alcohol detoxification process may suffer from hallucinations, delirium tremens and even convulsions that – if not immediately attended to – can be fatal.

You can manage patients with mild withdrawal symptoms (i.e. a CIWA-Ar score of 8 or less) and no increased risk for seizures without specific pharmacotherapy. Successful non-pharmacological treatments include frequent reassurance and monitoring by nursing staff in a quiet, calm environment. Patients who experience more severe withdrawal (i.e. a CIWA-Ar score of greater than 8) should receive pharmacotherapy to manage their symptoms and to lower the risk of seizures and delirium tremens.

Detoxification regime

- A starting point is completing a CIWA-Ar on admission to the ward, and then every eight hours for 24 hours.
- Record vital signs such as blood pressure, pulse, temperature, oxygen concentration and peak flow. On admission, determine blood alcohol concentration (BAC) using a breathalyser.
- Keep recording vital signs every four hours, and inform the doctor or the prescriber if the patient's diastolic blood pressure is greater than 120 mmHg or their systolic blood pressure is greater than 180 mmHg.

There are medicines available that can minimise withdrawal symptoms. However, it is important to carefully prescribe and administer the use of these medicines, so that in the event of the patient experiencing side effects it is possible to quickly treat them. Initial dosages of such medicines are usually high, and they can gradually be reduced during the detoxification programme. At present, benzodiazepines are the medicines of choice in the treatment of AWS because they have proven their efficacy in ameliorating symptoms and decreasing the risk of seizures and delirium tremens in patients withdrawing from alcohol. Benzodiazepines are usually administered for the first seven days of a detoxification programme.

Benzodiazepines

Theoretically, you can prescribe any benzodiazepine for detoxification. They are relatively safe and effective, as well as the preferred treatment for AWS. The best-studied benzodiazepines for alcohol withdrawal treatment are diazepam, chlordiazepoxide and lorazepam. The choice depends on the patient's circumstances. For example, if a patient has liver disease, it may be appropriate to prescribe a short-acting benzodiazepine such as lorazepam or oxazepam (see Chapter 10). Longer-acting benzodiazepines may be appropriate for those prone to seizures but may not be appropriate for older people. In people with mild dependence, only small amounts of chlordiazepoxide may be neccessary, or even managing the condition without medication. In moderate dependence, the patient may require larger doses of chlordiazepoxide; this can be up to 40 mg per day, then slowly reducing the dose to zero over a period of five to seven days. Severe alcohol withdrawal requires even larger doses of chlordiazepoxide under inpatient treatment. In most cases, it is not unusual for prescribers to prescribe a benzodiazepine immediately as a single dose (stat dose) after the patient has been seen by the prescriber during the admission process. Usually, the severity of the symptoms at the time and the concentration of alcohol shown by the breathalyser tend to determine the stat dose. In many cases, the stat dose is usually 5–50 mg of chlordiazepoxide. In extreme cases where a patient is experiencing severe alcohol withdrawal symptoms, chlordiazepoxide doses of up to 250 mg have been known, but this is only under the supervision of a specialist.

Table 11.3   Typical detoxification chlordiazepoxide (mg) regime for an individual who scores greater than 20 on the CIWA-Ar

Day	Time of day		
	09:00	13:00	17:00
1	40	40	40
2	30	30	40
3	30	30	30
4	20	20	30
5	20	20	20
6	10	10	20
7	10	10	10
8	10	-	-

After the initial period of assessment, which lasts for 24 hours, a reducing regimen of chlordiazepoxide is normally instituted, and this can last between five and seven days. We can give the medicine in divided doses (see Table 11.3), with higher evening and night-time doses to aid sleeping. In most cases, the dose is reduced by about 6 per cent of the original dose, but a longer period of reduction might be necessary, particularly for those patients suffering delirium tremens.

During the withdrawal stage, and particularly after the administration of chlordiazepoxide, it is important to continually observe and record the patient's physical and mental state. If necessary, you may need to rate withdrawal symptoms using the CIWA-Ar and record vital signs every four hours. Before you proceed further, try Activity 11.2.

Activity 11.2 Critical thinking

You have been asked to admit a 45-year-old man who suffers from depression to the ward. During the admission interview, he appears irritable and forgetful and shows fine tremors. He informs you that he has been drinking two bottles of whisky a day.

- Considering this information, what might you incorporate in the admission procedure?

An outline answer is provided at the end of the chapter.

Anticonvulsants

Though benzodiazepines are the medicines of choice for the treatment of AWS in most treatment settings, anticonvulsants may be suitable alternatives. There are several potential advantages to using anticonvulsant medicines. First, they decrease the probability of a patient experiencing a withdrawal seizure, thereby reducing the complications of AWS. Second, they reduce craving and have been shown to block kindling in brain cells (Silver et al., 1991). Third, they do not appear to have significant abuse potential and they have been effectively used to treat mood disorders, which share some symptoms with AWS, including depression, irritability and anxiety. Finally, the propensity of anticonvulsant medicines to cause sedation is much less in comparison with benzodiazepines.

Carbamazepine and its derivative oxcarbazepine inhibit voltage-gated sodium channels and enhance GABA neurotransmission. A Cochrane review shows some evidence in support of carbamazepine for treating withdrawal, with tentative advantages over benzodiazepines, particularly in mild to moderate symptoms of AWS (Barrons and Roberts, 2010). Furthermore, carbamazepine shows superiority in ameliorating global psychological distress and reducing aggression and anxiety in comparison to oxazepam (Hammond et al., 2015). Carbamazepine use, however, has been limited due to its interaction with multiple medications that undergo liver oxidative metabolism, making it less useful in older patients and patients with medical co-morbidities.

A systematic review including six studies and 281 subjects examined the efficacy and safety of sodium valproate for the treatment of AWS, but the evidence for its use is less convincing. Importantly, the use of sodium valproate may be limited by its unfavourable side effects profile, including somnolence, gastrointestinal disturbances, confusion and tremor, which are like alcohol withdrawal symptoms, making the assessment of improvement difficult (Hammond et al., 2015).

Gabapentin and the second-generation medicine pregabalin are of theoretical interest in AWS due to their ability to enhance the inhibitory effects of GABA and voltage-gated calcium channels. Gabapentin is structurally like GABA and its low toxicity makes it a promising medicine in the treatment of AWS. Other non-benzodiazepine anticonvulsants that show promise in the treatment of AWS are lamotrigine, topiramate, vigabatrin and levetiracetam. Overall, accumulating evidence supports the use of anticonvulsants in the management of AWS. Their use also supports the hypothesis that anticonvulsants redress the underlying neuroplastic changes responsible for both AWS and ongoing heavy drinking. This suggests a potential advantage for their use over benzodiazepines when used as a bridge between AWS and post-detoxification treatment.

Vitamin supplementation

People who misuse alcohol are likely to need more nutrients than the general population. This is because, first, they may substitute alcohol for food. Second, alcohol speeds up the metabolism of essential vitamin nutrients such as thiamine and riboflavin, so it is important to supplement these nutrients as they assist with blood circulation and glucose metabolism. Further, it is common practice to offer thiamine (vitamin B_1) to all patients going through an alcohol withdrawal programme to prevent Wernicke's encephalopathy (WE), which – when left untreated – can cause lasting brain damage. Normally, oral B_1 is prescribed for five days, followed by an oral vitamin B compound. In extreme cases of alcohol withdrawal, we can prescribe parenteral thiamine because the gastrointestinal tract poorly absorbs oral thiamine, particularly in those who have been drinking heavily. Long-term alcohol abusers are likely to have a deficiency of folic acid. Therefore, supplementing this nutrient (800–1,000 mcg per day) is important.

Long-term relapse prevention

If possible, we should carry out the long-term care of people with alcohol use problems in the community where benzodiazepines have no place beyond the detoxification stage. As previously mentioned, we should customise the treatment to meet individual needs. As a cautionary note, the use of medicines to treat substance-related problems without psychosocial intervention sends the wrong message to the patient. The substance abuser already leans heavily on substances to either escape or solve problems, and nurses should not collude in the dependence on substances to solve all problems. Nevertheless, medicines do play an important role in recovery.

Several medicines have market authorisation for the treatment of alcohol dependence in the long term. To understand how these medicines work, we need to understand how alcohol exerts its effects. The action of alcohol on the opiate postsynaptic receptors results in the release of dopamine into the reward circuit (see 'The dopamine theory of reward' on page 295). Alcohol may do this by acting directly on the μ-opiate receptors, or by releasing natural opiates such as enkephalin that stimulate the release of dopamine in the reward circuit.

Case study: Chris

Chris has been drinking heavily for over eight years since the break-up of his marriage. He accepts that his drinking has caused further problems in his life and he wants to stop. Having made several attempts to give up drinking in the past, Chris is aware of the difficulties of abstaining from alcohol. His doctor suggested that he could consider a medicine called naltrexone, which works by reducing his ability to enjoy alcohol. He was happy to try this medicine.

Medicines such as naltrexone work by blocking opiate receptors, therefore limiting dopamine release into the reward system. By limiting the amount of dopamine in the reward system, naltrexone effectively blocks the enjoyment of drinking. If Chris in the above case study drinks alcohol while taking naltrexone, he will not be able to enjoy the effects of drinking. The usual dose of naltrexone for alcohol dependence is 50 mg per day, although a few patients may require only 25 mg per day.

An alternative to daily oral naltrexone is a long-acting intramuscular injectable form of naltrexone that was first approved in the US in 2006 for the treatment of alcohol dependence. With this injection, naltrexone is released over the span of four weeks, effectively reducing some of the high-dose side effects we see with oral naltrexone while simultaneously maintaining therapeutic plasma levels for the duration of the four weeks. Furthermore, due to the infrequency of injections (only once per month), it offers a greater chance of increasing adherence in this population, ultimately increasing the beneficial treatment response. However, a drawback of using the injection is the occurrence of injection site-related side effects, such as necrosis, infection and inflammation. From an evidence perspective, a Cochrane systematic review of 50 randomised controlled trials with 7,793 patients found that naltrexone reduces the risk of heavy drinking (Rosner et al., 2010). The use of naltrexone is a good example of *interference therapy*. In other words, in the above case study, naltrexone is interfering with Chris's reward pathway. Another alcohol treatment takes the form of *aversion therapy*; the medicine disulfiram best exemplifies this approach.

Disulfiram

Case study: Jenny

Jenny is 33 years old and suffers from depression. She was physically and sexually abused as a young girl and has been drinking alcohol heavily since she was 15 years old. She drinks two to three bottles of spirits per day. In the past, she abstained from

---

> drinking alcohol on several occasions, but this never really lasted. Although she is determined to stop drinking, she is worried about the possibility of relapsing. After a discussion with her prescriber, she has agreed to have a medicine called disulfiram (Antabuse) implanted subdermally to help her abstain. Prior to Jenny taking disulfiram, the doctor explained the risks and benefits of disulfiram before conducting a full physical examination, as well as taking took blood samples for liver and thyroid tests and electrolyte levels.

In aversion therapy, the medicine makes the effects of using alcohol extremely uncomfortable. One such medicine is disulfiram, which discourages the patient from drinking by producing an aversive reaction if the patient does so. However, when a person abstains from alcohol, the medicine has minimal effects. In Jenny's case, if she drinks alcohol, it will react with the disulfiram, causing some very uncomfortable effects. Maintenance doses can range anywhere from 200 mg to 500 mg per day, with the average dose being 300 mg per day.

Disulfiram works by inhibiting *aldehyde dehydrogenase*, a liver enzyme responsible for breaking down aldehydes, which are alcohol **metabolites**. This allows aldehydes to accumulate in the body (acetaldehyde syndrome). The resulting increase in aldehydes causes severe facial flushing, a throbbing headache, nausea and vomiting, chest pain, palpitations, tachycardia, weakness, dizziness, blurred vision, confusion, and hypotension. Severe reactions include myocardial infarction, congestive heart failure, cardiac arrhythmia, respiratory depression and convulsions. Death can occur, particularly in vulnerable individuals.

A disulfiram reaction can occur up to two weeks after discontinuation of the therapy, but the time of risk is usually four to seven days. Even the small amount of alcohol in mouthwash, certain foodstuffs and medicines can cause a reaction. Although rare, a potentially fatal idiosyncratic liver toxicity reaction can occur with disulfiram. Therefore, it is important to carry out baseline liver function tests and an electrocardiogram (ECG), as well as monitoring the patient for liver toxicity (hepatoxicity) by monitoring symptoms and repeating the liver function tests at certain intervals. If a patient opts for disulfiram, explain all of the possible risks involved, including side effects and the effects of drinking alcohol while on the medication, so that the patient can make an informed choice, as the doctor did with Jenny in the above case study.

The most common side effects of disulfiram are transient, but occasionally patients may experience skin eruptions that can be controlled with an antihistamine. Another medicine we use in the long-term management of people with alcohol misuse problems is acamprosate.

Acamprosate

Acamprosate was first approved in the US in 2004 to treat alcohol dependence through preventing relapse and promoting abstinence. It is a synthetic compound that is structurally like the inhibitory neurotransmitter GABA, and it is neither a sedative nor an anxiolytic. More importantly, acamprosate is not addictive and it does not have reinforcing effects on humans. Unlike naltrexone, acamprosate does not reduce the rewarding effects of alcohol, nor does it precipitate aversive negative symptoms when co-ingested with alcohol as with disulfiram. Because withdrawal of alcohol following chronic usage can lead to excessive glutamate activity and a reduction in GABA activity, acamprosate appears to work by stimulating the GABA receptors and decreasing excitation at the glutamate (NMDA) receptors. It has been shown to suppress alcohol-stimulated increase of dopamine in the nucleus accumbens, a part of the reward circuit. It is supplied as an enteric-coated tablet for oral administration. It is important to advise patients to swallow the tablets whole and not to crush, cut or chew them. A dose of two 333 mg enteric-coated tablets three times per day with meals is recommended by the manufacturer to aid adherence. The patient should start acamprosate therapy as soon as possible after alcohol detoxification to maintain abstinence as part of a comprehensive psychosocial treatment programme. For patients with moderate renal impairment, the recommended dose is one 333 mg tablet three times per day. Patients with severe renal impairment should not receive acamprosate therapy. As stated earlier, the liver does not metabolise acamprosate to any known extent. Dosage adjustments are not necessary for older patients unless they have renal impairment. Acamprosate is well tolerated, with diarrhoea being the most common adverse side effect. In many cases, the care and management of people with alcohol misuse problems is similar for those with drug dependence, to which we now turn.

Care and management of drug abuse and dependence

As with alcohol-related problems, the treatment of people with drug problems requires that you consider the individual in their personal and social contexts, while being mindful of the complex interaction of these factors and how they affect the individual. Therefore, treatment will typically include social, psychological, educational and pharmacological therapies. Again, as with alcohol misuse, treatment should result in recovery and a health benefit. Consequently, we should tailor treatment goals towards the healthcare needs of the individual; for many patients, treatment will include abstinence as an explicit objective, while with other patients intermediate goals, such as a reduction of harmful injecting, may be more realistic and achievable.

There are different types of drugs that people misuse, and each of these classes may require different pharmacological approaches. The types we will look at are stimulants and opiates.

Psychostimulants

Case study: Obeng

Obeng is a 26-year-old man who has been treated for a psychotic disorder since he dropped out of university two years ago. At the time, he was using cannabis regularly, but soon moved on to crack cocaine because it was cheap and easily available. He particularly enjoyed the intense pleasurable feeling that he derived from the drug. He was admitted to hospital following deterioration in his mental state, and his mother stated that he was spending most of his time looking for drugs. Lately, he has not been able to get any drugs because he cannot find the money to finance his habit. On admission to hospital, Obeng stated that he feels irritable and depressed.

Psychostimulants are a group of drugs that people become dependent on or addicted to, as in Obeng's case. They excite the central nervous system and produce feelings of alertness and well-being. There are many naturally occurring psychostimulants, including caffeine, nicotine, ephedrine, amphetamine and cocaine.

Cocaine and amphetamines are the two major psychostimulants that people use globally for recreational purposes. Approximately 34 million people used amphetamines and 17 million people used cocaine in 2012 alone. Amphetamines are the second-most commonly used illicit drug type worldwide after cannabis, and they come in pill, powder or crystalline forms that vary in purity (Degenhardt et al., 2014). Cocaine is a water-soluble white powder with a short half-life that people take by snorting it or by injection. Like most stimulants, it increases levels of dopamine in the reward system in addition to increasing levels of serotonin and noradrenaline. Repeated use of the drug at increasingly high doses leads to a state of growing irritability, restlessness and paranoia, and this may develop into full-blown paranoid psychosis.

Another important psychostimulant is crack cocaine, a mixture of cocaine and baking soda (sodium bicarbonate). It is a hard, brittle crystalline substance that when taken is absorbed into the bloodstream faster than cocaine, making it a highly addictive stimulant. Initially, it causes a release of a large amount of dopamine in the reward system, inducing feelings of euphoria, supreme confidence, paranoia, insomnia, alertness, increased energy and loss of appetite. The euphoria usually lasts for up to ten minutes before dopamine levels in the brain's reward system plummet, leaving the user feeling low and depressed and craving more crack cocaine. This may partly explain why Obeng was feeling depressed and irritable upon admission to hospital in the above case study. Like most stimulants, crack cocaine causes physical health disorders, including constricted blood vessels, dilated pupils, increased temperature, rapid heart rate and high blood pressure. Unfortunately, there are no known pharmacological treatments with market authorisation for the treatment of psychostimulant dependence. However, current literature suggests that there is potential for the use of agonist replacement therapy for the management of stimulant use disorders, but the evidence for this is embryonic.

Stimulant drugs such as amphetamines, cocaine and ecstasy do not produce a major physiological withdrawal syndrome and can be stopped abruptly, as with Obeng in the above case study. However, people who have regularly used stimulant drugs may experience insomnia and depressed mood when they stop taking them. Like stimulants, *hallucinogenic* drugs such as LSD do not produce a physical withdrawal syndrome and can also be stopped abruptly. Care and management involve calming and reassuring the patient until the effects wear off. Occasionally, the person may need oral diazepam (10–20 mg) to help calm them; and in severe cases where symptoms do persist, the individual may need antipsychotic medication.

If a patient is experiencing low mood, they can use antidepressant medicines, but many stimulant users just need advice regarding the likely symptoms and reassurance that they will pass. In Obeng's case, the assessment of the severity of his depression is important, as well as looking out for suicidal ideation, which will require close observation.

Rarely, cocaine overdose can result in cardiovascular complications, including arrhythmia, hypertension and cardiac ischaemia. Seizures and hyperpyrexia can also occur. In such cases, treatment is supportive as there are no specific medicines at present to reverse the effects of cocaine. Some people experience severe distress during or after the use of hallucinogenic drugs and may need symptomatic treatment, such as a brief course of a benzodiazepine to reduce anxiety, as well as a safe place to be while the experience passes.

Opiates

In 2010, there were 15.5 million opiate-dependent people globally. The regions with the highest opioid dependence are North America, Eastern Europe and Australasia. Opiate dependence is a substantial contributor to the global disease burden. Its contribution to premature mortality varies geographically, with North America, Eastern Europe and southern sub-Saharan Africa most strongly affected. Opiates are naturally occurring **alkaloids** found in the opium poppy plant. The plant has at least 24 alkaloids, but only morphine, codeine and thebaine are psychoactive.

Opiates act as neurotransmitters in neurons that arise from the VTA to the nucleus accumbens in the brain. The body's own natural opiates, such as endorphins or enkephalins, which are stored in the opiate neurons, act on a variety of opiate receptors, which include the mu (μ), delta (δ) and kappa (ϰ) receptors. Opiate drugs of abuse, such as heroin, also act in a similar manner by mimicking the body's natural opiates (endorphins or enkephalins), particularly at the μ receptors. They induce a very intense but brief euphoria, sometimes called a 'rush', followed by a profound sense of tranquillity that may last several hours, followed by drowsiness, mood swings, mental clouding, apathy and slowed motor movements. In overdose, opiates act as respiratory depressants and can induce coma. When given chronically, opiates easily cause tolerance and dependence.

As with alcohol, one of the first obstacles that a nurse may face is how to assess opiate withdrawal symptoms. There are clear advantages to using a rating instrument that provides accurate and clinically relevant measurements, such as the shortened version of the opiate withdrawal scale (Gossop, 1990). This scale (see Table 11.4) provides a satisfactory and valid measure of the distress experienced by people withdrawing from opiates; it is a straightforward, clinically useful and easy-to-use instrument that takes less than a minute to complete.

Table 11.4 The shortened opiate withdrawal scale

Symptom	None	Mild	Moderate	Severe
Feeling sick				
Stomach cramps				
Muscle spasms/twitching				
Feeling of coldness				
Heart pounding				
Muscular tension				
Aches and pains				
Yawning				
Runny eyes				
Insomnia/problems sleeping				

The most commonly selected opioid for detoxification is methadone because it is most effective and absorbs well after oral administration. It has a relatively long half-life, so once or twice daily doses give an extended duration of cover against the more extreme aspects of withdrawal. It is important to always confirm opioid dependence by evidence of usage, such as positive urine results for opioids, recent sites of injection (depending on the route), and objective signs and symptoms of withdrawal, including nausea, stomach cramps, insomnia, muscular tension, muscle spasm/twitching, and aches and pains. Opioid withdrawal reactions are very uncomfortable but are not life-threatening, and it is important to ask the patient when they had their last dose as withdrawal symptoms tend to peak at around 32–72 hours after the last dose of opiates was taken. In general, symptoms tend to subside after five days.

As with anyone suffering from a mental health disorder, the issue of importance in treating opioid withdrawal symptoms is not so much treating the disease state as treating the individual. It is important to consider a patient's emotional and spiritual conditions as these play a key role in the recovery process. During the process of obtaining informed consent from the patient, providing detailed information about the detoxification procedure and any possible risks to the patient is important. It is also important to explain about the physical and psychological aspects of opioid withdrawal, such as the duration and intensity of symptoms and how these may be managed, including the use of non-medicinal approaches. Further, explain to the patient that there will be loss of tolerance to opioids following detoxification and an ensuing increased risk of overdose and death from illicit drug use that may be worse if the person uses of alcohol or benzodiazepines. Both benzodiazepines and alcohol facilitate the inhibitory effect of GABA at the $GABA_A$ receptor, while alcohol also decreases the excitatory effect of glutamate at NMDA receptors. Emphasise the importance of continued support, as well as psychosocial and appropriate pharmacological interventions, to maintain abstinence, treat co-morbid mental health problems and reduce the risk of adverse outcomes.

Traditionally, we tend to manage withdrawal from opiates by prescribing and administering reducing doses of either the opiate of dependence (e.g. diamorphine) or another opiate agonist (e.g. methadone). The choice is determined partly by the prescriber's judgement on the most suitable medicine for providing even cover, partly by the expressed wishes of the patient, and partly by the social and political context within which the treatment is provided. For example, diamorphine (heroin) is never prescribed as the drug for management of opiate withdrawal syndrome, largely because of the sense of public outrage that would ensue, as well as certain national prohibitions and restrictions.

It is important to offer patients advice on aspects of lifestyle that require attention during opioid detoxification, including a balanced diet, adequate hydration, sleep and hygiene, and regular physical exercise. You need to develop a care plan in agreement with the patient to establish and sustain a respectful and supportive relationship with them, to help them identify situations or states when they are vulnerable to drug misuse, and to explore alternative coping strategies, including the involvement of family and carers, so long as confidentiality is maintained. An important part of recovery from opioids is engagement with self-help groups, so you may provide the patient with information about groups such as Narcotics Anonymous.

NICE guidelines recommend prescribing methadone or buprenorphine as the first-line treatment in opioid detoxification (NICE, 2007). When deciding between these medications, healthcare professionals should consider whether the patient is receiving maintenance treatment with methadone or buprenorphine (if so, you should normally start opioid detoxification with the same medication), and the preference of the patient. Before you proceed further, try Activity 11.3.

Activity 11.3 Decision-making

Mavu is a 30-year-old man who has been using illicit drugs since he dropped out of university 11 years ago. He uses a variety of street drugs, including heroin. He informs you that he has been taking methadone as well as illicit drugs until 24 hours before he was admitted to hospital for depression.

- What should your admission assessment include?

An outline answer is provided at the end of the chapter.

Methadone

Case study: Doug

Doug is a 33-year-old man who spends an average of £200 per day on heroin. He is motivated to give up the habit and realises that he needs help. He has tried to give up many times in the past but relapsed. After seeing his GP, he now takes methadone medication.

Methadone is a typical example of *replacement therapy*. Replacement therapy is the use of substances that are like – but less addictive than – the abused drug. Methadone is probably the most most effective medicine currently in use for opiate detoxification. It is a synthetic opiate whose action is very similar to that of heroin, except that it has a longer half-life and does not produce the same euphoric effects. Methadone is a full agonist that has an affinity for opiate receptors; if a person takes it orally, parts of the body, such as the bones and liver, completely absorb the medicine. Its metabolism is slow, it reaches peak plasma levels within two to four hours after administration, and it has a half-life range of between 13 and 50 hours.

As with alcohol, opiate treatment starts with the detoxification stage. This is best carried out in a controlled environment as evidence suggests that the setting in which you provide the treatment has a profound effect, with much greater adherence and completion rates being seen within specialist inpatient services compared with general psychiatric ward settings.

We gradually increase the dose of methadone from an initial dose of 10 mg per day to 30 mg per day; it is important to increase doses slowly under supervision. It is not uncommon for people on methadone therapy to supplement their treatment with other illegal drugs, so conducting frequent urinary analyses is important. We can reduce doses of methadone over a period of 10–28 days. Recently, it has been demonstrated that it is possible to effectively manage the detoxification process within a shorter ten-day withdrawal regime in contrast to the previously widely used 21-day regime. Ultra-rapid detoxification takes place over a 24-hour period, typically under general anaesthesia or heavy sedation. Rapid detoxification may take one to five days, with a moderate level of sedation. Accelerated detoxification, which typically does not involve the use of sedation, uses limited doses of an opioid antagonist after the start of detoxification to shorten the process without precipitating full withdrawal (NICE, 2007).

Close monitoring of effects during the first two hours after ingestion is important because the slow methadone metabolisation may cause accumulation, which in turn may cause toxicity. Also, other drugs may interact with methadone and cause sedation and respiratory depression. There may be an increase in mortality risk during the first weeks of treatment. In the maintenance phase of treatment, meta-analyses conclude that flexible, high-dose strategies are most effective (Bao et al., 2009). The recommended dose range is 60–100 mg per day, sometimes up to 120 mg per day. Patients may continue to take methadone indefinitely, as may be the case with Doug in the above case study. The main reason for maintenance therapy using a replacement medication is that it is preferable to use monitored prescribed addictive medication than the uncontrolled use of a more highly addictive street drug. For example, in the above case study, if we maintain Doug on methadone, he is less prone to commit crime to support his habit or to contract a disease such as HIV or hepatitis. Before you read further, try Activity 11.4.

Activity 11.4   Critical thinking

It has been reported to you by another patient that Ravinder, a 30-year-old male who is on the fourth day of a heroin detoxification programme, has been secretly taking heroin in addition to the 120 mg of methadone that he was prescribed.

- How would you respond to this situation?

An outline answer is provided at the end of the chapter.

Buprenorphine

A Cochrane review of 31 trials and 5,430 participants found buprenorphine to be an effective medication in the maintenance treatment of people with heroin dependence, retaining people in treatment at any dose above 2 mg. It also suppresses illicit opioid use at doses of 16 mg or greater. Although it is less effective than methadone in retaining people in treatment, if prescribed in a flexible dose regimen, or at a fixed low dose (2–6 mg per day), its effects can last longer. However, at fixed doses of above 7 mg per day, it shows no difference from methadone prescribed at fixed doses of 40 mg or more per day in retaining people in treatment or in suppression of illicit opioid use (Mattick et al., 2014).

Buprenorphine is a synthetic partial agonist that binds to the μ-opioid receptor. As a partial agonist, the maximum effect of buprenorphine is less than that of full agonists such as methadone. It binds to the receptor almost irreversibly, and dissociation from the receptor is slow, which gives it a relatively long half-life. It will displace most other opioids from the receptor; and if a person takes buprenorphine, other opioids such as heroin will be unable to displace it, even in high doses. For these reasons, buprenorphine can precipitate withdrawal in users who have taken other opioids before buprenorphine, but buprenorphine maintenance may protect patients against overdosing with other opioids. The strong binding reduces the need for additional opioid use, but this may also cause problems in reversing the opioid effects with naltrexone or naloxone. Because it is a partial agonist (i.e. it partly stimulates the opioid receptors), it alleviates withdrawal and craving.

Side effects of opiates and their management

This section deals with the most commonly experienced side effects of opiates (buprenorphine and methadone). The major hazards are respiratory depression and, to a lesser degree, systemic hypotension. Respiratory arrest, shock, cardiac arrest and death have occurred with the use of methadone. Other common side effects, especially with methadone, include constipation, dizziness, drowsiness, dry mouth, headache, increased sweating, itching, light-headedness, nausea, vomiting and weakness (for the management of these side effects, see Chapter 12). In certain instances, patients may develop a severe allergic reaction to methadone, in which case inform the prescriber without delay. Some symptoms that suggest a person is experiencing a severe allergic reaction are skin rash, hives, itching, difficulty breathing, tightness in the chest, and swelling of the mouth, face, lips or tongue.

Also, call for medical help without delay if any of the following are present: confusion, excessive drowsiness, fainting, fast, slow or irregular heartbeat, hallucinations, loss of appetite, menstrual changes, mental or mood changes (e.g. agitation, disorientation, exaggerated sense of well-being), seizures, severe or persistent dizziness or light-headedness, shortness of breath, slow or shallow breathing, swelling of the arms, feet or legs, trouble sleeping, difficulty urinating, and unusual bruising or bleeding.

Opioid overdose management

In general, opioid adverse effects may be a chronic problem, in which case the main complaint will be constipation, and at times the person may complain of nausea, vomiting or just loss of appetite. The person may be sedated and craving for the next dose. In acute toxicity, the person presents with drowsiness, and this is more severe if alcohol has been ingested or if this involves other sedatives. Respiratory depression may be apparent, and other signs include hypotension, tachycardia and pinpoint pupils, but this sign may be absent if other drugs are involved. Evidence suggests that deaths from heroin overdose alone are uncommon; drug-related deaths from heroin usually involve other drugs too.

If there is a suspicion of an opioid overdose, the first thing is to try to arouse the patient; if unsuccessful, call for an ambulance straight away. While waiting for an ambulance and more help, establish a clear airway and adequate ventilation, or oxygen therapy if the patient's consciousness is impaired. If trained and competent, administer naloxone intravenous (IV) 0.4–2 mg if the person is in a coma or respiratory depression is present. Otherwise, give the naloxone intramuscularly if no vein is available. Repeat the dose if there is no response within two minutes; large doses of naloxone (4 mg) may be required in a severely poisoned person. If a person fails to respond to large doses of naloxone, this may suggest that another CNS depressant or brain damage are present. It is important to stay with the patient until help arrives.

Some dos and don'ts in nursing people with drug misuse problems

- Always ensure that you assess the patient's level of motivation and offer brief interventions focused on motivation to change.
- It is important that before withdrawal treatment commences, you should agree an enforceable contract with the patient about the terms and conditions of treatment.
- Never commence treatment before you do a thorough assessment of the level of substance misuse, symptoms experienced and how frequently, coexisting mental health problems, and family and social support. If a patient withdrawing from opioids reports current use of maintenance medication, you should confirm this with the treating doctor or dispensing pharmacy. Confirmation is usually in the form of a faxed letter, an email or a prescription.
- Always confirm the use of drugs by a patient by performing a urine test to ascertain the main drug of abuse, as well as other drugs that the patient may have not reported.
- Methadone should not be given to patients taking respiratory depressants, such as alcohol and benzodiazepines, because the risk of overdose is greatly increased.
- If a patient has liver function problems, you should withhold giving methadone and report this to the doctor. Renal or hepatic dysfunction interferes with the breakdown of methadone and can result in the accumulation of methadone in the plasma, potentially causing an overdose.
- You should be aware that medications used in detoxification are open to misuse and diversion, and therefore you need to be vigilant during supervised consumption to limit the risk of concealment.
- For patients on methadone, an ECG should be recorded at regular intervals. Some authorities recommend an ECG prior to methadone commencement, then again after four weeks (period of stabilisation), and then at 6–12 months thereafter (Taylor et al., 2007).

What the patient needs to know

- Before starting detoxification, you should provide the patient with detailed information about the treatment and its benefits and risks, including the risk of seizures for alcohol detoxification, or – if the patient is taking opiates – the risks of interaction between opiates and other respiratory depressants.
- You should routinely provide the patient with information about self-help groups to assist with recovery after detoxification.
- You should give the patient the option for relatives and carers to get involved in their care plan, but you should also respect the patient's right to confidentiality.
- You should provide information to the patient about the physical effects of drugs or alcohol.
- For patients taking opiates (methadone or buprenorphine), you should inform them that the medicine can make them feel sleepy and drinking alcohol will make them even sleepier. It will obviously affect their ability to operate machinery and drive.
- Patients must not take opiates within two weeks of taking monoamine oxidase inhibitors (MAOIs) or if they are having an asthma attack.

Chapter summary

The non-therapeutic use of psychoactive substances is very common and accounts for a significant proportion of the global burden of disease. The most commonly used substance is alcohol, although the use of stimulants and opiates poses a significant challenge to society because users tend to be involved in criminal acts to finance their habit. Much controversy surrounds the classification of substance use disorder as a disease; but whatever one's viewpoint, there is no denying the huge personal, social, economic and health implications for the user. For this reason, people who abuse substances are entitled to the same treatment as everyone else.

Dopamine in the mesolimbic region has been implicated in addiction. A pleasurable experience is accompanied by an increase in dopamine levels in the limbic region, resulting in the reward process. The dopamine mesolimbic pathway interacts with CRF in driving addiction. Care and management of people with substance use disorders should always include psychosocial interventions. The treatment of substance misuse is usually in two stages, namely detoxification and maintenance or rehabilitation. In alcohol dependence, benzodiazepines are the medicines of choice during detoxification, and disulfiram, acamprosate or naltrexone are used during the maintenance phase. With regard to opiates, either methadone or buprenorphine is used for both withdrawal and maintenance. Opioid overdose can be fatal, and naloxone is used to counteract the effects.

Activities: brief outline answers

Activity 11.1 Critical thinking (page 297)

The starting point is to go and see your patient as a matter of urgency. Check his level of commitment to giving up drinking. The fact that he has called you is an indication that he has made some sort of commitment to giving up but may be unsure if he can. Explore ambivalence with him and offer information and treatment options. Offer detoxification, probably as an inpatient if possible. Contact his doctor and arrange for admission if needed.

Activity 11.2 Critical thinking (page 304)

Obtain a full history of his drinking and his reasons for drinking. Ask how it was financed as this may lead to further revelations of financial difficulties. Elicit symptoms using a scale, discuss detoxification options and inform a doctor. Most importantly, provide support and reassurance and make sure documentation is full and complete.

Activity 11.3 Decision-making (page 313)

You need to assess for symptoms of withdrawal, possibly using a rating scale. You need to take a history of drug usage that includes the type of drug, the quantity taken per day and approximately how much the patient spent per day on drugs. Take a history of his methadone use, including the prescribing doctor and the dispensing pharmacy; it is vitally important to confirm the prescription or dispensing record. Lastly, you need to confirm which drugs the patient has been taking by undertaking a drug urine analysis.

Activity 11.4 Critical thinking (page 314)

The supplementation of opiates with illegal drugs is not only a common problem, but also hazardous. Many overdoses in people with substance misuse problems are a result of an interaction between prescribed opiates and other drugs. You should therefore ask Ravinder for a urine sample to test for the presence of other drugs. If the urine test is positive for heroin or other unprescribed illegal substances, you need to inform Ravinder of this, withhold giving methadone and notify the prescriber.

Further reading

Mutsatsa, S. (2015) *Physical Healthcare and Promotion in Mental Health Nursing.* London: SAGE.

Chapter 7 of this book discusses the physical problems of substance misuse in more detail and outlines possible nursing care and management.

National Institute for Health and Care Excellence (NICE) (2010) *Alcohol Use Disorders: Physical Complications.* London: NICE.

NICE produces guidelines on all types of substance misuse and their management, easily available through their website (see the useful websites section below).

Stahl, S.M. (2013) *Stahl's Essential Psychopharmacology: The Prescriber's Guide,* 4th edition. Cambridge: Cambridge University Press.

This is a comprehensive guide to psychopharmacology that is clearly written and has good illustrations.

Taylor, D., Paton, C. Barnes T.R.E. and Young A.H. (2018) *The Maudsley Prescribing Guidelines in Psychiatry,* 13th edition. London: Informa Healthcare.

This is a very useful, easy-to-understand, evidence-based prescribing and general medicines management manual. It is particularly useful for prescribers.

Useful websites

www.alcoholics-anonymous.org.uk

The UK Alcoholics Anonymous website provides information from people who share their experiences, strength and hope with each other that they may solve their common problem and help others to recover from alcoholism.

www.drugs.com

This very useful website has information on virtually all medicines, side effects, preparations and interactions, as well as the latest drug warnings and reported adverse effects.

www.nice.org.uk

The NICE website was launched to manage the synthesis and spread of evidence-based practice, particularly in the NHS. Its introduction has ensured that everyone working in health and social care has free access to the quality-assured best practice information required to inform evidence-based decision-making quickly and easily.

www.ukna.org

The UK Narcotics Anonymous website enables people with drug problems to share their experiences and assist each other towards abstaining from drugs.

Chapter 12   Adverse drug reactions and the management of medicine side effects

Chapter aims

By the end of the chapter, you should be able to:

- describe the different types of adverse drug reactions (ADRs);
- manage ADRs and side effects, both routine and in emergency situations;
- advise patients on how to manage psychotropic side effects.

Introduction

Before a medicine gets market authorisation for use, evidence of its safety and efficacy is limited to the results from clinical trials. This means that at the time of a medicine's authorisation, it has only been tested in a relatively small number of selected patients under strictly controlled conditions and for a limited time. After authorisation, however, the medicine may be used in the rest of the population with other medicines and for a long time. Some side effects may emerge in such circumstances. It is therefore important to identify any new or changing risk of a medicine as quickly as possible, and to take measures to minimise and promote safe and effective use (EMA, 2018). The company that holds the marketing authorisation for a medicine has a legal obligation to continuously collect data and conduct pharmacovigilance. Pharmacovigilance is the science and activities relating to the detection, assessment, understanding and prevention of adverse effects or any other medicine-related problem. Many countries have official bodies that monitor medicine safety and reactions. At an international level, the World Health Organization (WHO) runs the Uppsala Monitoring Centre (UMC) and the EU runs the European Medicines Agency (EMA). In the US, the Food and Drug Administration (FDA) is responsible for monitoring post-marketing studies. In the UK, the Medicines and Healthcare Products Regulatory Agency (MHRA) runs the Yellow Card Scheme, which was established in 1963.

Adverse drug reactions

The WHO defines an ADR as 'a response to a drug that is noxious and unintended and can occur in doses normally used in man for the prophylaxis, diagnosis or therapy of disease, or for modification of physiological function' (WHO, 1972). However, the WHO definition of an ADR has been criticised for several reasons, and a new definition of ADR was proposed in 2000 thus:

An appreciably harmful or unpleasant reaction, resulting from any intervention related to the use of the medicinal product, which predicts hazard from future administration and warrants prevention or specific treatment, or alteration of the dose regimen, or withdrawal of the product.

(Edwards and Aronson, 2000)

Research in the UK and the US has shown that ADRs are a common feature in clinical practice and are the cause of many unplanned hospital admissions. Though most ADRs do not cause serious harm, the incidence of ADRs has remained relatively unchanged over time, with research suggesting that between 5 and 10 per cent of patients may suffer from an ADR during admission to or discharge from hospital, despite various preventative efforts (Coleman and Pontefract, 2016). Whether we consider an effect to be harmful depends on both the medicine's beneficial effects and the severity of the disease for which it is treating. To call an event an ADR, it is only necessary to suspect a causal relationship between the medicine and adverse reaction, and there is no need to prove a pharmacological mechanism action. This is central to the definition of an ADR. The terms 'adverse drug reaction' (ADR) and 'adverse drug effect' (ADE) have been used interchangeably but they are not the same. While an adverse reaction applies to the patient's point of view, the term 'adverse effect' includes all unwanted effects; it makes no assumptions about mechanism of action and suggests no ambiguity. It therefore follows that all ADRs are ADEs, but not all ADEs are ADRs, and this distinction is important in the assessment of the medicine's safety. Medicines that have been particularly implicated in ADR-related hospital admissions include antiplatelets, anticoagulants, cytotoxics, immunosuppressants, diuretics, antidiabetics and antibiotics. Fatal ADRs, when they occur, are often attributable to haemorrhage, the most common suspected cause being an antithrombotic/anticoagulant co-administered with a non-steroidal anti-inflammatory drug (NSAID) (Wester et al., 2008). Conventionally, we classify ADRs into two types:

Type A reactions: Sometimes referred to as augmented reactions, which are 'dose-dependent' and predictable because of the pharmacology of the medicine (e.g. insulin-induced hypoglycaemia).

Type B reactions: Bizarre reactions, which are idiosyncratic and not predictable based on the pharmacology (e.g. pencillin-induced anaphylaxis).

Although this system of classification is still widely referred to, it does not apply to all ADRs, such as those associated with cumulative medicine exposure (e.g. osteoporosis with long-term corticosteroid treatment) or withdrawal reactions (e.g. rebound syndrome from antidepressants). Another example is that some reactions, such as asthma from β-adrenoceptor antagonists, do not occur in all patients. In this method, the properties of the medicine alone define the classification – its known pharmacology and the dose dependence of its effects. However, we should take into account other criteria in a comprehensive classification, including properties of the reaction (the time course of its appearance and its severity) and properties of the individual (the genetic, pathological and other biological differences that confer susceptibility).

An alternative and perhaps more comprehensive classification scheme is the 'DoTS' system. This system classifies reactions dependent on three factors: (1) the *dose* of the medicine; (2) the *time* course of the reaction; and (3) relevant *susceptibility* factors (such as genetic, pathological and other biological differences). According to the DoTS

Table 12.1 The DoTS system

Dose relatedness	Time relatedness	Susceptibility
Toxic effects: ADRs that occur at doses higher than the usual therapeutic dose (e.g. lithium toxicity or serotonin syndrome due to serotonergic medicines). *Collateral effects:* ADRs that occur at standard therapeutic doses in some patients (e.g. neuroleptic malignant syndrome or the development of dystonia due to use of high-potency antipsychotics). *Dose hypersusceptibility reactions:* ADRs that occur at subtherapeutic doses in some patients (e.g. anaphylaxis in individuals allergic to penicillins is encountered at doses much lower than the therapeutic dose).	*Time-independent reactions:* ADRs that occur at any time during the treatment (e.g. neuroleptic malignancy syndrome or digoxin toxicity). *Time-dependent reactions:* Rapid reactions that occurr when a medicine is administered too rapidly (e.g. development of red man syndrome due to rapid administration of the antibiotic vancomycin). *First dose reactions:* These occur after the first dose of a course of treatment and not necessarily thereafter (e.g. hypotension after the first dose of an angiotensin-converting enzyme inhibitor such as ramipril). *Early reactions:* These occur early in treatment then abate with continuing treatment. These are adverse drug reactions to which patients develop tolerance (e.g. nitrate-induced headache). *Intermediate reactions:* These occur after some delay; however, if a reaction has not occurred after a certain time, there is little or no risk that it will occur later (e.g. elevated risk of neutropenia with carbimazole and venous thromboembolism with antipsychotics). *Late reactions:* These occur rarely or not at all at the beginning of treatment, but the risk increases with continued or repeated exposure (e.g. many of the adverse effects of corticosteroids and tardive dyskinesia with dopamine receptor antagonists). Withdrawal reactions are late reactions that occur when a medicine is withdrawn, or its dose is reduced after prolonged treatment. They include opiate and benzodiazepine withdrawal syndromes, hypertension after withdrawal of clonidine or methyldopa, and acute myocardial infarction after withdrawal of beta blockers. *Delayed reactions:* These occur some time after exposure, even if the medicine is withdrawn before the reaction appears (e.g. carcinogenesis due to diethylstilbestrol *in utero* and phocomelia due to thalidomide).	Raised susceptibility may be present in some individuals but not others. Susceptibility may be related to factors such as age, genetic variation, sex, altered physiology, interactions and disease. For example, poor renal function is related to lithium toxicity or Stevens–Johnson syndrome, and is common in some ethnicities such as the Han Chinese and Thai populations.

system, we can classify ADRs as: (1) supratherapeutic reactions (occurring at higher doses than recommended); (2) collateral reactions (usually occurring at the recommended dose); or (3) hypersensitivity reactions (occurring at lower doses than are recommended). We can also classify ADRs as either time-independent or time-dependent reactions.

Apart from classifying reactions, the DoTS system has the advantage of being helpful in considering the diagnosis and prevention of ADRs in practice (see Table 12.1).

While some ADRs are unpredictable, such as anaphylaxis in a patient after one previous uneventful exposure to a penicillin-containing antibiotic, other ADRs are preventable with adequate foresight and monitoring. Studies tend to find that between one-third and one-half of ADRs are – at least potentially – preventable (Ferner and Aronson, 2010). Interventions that reduce the probability of an ADR or side effect occurring can be an important way to reduce the risk of patient harm. We use the terms 'ADRs' and 'side effects' interchangeably, though there may be subtle differences. ADRs are harmful effects that make no assumptions about the way the medicine works, and may be unexpected or inexplicable. Side effects, on the other hand, can be expected and are related to the way the medicine works. The effects may be beneficial or harmful. The management of side effects is an important nursing role in mental health, and the following section focuses on key strategies for alleviating side effects in people with mental health problems.

The management of psychotropic side effects

Case study: Jessie

Jessie is a 28-year-old married woman who works in a demanding and stressful job. She has very high standards for herself and can be very self-critical when she fails to meet them. Lately, she has struggled with significant feelings of worthlessness and shame due to her inability to perform as well as she always has in the past. At home, she has been finding it difficult to fall asleep at night, and her insomnia has been keeping her husband awake as she tosses and turns for an hour or two after they go to bed. She was subsequently diagnosed with depression and prescribed 20 mg of citalopram once per day by her GP. After about a week of taking the antidepressant, she suffered a common cold and treated this with a cough suppressant she bought from a local pharmacy. However, she started feeling restless and confused, and had rigid muscles and twitching. She was diagnosed with serotonin syndrome and her antidepressants were discontinued.

The use of psychotropic medicines in mental health is now so common that it is difficult to imagine treatment without these medicines. They have dramatically altered the theory and practice of mental health nursing. Psychotropic medication has been available for over five decades; but despite universal use, these medicines have several problems regarding their safety and tolerability. Like any other medicine, they can induce side effects, as the above case of Jessie demonstrates. In most cases, psychotropic side effects are mild, transient and tolerable; however, some are profound or can even be fatal. They can affect neurotransmitter systems, and this effect can extend beyond the brain to other systems and organs in the body. In the above case of Jessie, the primary aim of the citalopram was to treat Jessie's symptoms of depression; but when Jessie took a cough suppressant, she may not have been aware that most cough suppressants contain the compound dextromethorphan. Unfortunately, dextromethorphan can increase blood serum serotonin to unusually high levels, leading Jessie to suffer serotonin syndrome (see page 187). To minimise side effects, the careful prescribing and management of psychotropic medication is an important part of the treatment plan. The treatment plan should include the evaluation of side effects, which is frequently a part of the quality of life assessment. This is because the frequency and severity of side effects may play a role in the effectiveness and cost analysis of the treatment with psychotropic medications. Thus, Jessie is unlikely to enjoy the full benefit of medication treatment if she is restless and confused for a significant portion of the day. Not only does this make the correct diagnosis and assessment of side effects a vital part of quality of life assessment; it is also an essential skill for the mental health nurse. However, many side effects and symptoms of psychotropic medication can mimic symptoms of mental health disorders, and this poses specific problems, which we will turn to next.

The overlapping nature of mental health pathology and treatment of side effects

One of the greatest challenges in the treatment of mental health disorders is discriminating between symptoms intrinsic to a person's illness and potential treatment side effects. For example, treatment with antipsychotic medication can induce akathisia, but akathisia is difficult to distinguish from psychotic agitation, anxiety or manic symptoms. In the case of depression, it is easy to mistake symptoms such as lethargy and lack of sleep, which are typical of depression, for antidepressant side effects.

One area of difficulty is when a patient experiences a worsening of symptoms after commencement of treatment. In such a case, it may be difficult to decide if the worsening of symptoms is due to adverse medication side effects or simply a worsening of the illness symptoms. For example, a depressed patient may present with agitation, insomnia and suicidal ideation after a period of treatment.

In drug trials research, it has been known for some time that some patients taking placebos complain of side effects from placebos. In a similar vein, the act of informing patients about possible side effects of a medication can dramatically increase the likelihood of a patient complaining about them. This is best supported by an early study, which found that patients who were informed that they might experience sexual side effects after treatment with beta blocker medication reported these symptoms between three and four times more often than patients in a control group who were not informed about these symptoms (Mondaini et al., 2007). This presents a challenge to the informed consent process, which expects the nurse to explicitly mention medication side effects to the patient during the treatment process.

Similarly, in clinical practice, some patients complain of medication side effects that are not consistent with the medicine's pharmacological profile, and this provokes a unique type of concern that a person might have for their physical health. Even though physical side effects from placebos are not pharmacodynamic in origin, if a person can attribute these to treatment this can provide validation and legitimacy to the individual's subjective sense of suffering. In any event, a patient who is complaining of side effects is communicating important information about themselves that you must take seriously.

Scenario

Imagine you are nursing Jim, who is 47 years old. He reports experiencing diarrhoea after taking olanzapine and attributes this to a side effect to the medication. Should you challenge the validity of this dubious self-reporting? You decide to assure Jim that the condition poses no serious medical hazard. Jim later complains of distress arising from the adverse effect, and you decide to advocate an alternative treatment because if Jim continues with olanzapine he may have a negative therapeutic experience.

Negative therapeutic reaction and experience

From a psychodynamic perspective, a negative therapeutic experience occurs when a patient develops an incongruous worsening of symptoms in response to accurate treatment interventions. Although any treatment regimen can result in adverse side effects at any time, there are times when we see patients whose symptoms clearly worsen in response to a medication that aims to improve their condition. An intensification of depression, mood and feelings of guilt during antidepressant therapy is a useful example. It is therefore tempting to think that this is due to lack of medication efficacy, but a psychodynamic perspective is equally valid. Freud, as cited by Levy (1982), describes the above phenomenon as 'an unconscious expression of guilt or masochism on the part of the patient whose symptoms worsen because the prospect of improvement is contrary to an unconscious investment in the person's own suffering'.

In the above scenario, Jim might describe a seemingly endless stream of physical ailments that he links to treatment, while at the same time he develops a parallel sense of frustration, resentment and loss of sympathy from the healthcare team. This will evidently make interactions between Jim and the nurses personally and psychodynamically complex. Therefore, it is necessary to appreciate the psychological context of Jim's presenting symptoms to avoid his treatment becoming a relentless and seemingly fruitless effort to combat side effects or to identify less harmful medicines while the patient is receiving no tangible treatment benefits.

To break this cycle, seeking consultation is important, or in certain instances it might be necessary to honestly acknowledge to the patient that existing treatments may not be capable of providing tangible benefits that outweigh side effects. In such circumstances, it is important to discuss alternative therapies with the patient, including psychotherapy, as these may hold greater prospects for success (Goldberg and Ernst, 2018).

The general principles of side effects management

The person who is under treatment has important and clinically relevant characteristics that will have an impact on the course of their illness and treatment behaviour. Therefore, it is important to collaborate with the person to facilitate the implementation of a successful treatment plan. This is likely to involve proactive strategies for managing side effects as they are a major obstacle to treatment adherence, and this compromises treatment effectiveness. Furthermore, patient education must be ongoing, and it is not possible to accomplish this in a single encounter or a single handout. We will look at the role of the nurse in educating the patient about their medication in later sections.

Before the commencement of treatment, it may be helpful to ask the patient to make a list of troublesome symptoms that the medication should target. Second, and perhaps critically, when a patient complains of adverse side effects, it is important to establish whether they were present or absent before treatment. If the problem was absent before treatment, it is likely that it is a medication side effect. In the case of illness symptoms that intensify during treatment with medication, this differentiation can be particularly difficult. For example, insomnia that predates the initiation of some antidepressants such as selective serotonin reuptake inhibitors (SSRIs), which then worsens after commencement of treatment, may be particularly difficult to attribute either to side effects or to a worsening in mental state. Third, it is important to gather information about the patient's previous medication and past adverse side effects, and to then make a summary of past medications, dates taken, dosages, benefits and side effects. This information will help us to understand previous treatment complications or failures, reasons for non-adherence, and the patient's ability to tolerate side effects. It will also help us to recognise potential patterns or sensitivities that may heighten the patient's expectations about future potential side effects or concerns. Before you read further, try Activity 12.1.

Activity 12.1   Critical thinking

What factors might influence intolerance to side effects?

An outline answer is provided at the end of the chapter.

From a nursing care viewpoint, the assessment of the patient's attitudes and beliefs about medicines, both beneficial and harmful, is important to tailor a discussion accordingly. You are likely to ill-serve those patients with anxiety about possible treatment side effects by cognitively flooding them with a listing of all possible side effects. Such individuals are likely to benefit from the fostering of an emotionally safe and secure environment in which the nurse projects an image of care for the patient, guarding them against the intrusion of side effects.

Obsessional and paranoid patients benefit most when they are reassured about their safety concerns, allowing them to be their own watchmen having to safeguard their own welfare. In this regard, they are likely to research all possible side effects, regardless of the likelihood of occurrence. Individuals who present themselves in a histrionic or dramatic way may exaggerate their experiences of suspected adverse side effects. Wisdom often demands that the nurse explores with such patients their subjective complaints and concerns beyond their face value.

For most patients, an honest and reasonable approach for anticipating side effects is to proactively inform patients of the most common and important ones. The discussion about side effects should be positive, minimise over-concern, and provide a sense of context and proportion about their likelihood, seriousness and time course. It is important to discuss common side effects with the patient, as well as what to do if these occur, but it is not necessary to read out all the possible side effects that are in the *British National Formulary* (BNF). Merely listing the side effects is likely to increase the patient's anxiety. Rather, for those who have sleep problems, present sedation as a beneficial effect. Alternatively, suggest that if daytime sedation becomes a problem, then the patient should let the treating staff know, with a view to reviewing the medication.

In some situations, the nurse may say, 'Nausea is the most common side effect of SSRIs and passes shortly after starting the medicine. It is less likely to occur if the medicine is taken with food than on an empty stomach. If it occurs and is bothersome, an over-the-counter medication such as famotidine may be helpful until the nausea goes away.' Sometimes such information can help to empower the patient to know the circumstances under which side effects may occur. It gives a sense of predictability to what is seemingly an unpredictable event.

Another useful example is with the prescription of lamotrigine. The nurse might inform the patient, 'The greatest risk window for developing a serious rash during treatment is from two to eight weeks. The rash has a characteristic appearance, and the risk can be minimised by avoiding new environmental exposures.' Where anticholinergic side effects such as blurred vision and dry mouth are concerned, the nurse could describe these as usually bothersome and can advise the patient that these effects are usually worse during the first two weeks of treatment, with some tolerance developing if they stay on the same dosage.

In some situations where a patient is experiencing side effects, the prescriber can taper the medicine off and introduce an alternative. For some patients, however, medication dose reduction or tapering off is not a clinically viable option, given the seriousness of some mental health problems and the high risk of relapse and significant harm to self or others.

Overall, there are different ways to inform a patient about side effects, but the key part of the process is the discussion of the risks and benefits that treatment poses, as well as obtaining informed consent. Always document the discussion with patients regarding side effects and consent issues.

It is important to be alert to the presence of pharmacodynamic inconsistencies when a patient is complaining about adverse side effects such as co-occurring problems that have an opposing mechanism of action. For example, the co-occurrence of dry mouth with diarrhoea or excessive salivation with constipation should alert the nurse to the need to probe the patient further to elicit other underlying problems that the patient may have. In this case, it is important to validate the patient's experience rather than to say that it is impossible as the medicine has no cholinergic effects.

In the assessment of side effects, a good starting point is to establish whether the side effects bear any relationship to treatment. The best approach is to use a method devised by Naranjo et al. (1981). The Naranjo Adverse Drug Reaction Probability Scale (NADRPS) is a simple and widely used non-specific scale (see Table 12.2).

Table 12.2 The NADRPS (adapted from Naranjo et al., 1981)

	Question	**Yes**	**No**	**Do not know**	**Score**
1	Are there previous *conclusive* reports on this reaction?	+1	0	0	
2	Did the adverse effect occur after the suspected drug was administered?	+2	−1	0	
3	Did the adverse reaction improve when the drug was discontinued or a *specific* antagonist was administered?	+1	0	0	
4	Did the adverse reaction reappear when the drug was readministered?	+2	−1	0	
5	Are there alternative causes (other than the drug) that could have on their own caused the reaction?	−1	+2	0	
6	Did the reaction reappear when a placebo was given?	−1	+1	0	
7	Was the drug detected in the blood (or other fluids) in concentrations known to be toxic?	+1	0	0	

	Question	Yes	No	Do not know	Score
8	Was the reaction more severe when the dose was increased or less severe when the dose was decreased?	+1	0	0	
9	Did the patient have a similar reaction to the same or similar drugs in *any* previous exposure?	+1	0	0	
10	Was the adverse effect confirmed by any objective evidence?	+1	0	0	
	Total score				

Scoring

9 or more = definite ADR

5–8 = probable ADR

1–4 = possible ADR

0 = doubtful ADR

In addition to the use of this scale to assist with adverse side effects management, the 'Ten Commandments' of wise medicine management maybe helpful in minimising adverse side effects. These are:

1. Know your patient well.

2. Work on offering a treatment package, not just a medicine.

3. Educate the patient.

4. Assist the patient in choosing the right medicine.

5. Ensure that the patient takes the medicine correctly.

6. Ensure that the patient is on as few drugs as possible.

7. Assist in ensuring that treatment is tailored to the patient's needs.

8. Have a good knowledge of the medicine that the patient is taking.

9. Be vigilant of side effects.

10. Always consider the patient's viewpoint as it is critical.

We can now turn to specific side effects of psychotropic medication and their management; we will start with extrapyramidal side effects.

Extrapyramidal side effects and their management

Extrapyramidal side effects are various movement disorders that are caused by the antagonistic action of psychotropic medication on the extrapyramidal system or the nigrostriatal dopamine pathway (see Chapter 8). Dopamine antagonists that cause extrapyramidal side effects are metoclopramide and most types of antidepressants, including SSRIs, tricyclic antidepressants (TCAs) and tetracyclic antidepressants. The most common cause of extrapyramidal side effects is antipsychotic medication. Extrapyramidal side effects can take several forms, including dystonia, akathisia, Parkinsonism and tardive dyskinesia. We will now turn to the management of these side effects.

Dystonia

As explained in Chapter 8, the key features of dystonia are involuntary contractions or spasms of the muscles affecting the head, spine and extremities, as well as the facial, laryngeal and neck muscles, which can be painful and frightening. For example, the jaw may open involuntarily, which can result in dislocation. Laryngeal spasms can result in difficulties in swallowing, which can be life-threatening. Acute dystonic reactions typically occur within hours of initiating treatment, particularly with intramuscular injections of high-potency antipsychotics. An oculogyric crisis is a type of dystonic reaction that involves a sustained involuntary upward deviation of the eyes. The early symptoms of the condition include restlessness, agitation, malaise or a fixed stare. This is followed by extreme and sustained upward deviation of the eyes. The eyes may converge, deviate upward and laterally, or deviate downward. All classes of antipsychotics have an association with an oculogyric crisis. Other types of medication such as SSRIs, lithium, carbamazepine, amantadine, benzodiazepines and propofol can also cause an oculogyric crisis. Although the diagnosis of acute dystonia is relatively straightforward, there are situations when the condition has been mistaken for hysterical reactions, tetanus or even meningitis.

In the event of an acute dystonic reaction, the nurse can start by reassuring the patient and take the necessary steps to alleviate the condition. Dystonic reactions generally respond dramatically well to anticholinergic medication such as an intramuscular injection of procyclidine, and this is the treatment of choice. Most patients respond within five minutes and are symptom-free by 15 minutes. If there is no response, repeat the dose after ten minutes, but if that does not work then the diagnosis is probably wrong. Before reading further, try Activity 12.2.

Activity 12.2   Critical thinking

We treat a severe dystonic reaction with an intramuscular dose of an anticholinergic medication. Why is it not advisable to give an oral tablet of an anticholinergic in severe dystonia?

An outline answer is provided at the end of the chapter.

Some patients can respond well to benzodiazepines, diphenhydramine or biperiden. Apart from prescribing and administering medication to ameliorate the condition, the role of the nurse during acute dystonia is to provide as much reassurance as possible. Many patients rightly find the condition frightening, and it is important to emphasise that it is temporary and will ameliorate after treatment. However, in some patients, persistent dystonia (tardive dystonia) may occur due to chronic exposure to antipsychotics. If what appears to be chronic dystonia does not respond to standard treatment, the condition might not be due to antipsychotics, and such illnesses might include Wilson's disease, Huntington's disease or **idiopathic** torsion dystonia. Another troublesome extrapyramidal side effect is akathisia, which we will look at next.

Akathisia

Akathisia often develops in patients taking all types of antipsychotics or during rapid dose escalation. To a lesser extent, akathisia can develop with all types of antidepressants and lithium. As we discussed in Chapter 8, high-potency second-generation antipsychotics such as risperidone, ziprasidone and aripiprazole possess a higher risk than olanzapine, whereas low-potency second-generation antipsychotics such as quetiapine and clozapine present the lowest risk.

The first line of managing akathisia is the discontinuation of the offending medication. However, an atypical antipsychotic with a lower propensity to induce akathisia may be a better alternative. In cases where this is not possible, benzodiazepines such as diazepam or beta blockers such as propranolol are first-line treatments for akathisia. If the akathisia appears to have its roots in the imbalance of the noradrenergic system, then a beta blocker usually works better. Patients who have symptoms of Parkinsonism together with akathisia (approximately 65 per cent of patients) may respond to anticholinergic medication such as procyclidine.

By far the most promising treatment for akathisia is the use of antidepressants such as mirtazapine, trazodone and mianserin, which antagonise the serotonin (5-HT_{2A}) receptor. A systematic review of six randomised controlled trials found that 5-HT_{2A} antagonists are effective in the treatment of antipsychotic-induced akathisia (Laoutidis and Luckhaus, 2014). Apart from prescribing, the nurse is likely to be responsible for administration of medication and observation of further side effects. Because of the disabling nature of akathisia, it is important to provide adequate support and reassurance to the patient.

Drug-induced Parkinsonism

Parkinsonism is a complication of antipsychotics treatment, as well as antidepressants, calcium channel antagonists, gastrointestinal prokinetics such as domperidone, some anti-epileptic medicines, and many other compounds that interfere with the dopamine system. It occurs in about 15 per cent of patients and it usually develops within 5 to 90 days of treatment initiation (see Chapter 8).

The three critical steps in the management of drug-induced Parkinsonism include the reduction in the medication dosage, administering anticholinergic medication, and changing the antipsychotic medication. The first step is to reduce the dosage of the medicine or administer a concomitant anticholinergic dose of procyclidine trihexyphenidyl, benztropine or amantadine. Except for amantadine, which offers a more cognitively benign remedy, most anticholinergic medications block acetylcholine receptors (antimuscarinic) and cause uncomfortable side effects such as dry mouth, constipation and blurred vision. In this regard, we need to encourage the patient to drink enough fluids to counteract these effects. If the symptoms persist and the patient finds them intolerable, it is then imperative to review the medication with a view to switching to another medication that has a lower propensity for causing Parkinsonian side effects. For example, if a patient develops Parkinsonism on risperidone, it might be reasonable to switch to a less offending medicine such as clozapine or quetiapine. Quetiapine may produce fewer Parkinsonian effects than high-potency medicines such as paliperidone, aripiprazole and risperidone (Asmal et al., 2013). We now turn our attention to tardive dyskinesia.

Tardive dyskinesia

Case study: Deidre

Deidre is a 42-year-old woman with a 16-year history of suffering from paranoid schizophrenia. After ten years of treatment with haloperidol deaconate, a first-generation antipsychotic medicine, she developed involuntary movements with tongue chewing, lip puckering, jaw stiffness and finger piano playing.

Haloperidol decanoate was therefore gradually tapered off and replaced with Risperidal consta, a depot injection formulation of risperidone. The dyskinetic movements largely resolved over the following three months and Deidre's condition remained stable for four years.

Tardive dyskinesia (TD) is a complex involuntary movement disorder that typically occurs in patients taking psychotropic medication, particularly antipsychotics and TCAs (see Chapter 8). TD consists of abnormal involuntary, irregular choreoathetoid movements of the muscles of the head, limbs and trunk. Perioral movements are the most common, and they include darting, twisting and protruding movements of the tongue, chewing and lateral jaw movements, lip puckering, and facial grimacing. Finger movements and hand clenching are also common (see Chapter 7).

The management of tardive dyskinesia starts with the correct assessment of symptoms, which can be done by using a rating scale. The abnormal involuntary movement scale (AIMS) (Guy, 1976) is probably the scale with the widest use for the assessment to establish the presence of tardive dyskinesia. This 12-item scale records details of the occurrence of dyskinesia in patients; each item is rated on a five-point scale (0 = none to 4 = severe).

The treatment of TD includes gradual reduction of any anticholinergic co-medications as the primary step before switching from the offending medicine to an atypical antipsychotic. Switching to a low-potency second-generation antipsychotic remains the most effective treatment of antipsychotic-induced tardive dyskinesia, as we saw in the above case of Deidre. Determining which second-generation antipsychotic to use depends on the patient's clinical profile and the specific second-generation medication's pharmacological profile. If switching medication fails to improve TD symptoms, it is usual for the prescriber to consider another second-generation medicine. Clozapine has a lower risk of TD and reduces dyskinetic movements in patients with TD. A review of 15 randomised controlled trials and 28 case reports concluded that clozapine is useful for reducing TD syndromes in the dose range of 200–300 mg/day and the beneficial effect usually shows within 4–12 weeks of treatment initiation (Hazari et al., 2013). Next, there is emerging evidence that tetrabenazine is effective for the treatment of movement disorders, including tardive dyskinesia. A review of the literature concludes that tetrabenazine is a credible alternative for the treatment of dystonia, TD and Huntington's disease. Preliminary results from randomised controlled trials suggest a place in the treatment of TD for vitamin E. A Cochrane review of 13 randomised controlled trials concluded that vitamin E may protect against deterioration of TD, but there is no clear-cut evidence that vitamin E improves symptoms of TD once the condition is established (Soares-Weiser et al., 2018). Therefore, new and better-designed trials are needed to conclusively demonstrate its effectiveness. The use of the extract ginkgo biloba seems to hold promise in the treatment of TD. A meta-analysis of three randomised controlled trials with a total population of 299 participants found ginkgo biloba to be superior to placebo in the allevaiating symptoms of TD (Zheng et al., 2016). However, as with vitamin E, more and better-designed studies are required to conclusively demonstrate its efficacy and safety. Other treatment options that hold promise in the treatment of TD are vitamin B_6/branched-chain amino acids, donepezil, melatonin levetiracetam and amantadine.

A Cochrane review of three studies concluded that pyridoxal 5 phosphate (vitamin B_6) may have some benefits in reducing the severity of TD symptoms among individuals with schizophrenia. However, due to the low number of participants, further studies are needed to conclusively demonstrate the utility of this compound in treating TD (Adelufosi et al., 2015). It is important to remind patients that none of the available pharmacological options for the treatment of TD reduces symptoms dramatically or halts symptom progression significantly. This condition remains intransigent and there is no reliable or well-proven treatment.

Cardiovascular effects

As previously mentioned, there is current concern and focus on the prevalence of cardiovascular disease (CVD) in people with mental health problems (Mutsatsa, 2015). Although this high prevalence is due to a combination of factors, both biological and lifestyle, it has been known for a long time that psychotropic medication, and specifically antipsychotics have an association with cardiovascular disorders.

As discussed in Chapter 8, most psychotropic medicines that have an affinity for the acetylcholine receptors (antimuscarinic) can cause cardiovascular complications. These psychotropics include low-potency antipsychotics, TCAs, non-selective monoamine oxidase inhibitors (MAOIs) and all anti-Parkinsonian medicines.

Prevention is better than cure for any disease, and this is particularly true for CVD. To minimise the cardiovascular effects of antipsychotic medication, it is important to check the patient's baseline vital signs, electrolytes and electrocardiogram (ECG) prior to commencing medication. It is imperative to check these regularly and inform the patient about the potential for cardiac problems (Mutsatsa, 2015). A further measure that should be taken to prevent CVD is to encourage the patient to establish and maintain conditions that minimise the development of the condition. This will involve the creation of environmental, economic, social and behavioural conditions conducive to health. Key activities that are conducive to good cardiac condition are exercise and an appropriate diet. For example, encouraging overweight people to lose 15 per cent or more of their body weight can significantly reduce the risk of cardiovascular disease by up to 45 per cent. We will now turn our attention to the endocrinological side effects of psychotropic medication.

Endocrinological effects

Psychotropic medicines induce a wide range of adverse hormonal (endocrinological) and metabolic effects. Some of these psychotropic medicines include antipsychotics, mood stabilisers and antidepressants. Common metabolic and hormonal effects that these medicines induce include elevated levels of prolactin, calcium and glucose, ketoacidosis, and weight gain. These effects are mainly due to the antagonistic effects of psychotropic medication on the tuberoinfundibular dopamine pathway (see Chapter 8). Further, the experience of orgasmic dysfunction and reduced libido is possibly due to alpha-adrenergic activity of antipsychotics and calcium channel blockade.

In addition to the antipsychotic action in causing hormonal side effects, SSRIs can cause various forms of sexual dysfunction, such as the inability to achieve an orgasm, erectile dysfunction and diminished sexual appetite. Before you read further, try Activity 12.3.

Activity 12.3   Critical thinking

Sophie, a 26-year-old woman who suffers from schizophrenia, is prescribed a depot injection of Risperidal consta. Recently, she stated that she has given birth to a child, although this is untrue. This belief, which she holds firmly, is outside her delusional system; the treatment team feels that the current depot dose is not enough, and therefore the dose should be increased.

- Do you have any misgivings about this?

An outline answer is provided at the end of the chapter.

When a patient appears to be suffering from hyperprolactinaemia-related side effects such as sexual dysfunction, the prescriber should discuss this with the patient. A starting point is to test prolactin levels to ascertain if this is above the threshold (ranges of 32–309 mIU/L for males and 39–422 mIU/L for females). It is important to provide explanation and reassurance to the patient where this is necessary. If prolactin levels are high, then the prescriber should discuss this with the patient with a view to reducing the dose of the offending medication if possible. If this is not possible, then it is important to advise the patient that there are other types of medication which have less propensity for causing sexual dysfunction, such as aripiprazole, clozapine, quetiapine or moderate doses of olanzapine.

In some instances, it may be possible to prescribe dopamine agonists that suppress prolactin secretion, such as bromocriptine, cabergoline or pergolide. However, advise the patient that these dopamine agonist medications can increase agitation, psychosis or mania, particularly if the patient does not continue with adequate treatment with an antipsychotic or mood stabiliser. Weight gain is another important side effect of psychotropic medication, and we will turn to its management next.

Weight gain

One of the most common adverse side effects of treatment with medicines that block the dopamine receptor system is weight gain. Excessive weight gain renders the patient vulnerable to metabolic illnesses. Such illnesses include cardiovascular diseases and non-insulin dependent diabetes. The most recommended interventions are the provision of dietary advice, physical activity, and psychoeducation of the patient and family.

It is important to note that, although commendable, the provision of advice alone does not ensure that patients most in need of intervention receive any. Moreover, due to physical and psychological challenges, people with mental health problems may require both a tailored exercise prescription and ongoing clinical monitoring. At the most basic level of exercise, encourage the patient to take part in leisure activities that include going out to places of interest or to parks. There is evidence to suggest that exercising in natural environments offers greater benefits than exercising indoors – this is the basis of ecotherapy. Ecotherapy is the implementation of interventions such as walking, relaxation and creative activity, which aims to improve physical, psychological and social functioning using green spaces. A review of studies concludes that in comparison with exercising indoors, exercising in natural environments such as parks or taking country walks has a greater association with feelings of revitalisation and positive engagement, and a decrease in tension, confusion, anger, depression and increased energy.

Exercising in green spaces may be ideal for beginners or for older persons who may be physically frail. In formulating exercise for patients, take into consideration whether the patient understands the types of exercise available and the importance of exercise; most importantly, there is a need to establish the individual's fitness level to be able to tailor activities. It is important to provide information to the patient about the benefits of exercise, and then help them to decide whether they want to carry out exercise as part of a group or on their own.

Individual activities or exercises for consideration may include walking in open spaces, gardening, a one-mile brisk walk, a half-mile run, a bike ride or low-impact aerobics. Enjoyable group activities or exercises include rounders, baseball, tag, badminton, volleyball, basketball or bike riding.

High-intensity exercise should raise the heart rate and make the person breathless. The Department of Health and Social Care recommends that people should exercise for at least half an hour, five times per week. This does not have to be done all at once as short bursts of exercise are just as beneficial. For example, instead of exercising continuously for 30 minutes, the individual can split it into three ten-minute sessions of high-intensity exercise. Evidence suggests that very brief high-impact exercise makes the heart and lungs stronger. It burns more energy and improves insulin sensitivity. In addition to exercise, an important role in maintaining a low weight is played by our diet.

Restriction of calorie intake is among the most robust interventions for extending lifespan. In a discouraging trend, modern societies seem to be converging on a common dietary pattern – one that is not ideal for our weight or healthy ageing. The key characteristics of this diet consist of high calorie intake, high in saturated fat, sugar and refined carbohydrates, a high intake of meat (especially red and processed meats), and a low intake of fruits, vegetables, fibre and phytonutrients. We often call this the 'Western diet', and it is common in the UK. Unfortunately, it is also a dietary pattern that modernising societies are adopting. There is good evidence that the Mediterranean dietary pattern, rich in food groups such as fruits, vegetables, whole grains and fish, can be beneficial for maintaining a healthy weight, as well as helping to reduce incidences of many physical and mental health problems.

Another common side effect of psychotropic medication is haematological-related disorders, and we will discuss their management next.

Haematological and hepatic effects

A variety of blood disorders (dyscrasias) may be present in people with mental health disorders taking psychotropic medication, including an abnormal reduction in white blood cells (leucopenia), a decrease in the number of neutrophils (neutropenia), a marked reduction in leucocytes (agranulocytosis) and a decrease in the number of blood platelets (see Chapter 8). These blood disorders are mainly because of psychotropic medications such as antipsychotics, anti-epileptics (especially carbamazepine), benzodiazepines and antidepressants. Most blood-adverse effects of medication usually disappear after stopping the offending medicine, although drug-induced aplastic anaemia may not resolve upon medicine withdrawal. Neutropenia and agranulocytosis are the most clinically important and common medicine-related blood disorders.

If a patient who is on medication that can cause blood dyscrasias develops an infection, then there is justification in suspecting that this may be due to the medication. In many instances, the patient may develop a fever that can be the only sign of an infection, and therefore you should investigate all episodes of pyrexia in patients who are on these medicines. There is a need to report such occurrences promptly and as a matter of course.

From a treatment management perspective, it is good practice to measure the leucocyte count before treatment so that there is a baseline value in case problems occur later. The monitoring of the leucocyte and neutrophil counts during treatment is also important, especially in highly vulnerable groups such as older persons and females. If the leucocyte count drops significantly, it is normal to withdraw the medicine promptly. This is because a marked drop in leucocytes may result in life-threatening infection. To counter this threat, it is normal to administer intravenous prophylactic broad-spectrum antibacterial and antifungal therapy to the patient if they have a low leucocyte count. Nurses play a critical role not only in prescribing, but in the whole treatment process, including administering medication, providing explanations for the patient, and reassuring the patient where necessary.

Though rare, we may encounter a patient who develops neutropenia on a range of different antipsychotics. In this case, the treatment of choice is amisulpride or sulpiride as there are no published reports of these medicines causing blood disorders. Apart from blood disorders, many psychotropic medications can cause neuroleptic malignant syndrome (NMS), which we will turn to next.

Neuroleptic malignant syndrome

Case study: Chris

Chris is a 25-year-old man who was recently diagnosed with paranoid schizophrenia. While on the ward, he was involved in a fight with another patient. He was physically restrained, and as part of the management plan he was administered an intramuscular injection of 10 mg of haloperidol and 2 mg of lorazepam. A day later, a nurse noticed that Chris was still restless but with notable differences: he showed more confusion and signs of muscle rigidity, his blood pressure was 160/100, and his temperature was 41°C.

NMS was described in Chapter 8. Like agranulocytosis, it is a potentially fatal side effect of psychotropic medications and it can occur at any time during treatment. The main symptoms of NMS are hyperthermia, muscle rigidity, mental status changes, slow movements (bradykinesia) and muscle rigidity, blood pressure instability, profuse perspiration (diaphoresis), tachycardia, and altered consciousness, as in the above case of Chris.

The symptoms of NMS usually evolve over 72 hours, and if there is no treatment they can last 10–14 days. Quite often it is possible to miss this diagnosis during the early stages as the symptoms are frequently mistaken for agitation or an increase in psychosis.

The key to a successful intervention to prevent mortality for an individual with NMS is early detection and stopping the offending medicine. In the above case study, it would be preferable to transfer Chris to an adult medical ward as soon as possible. It is important to encourage the patient to take fluids, and electrolyte restoration is vital. Where a patient is not able to take oral fluids, consider administering fluids nasogastrically or intravenously, depending on the ability of the nurse. Encourage the patient to use a cooling fan to reduce peripheral body temperature. Before reading further, try Activity 12.4.

Activity 12.4 Decision-making

You notice that a patient who was previously withdrawn is unusually aggressive and restless after an injection of a depot antipsychotic.

- What action would you take, and why?

An outline answer is provided at the end of the chapter.

It is likely that the patient will be started on bromocriptine, a dopamine agonist, to improve the hypodopaminergic state that is postulated as the underlying pathophysiology of NMS. Apomorphine may have greater efficacy and faster action than bromocriptine. Another key element of the care of NMS is continual reassurance and orientation of the patient. We now need to discuss another important and common side effect of psychotropic medicines: sedation.

Sedation

Case study: Olu

Olu is a 22-year-old university student who suffers from bipolar affective disorder. Over the past few weeks, his family and friends have noticed increasingly elated behaviour; therefore, his sodium valproate was increased to 800 mg per day and his quetiapine was increased to 600mg per day. Recently, he has been complaining of being unable to stay awake during the day and this is affecting his studies. His medication dose was altered to enable him to have 200 mg of sodium valproate in the morning and 600 mg at night. In respect of quetiapine, the dosage was altered so that he had 200 mg in the morning and 400 mg at night. He was encouraged to drink plenty of fluids and to exercise more.

We can define sedation as a decrease in psychomotor and cognitive performance, and it is a property of many psychotropic medicines, including antipsychotics, antidepressants, anticonvulsants, antihistamines and anxiolytics. Second-generation antipsychotics such as clozapine, olanzapine and quetiapine are particularly sedative. In the case study above, Olu took the second-generation antipsychotic quetiepine and a mood stabiliser. Unsurprisingly, he experienced daytime sedation. First-generation tricyclic medicines such as amitriptyline induce similar effects in patients.

Sedative medicines do not have a common pharmacology but can act on several inhibitory pathways in the brain. Sedation may be beneficial during the initial stages of treatment, particularly for patients who are highly agitated. In the long term, however, it can interfere with rehabilitation and social functioning. For example, in the above case study, sedation may have been useful during the early stages when Olu was experiencing symptoms of elation, but during the later stages it was interfering with his studies. Sedation can be difficult to distinguish from the mental slowing of cognitive impairment.

The treatment of drowsiness depends on the individual's diagnosis and age, the medicine causing the drowsiness, and other factors. Treatment generally involves a multifaceted plan that addresses the underlying cause and helps to minimise the abnormal drowsiness so that a person can sleep well at night, be alert during the day, and lead an active, normal life. One way of achieving this is to prescribe a relatively low dose of the medicine in the morning and a large dose at night, as in the above case of Olu. A low dose in the morning is likely to minimise daytime drowsiness, and a large dose at night is likely to cause drowsiness and aid sleep during the night. Other measures may include drinking extra fluids, good nutrition and a short period of sleeping, but avoiding excessive sleeping during the daytime. In some cases, the use of small amounts of caffeine can temporarily relieve drowsiness. However, ongoing or excessive use of caffeine can lead to rebound drowsiness in some people. It can also result in disturbance of sleep, resulting in an increase in daytime drowsiness. Next, we turn our attention to serotonin syndrome.

Serotonin syndrome

Serotonin syndrome is a potentially life-threatening adverse reaction that may occur following therapeutic use of antidepressants or some antipsychotics. It is not an idiosyncratic medicine reaction, but predictable if there is excess serotonin in the central nervous system, and this will in turn excessively stimulate the $5HT_2$ receptors. Numerous medicines and medicine combinations produce serotonin syndrome. These medicines include most types of antidepressants, serotonin-releasing agents such as amphetamines, opioid analgesics, anti-migraine medicines, and lithium. Serotonin syndrome or toxicity starts within hours of ingesting serotonergic medicines (for its clinical features, see Chapter 6). We make the serotonin syndrome diagnosis using the Hunter Serotonin Toxicity Criteria (Dunkley et al., 2003), which requires the presence of one of the following classical features or groups of features: spontaneous clonus; inducible clonus with agitation or profuse perspiration (diaphoresis); ocular clonus with agitation or diaphoresis; tremor and hyperreflexia; or hypertonia, temperature above 38°C and ocular or inducible clonus.

Patients with moderate or severe cases of serotonin syndrome require hospitalisation. Critically ill patients may require neuromuscular paralysis, sedation and intubation. Supportive care mainly consists of giving a sedative to the patient if necessary, ensuring that the patient has adequate fluid intake, and carefully monitoring vital signs and urine output. Preventing hyperthermia and subsequent multi-organ failure is a key goal if the patient has severe serotonin toxicity. An additional benefit of lowering temperature is that this indirectly decreases (downregulates) the activity of the serotonin ($5HT_{2A}$) receptors in the central nervous system. In treating serotonin syndrome, we should aim to reduce or prevent hyperthermia by using cooling fans with water sprays, ice packs or cooling blankets. Serotonin antagonists, particularly $5HT_{2A}$ receptor antagonists, reduce hyperthermia and other severe manifestations of serotonin toxicity. Serotonin antagonists that are in common use are sublingual olanzapine or intravenous chlorpromazine, but intravenous fluid loading is essential to prevent hypotension with the use of chlorpromazine. We can consider the use of the antihistamine cyproheptadine, which is also a $5\text{-}HT_{2A}$ antagonist, in moderate and severe cases of the condition. Currently, it is available only as an oral preparation, and the initial dose is 12 mg, then adjusted to 2 mg every two hours until symptoms improve.

There is a limited role for traditional antipyretics as the mechanism of serotonin syndrome is due to muscle tone rather than central thermoregulation dysfunction. It is important to avoid physically restraining the patient if possible as this can increase hyperthermia, lactic acidosis and rhabdomyolysis. From a preventative point of view, an awareness of medicines with potent serotonergic effects is the key to preventing the condition. We now turn our attention to serotonin discontinuation syndrome.

Serotonin discontinuation syndrome

Serotonin discontinuation syndrome is a condition that can occur following the dose reduction, discontinuation or interruption of mainly SSRIs or selective noradrenaline reuptake inhibitors (SNRIs). The condition typically starts from the time of reduction in dosage or complete discontinuation, depending on the half-life of the medicine and the patient's metabolism. Serotonin discontinuation syndrome affects approximately 20 per cent of patients following inappropriate and/or sudden discontinuation of their medication or at the start of medication being tapered off. The symptoms of the condition may include dizziness, electric shock-like sensations, sweating, nausea, insomnia, tremor, confusion, nightmares and vertigo (see also Chapter 6).

You can alleviate most symptoms of serotonin discontinuation syndrome by immediately reinstating the original antidepressant or one with a similar mechanism of action. SSRIs with a short half-life such as paroxetine are more likely to cause serotonin discontinuation syndrome. Those SSRIs with a long half-life such as fluoxetine are associated less with serotonin discontinuation syndrome, and you can use these for its treatment. You can do this either by administering a single 20 mg dose of fluoxetine or by starting the patient on a high dose of fluoxetine and slowly titrating down. From a preventative perspective, serotonin discontinuation syndrome can be overcome by a gradual tapering of the medicine or prescribing a medicine with a longer half-life. Furthermore, it has been suggested that antidepressants administered for longer than eight weeks should be tapered, although some advocate a more cautious approach.

Postural hypotension

Postural hypotension is low blood pressure that causes dizziness, especially on standing up quickly, and is more common in older patients and those with diabetes (Bouhanick et al., 2014). Historically, postural hypotension has mainly been caused by antihypertensive therapy. Other medicines that induce postural hypotension are those that bind to the alpha-adrenergic receptors such as antipsychotics and TCAs.

It is important to prospectively monitor for changes in postural blood pressure, particularly for those with psychotic disorders as they do not articulate symptoms of orthostasis. From a non-pharmacological management strategy, the nurse may employ patient education by most notably advising the patient to rise slowly from the supine position and to drink plenty of fluids. In some cases, we can give special nylon stockings to promote arterial constriction in the legs. In severe cases, we can administer medication such as noradrenaline or phenylephrine 9-a-fluorohydrocortisone, which can be given orally.

Sexual dysfunction

Sexual dysfunction includes difficulties during any stage of normal sexual activity, including desire, arousal or orgasm. Many psychotropics, including most SSRIs and second-generation antipsychotics such as risperidone, can cause sexual dysfunction. Antidepressants such as SSRIs induce sexual dysfunction through a different mechanism (see Chapter 6).

From a management viewpoint, the prescriber should switch to other antidepressant medication such as bupropion or trazadone if this side effect proves to be intolerable. However, it is also important to note that trazadone can cause priapism. For the improvement of erectile dysfunction, data support the use of phosphodiesterase inhibitors such as sildenafil (Viagra) and tadalafil (Cialis) as they indicate that these compounds lead to a greater improvement in erectile function than placebo, though their efficacy in women is unknown.

Constipation

There is no generally accepted international definition of the diagnosis of constipation, though symptoms include a reduction in the frequency of defecation, hard and dry stool, and difficulties in defecation. Functional constipation is defined by the internationally acknowledged Rome III criteria (Dal Molin et al., 2012). However, in contrast to the clear definition in the Rome III criteria, people tend to make their own individual definition of constipation that they base on a subjective assessment. A variety of physical, physiological, social and pathological factors can cause the condition. Constipation manifests itself in a range of physical symptoms such as abdominal pain, straining, bloating and nausea. Many psychotropic medicines, including second-generation antipsychotics, most antidepressants and anticholinergic medicines such as procyclidine, induce constipation.

As has been established above, constipated patients present with several symptoms, so it is important to ascertain the patient's complaint relating to what they mean by constipation. The nurse should conduct a careful history noting physical health conditions and medications that affect colonic transit. The history should also include an assessment of stool frequency, stool consistency, stool size, degree of straining during defecation, and a history of ignoring a call to defecate. Conducting a dietary history is important to assess the amount of fibre and water intake, as well as the number of meals and when they were consumed. Further, the history may include the number, type and frequency of laxatives the patient has used in the past. Finally, information about the patient's activities of daily living (ADLs), such as dressing and eating, and their instrumental ADLs, such as grocery shopping and housework, can provide clues on the patient's functional capacity and level of cognition.

Be aware that patients who have a normal bowel pattern usually move their bowels at the same time every day, suggesting that defecation is partly a conditioned reflex. Likewise, colonic motor activity increases after waking and after a meal (gastrocolic reflex). These suggest that a patient with constipation may establish a regular pattern of defecation by ritualising a bowel habit that takes advantage of this normal physiological stimulus. Using the same principle, it may be necessary to educate patients to attempt a bowel movement at least twice a day, usually 30 minutes after meals, and to strain for no more than five minutes.

Evidence shows that a high-fibre diet increases stool weight and decreases colon transit time, while a low-fibre diet leads to constipation. A fibre intake of 20–30 g per day is generally recommended. A relatively early randomised controlled trial showed that dried plums were more effective than the fibre supplement psyllium in the management of mild to moderate constipation (Rao et al., 2009). Other foods rich in fibre are fruits, green vegetables and bran. Advise the patient to take plenty of fluids, regular meals and regular exercise, especially walking. If this does not help, the patient may have to be prescribed a laxative on a short-term basis.

It is good practice to individualise the use of laxatives with special attention paid to the patient's medical history (cardiac and renal co-morbid conditions), medicine interactions, costs and side effects. Laxatives in common use in clinical practice include milk of magnesia, lactulose, senna compounds, bisacodyl and polyethylene glycol (PEG) preparations. Although widely used, stool softeners have limited clinical efficacy. The patient may use suppositories with obstructed defecation to help with rectal evacuation. Similarly, you may use enemas in older patients to prevent faecal impaction. However, side effects such as electrolyte imbalances have been noted with phosphate enemas and rectal mucosal damage with soapsuds enemas. When necessary, you should use tap water enemas as they are safer.

Blurred vision

Blurred vision is usually due to the anticholinergic effects of many psychotropic and other medications used to treat extrapyramidal side effects. These medicines include most antipsychotic medicines, TCAs, anticholinergics, bronchodilators, antispasmodics, antiemetics, antiulcer, mydriatics and some SSRIs. These medications can cause the patient to have difficulty focusing, with things looking fuzzy.

Advise the patient not to drive. In some cases, pilocarpine eye drops can be prescribed. Advise the patient to drink plenty of fluids. In severe cases, physostigmine can be prescribed, but evidence for its use is embryonic. Reassure the patient that the effect is transient.

Xerostomia (dry mouth)

The most frequently reported cause of xerostomia, or dry mouth, is the use of xerostomic medications. Several commonly prescribed medicines that block choline receptors, such as antipsychotics, antidepressants and lithium, can all cause xerostomia. Other medicines that can cause xerostomia include those that we use to control allergies, cold symptoms or blood pressure, as well as some painkillers.

In xerostomia, there is a reduction in salivary flow due to the blockade of cholinergic receptors; however, symptoms may occur without a measurable reduction in salivary gland output. Additionally, xerostomia is often associated with Sjögren's syndrome, a disorder in which the body's immune system mistakenly attacks its own moisture-producing glands, including the salivary glands. This impairment results in dry mouth due to a lack of saliva. Strategies that a patient can use to improve salivary flow may include:

- chewing sugar-free gum or sucking on sugar-free hard candies to stimulate salivary flow;
- sucking on ice chips;
- sipping water with meals to aid in chewing and swallowing food;
- using alcohol-free mouthwash;
- avoiding carbonated drinks (e.g. soda), caffeine, tobacco and alcohol;
- using a lanolin-based lip balm to soothe cracked or dry lips.

If the patient is developing cavities in their teeth, they might use a toothpaste or mouthwash that has fluoride in it to help protect their teeth. They might also apply a fluoride gel or use a fluoride-containing rinse. Most importantly, advise the patient to pay careful attention to oral hygiene and use sugarless fluids frequently. In some instances, the use of pilocarpine and oxidised glycerol triesters treatment may be helpful.

Psychotropic drug-induced DRESS syndrome

Drug rash with eosinophilia and systemic symptoms (DRESS) syndrome is a severe cutaneous eruption that has been linked to several common medicines and medicine categories, including anti-epileptics, allopurinol, sulphonamides and various antibiotics. It was originally observed in patients treated with anticonvulsants in the early 1930s, when phenytoin first became available. However, because of several recent case reports linking psychotropic medications to this condition, DRESS syndrome is increasingly recognised in mental health settings. Many psychotropic medicines, including carbamazepine, lamotrigine, phenytoin, valproate and phenobarbital, have been identified as causative of the condition. The list of potential causative agents of DRESS syndrome is considerable, but carbamazepine is the most frequently reported. The onset of symptoms typically occurs two to six weeks after medicine administration, though symptoms may occur more rapidly and be more severe upon re-exposure (Husain et al., 2013). The condition is characterised by fever, rash, **lymphadenopathy**, internal organ involvement and haematological abnormalities. The most affected organs are the liver, the lungs and the kidneys, and characteristic blood abnormalities include **lymphocytopenia**, atypical lymphocytes and **eosinophilia**. DRESS syndrome can be difficult to diagnose because of its non-specific presentation. Moreover, it is often asymptomatic until a considerable amount of time has passed after the initial medicine exposure. The appropriate management of DRESS syndrome is important because the condition is associated with significant morbidity and mortality. Although most patients recover from the condition, some patients suffer from chronic complications, and approximately 10 per cent die, primarily from visceral organ compromise.

We should manage patients with DRESS syndrome in an intensive care or burns unit for appropriate care and infection control. In addition, it is important to consult an appropriate specialist based on the affected organ systems. Upon clinical diagnosis of DRESS syndrome, the cornerstones of clinical management of the condition include prompt withdrawal of the implicated medicine and administration of corticosteroids, most commonly prednisolone, which can be initiated and then tapered over six to eight weeks to prevent relapse of organ involvement. Other treatments can involve intravenous methylprednisolone and plasmapheresis.

For cases of corticosteroid-resistant DRESS syndrome, intravenous immunoglobulin, cyclophosphamide, cyclosporine and immunosuppressants show efficacy. Management of co-morbid psychiatric illness includes strict avoidance of the implicated medicine and other medicines in the same class, as well as identification of a replacement medicine (e.g. valproate for carbamazepine-induced DRESS syndrome).

Fluid and electrolyte replacement and nutritional support are required for those with **exfoliative dermatitis**. A warm and humid environment with gentle skincare (e.g. warm baths, wet dressings) is indicated. We can also treat patients symptomatically if they have no clinical, laboratory or imaging evidence of renal or pulmonary involvement and only modest elevations of liver enzymes.

Stevens–Johnson syndrome and toxic epidermal necrolysis

Skin rash is a common side effect of many anti-epileptic medicines also used as mood stabilisers. This side effect has been the leading cause of withdrawal from some drug trials. Anti-epileptic medicines that can cause skin rash include carbamazepine, phenytoin, phenobarbital, sodium valproate, pregabelin and lamotrigine. Whereas most anti-epileptic medicines are associated with benign skin rash, serious rashes, including Stevens–Johnson syndrome (SJS) and toxic epidermal necrolysis (TEN), can occur (see Chapter 7). The characteristics of Stevens–Johnson syndrome are severe weeping conjunctivitis and severe stomatitis with extensive mucosal necrosis and purpuric macules, which can be accompanied by the development of large areas of epidermal detachment.

The management of SJS/TEN in the acute stage involves successively assessing the severity and prognosis of disease, prompt identification and withdrawal of the culprit medicine, and rapidly initiating supportive care in an appropriate setting. Evidence shows that the earlier the causative medicine is withdrawn, the better the prognosis, and that patients exposed to causative medicines with long half-lives have an increased risk of dying (Garcia-Doval et al., 2000). To identify the culprit medicine, it is important to consider the chronology of administration of the medicine and the reported ability of the medicine to induce SJS/TEN. The chronology of administration of a culprit medicine, or the time between first administration and development of SJS/TEN, is between one and four weeks in most cases.

Because SJS/TEN is a life-threatening condition, supportive care is an essential part of the therapeutic approach. A critical element of supportive care is the management of fluid and electrolyte requirements. Giving intravenous fluid to maintain urine output of 50–80 mL per hour with 0.5 per cent sodium chloride (NaCl) supplemented with 20 mEq of potassium chloride (KCl) is critical. Appropriate early and aggressive replacement therapy is necessary in the case of **hyponatraemia, hypokalaemia** or **hypophosphataemia**, which quite frequently occur. It is important to treat wounds conservatively without skin debridement, which is often performed in burns units as blistered skin acts as a natural biological dressing that favours re-epithelialisation. Use non-adhesive wound dressings where they are required and avoid topical sulphamide-containing medications. Further, there may be a benefit of using high-dose intravenous immunoglobulins (IVIG), tumour necrotic factor antagonists (TNF-α) and cyclophosphamide (CPP) in the treatment of TEN, but firm conclusions cannot be drawn at this stage because of the embryonic nature of the evidence. Most patients recover without major harm from the disease. However, even with prompt management with close observation, SJS/TEN poses a significant risk of mortality that correlates with the extent of skin descaling.

Urinary retention

Urinary retention, the inability to void despite a full bladder, is usually transitory but can be prolonged in some cases. It can lead to several complications, including urinary tract infection, long-term bladder dysfunction, and kidney damage leading to chronic kidney disease. Catheterisation, generally regarded as the optimal management method, is associated with risks, and so pharmacological treatment of post-operative urinary retention that could remove or reduce the need for catheterisation is desirable. Urinary retention is characterised by a poor urinary stream with intermittent flow, straining or a sense of incomplete voiding, and hesitancy. Arrange for the patient to see a doctor to review their medication. While it may appear that cholinergic agents and intravenously administered prostaglandin offer the most promise in the treatment of urinary retention, the evidence is weak. Bethanechol is sometimes given to relieve the symptoms.

Chapter summary

ADRs are a common feature in clinical practice and are a cause of many unplanned hospital admissions, but many do not cause serious harm. Only between 5 and 10 per cent of patients suffer from an ADR during admission to or discharge from hospital. Historically, ADRs have been classified into two types: type A reactions, which are dose-dependent and type B reactions, which are bizarre or idiosyncratic. Interventions that reduce the probability of an ADR occurring can be an important way to reduce the risk of patient harm. There are various strategies for managing these side effects, but basic approaches may include discontinuation of the medication and switching to a more tolerable alternative, or the use of other medications to counteract the effects of the primary medicine.

Activities: brief outline answers

Activity 12.1 Critical thinking (page 327)

Age, type of medication, weight, gender, genetics and cultural values might influence intolerance to side effects.

Activity 12.2 Critical thinking (page 330)

People going through severe dystonia also experience difficulties in swallowing (dysphagia); therefore, giving oral medication is inadvisable.

Activity 12.3 Critical thinking (page 334)

It may be too soon to increase the dose of risperidone as it is quite likely that Sophie's delusions may be of a secondary nature, and it is therefore important to explore her beliefs beyond their face value. It is quite likely that Sophie is experiencing hormonal side effects of the depot such as lactating. If this is the case, it might explain her delusions. In any event, it is important to test for prolactin levels to exclude the possibility of sexual side effects.

Activity 12.4 Decision-making (page 338)

A good starting point is to speak to the patient and express your observation, and then take a note of the patient's response. If the restlessness is due to NMS, then the patient is unlikely to give you a coherent or rational reason why. In any event, check what medication the patient is taking and when it was last administered – and by what route (i.e. intramuscular or oral). Take vital signs and observe for rigidity and high temperature. If one of these is present, call the doctor without delay.

Further reading

Balon, R. (2007) *Practical Management of the Side Effects of Psychotropic Drugs.* New York: Marcel Dekker.

This is an easy-to-follow book that gives practical guidance on how to manage the side effects of different psychotropic medications.

Cunningham Owens, D.G. (2014) *A Guide to the Extrapyramidal Side-Effects of Antipsychotic Drugs.* Cambridge: Cambridge University Press.

This book discusses extrapyramidal side effects and their management in more detail.

Goldberg, J.F. and Ernst, C.L. (2018) *Managing the Side Effects of Psychotropic Medications.* Arlington, VA: APA Publishing.

This book discusses different types of side effects and how to manage them comprehensively. It is useful for prescribers and those who administer medication.

Useful websites

http://psychcentral.com/lib/coping-with-atypical-antipsychotic-side-effects/0002823

This website gives useful advice on how to cope with antipsychotic side effects and provides useful tips.

www.webmd.com/depression/managing-the-side-effects-of-antidepressants

This is a useful website that gives advice on how to manage the side effects of antidepressants.

Glossary

agranulocytosis A marked decrease in the number of white blood cells called granulocytes that are responsible for fighting infection.

akinetic The loss or impairment of the power of voluntary movement.

aldolase An enzyme in humans that helps to convert glucose (sugar) into energy (also known as fructose-bisphosphate aldolase).

alkaloids Any of a class of naturally occurring organic nitrogen-containing bases. Alkaloids have diverse and important physiological effects on humans and other animals. Well-known alkaloids include morphine, strychnine, quinine, ephedrine and nicotine.

Alpers-Huttenlocher syndrome A progressive, neurodevelopmental, mitochondrial disease most often associated with mutations in the mitochondrial DNA replicase. It is characterised by three co-occurring clinical symptoms: psychomotor regression (dementia), seizures and liver disease.

ambivalence Feeling two ways about something; ambivalence is a natural phase in the process of change and must be resolved for change to occur.

amyotrophic lateral sclerosis (ALS) A group of rare neurological diseases that mainly involve the nerve cells responsible for controlling voluntary muscle movement such as chewing, walking and talking. The disease is progressive; currently, there is no cure for ALS and no effective treatment to halt or reverse the progression of the disease.

anabolic steroids Drugs that mimic the effects of the male sex hormones. They enhance protein synthesis within cells, which results in the build-up of cellular tissue, particularly muscles.

anhedonia Loss of the ability to experience pleasure from normally pleasurable experiences.

aplastic anaemia A condition where bone marrow does not produce sufficient new cells to replenish blood cells. Patients with aplastic anaemia have lower counts of all three blood cell types (red and white blood cells and platelets).

autoreceptors Types of receptors located in the membranes of presynaptic nerve cells. They serve as part of a negative feedback loop in signal transduction. They are only sensitive to the neurotransmitters or hormones released by the neuron on which the autoreceptors sit.

basal ganglia A collection of nuclei found on both sides of the thalamus. It is mainly in the basal ganglia that the neurotransmitter GABA plays an important role.

Bolam principle Established that a medical practitioner is to be judged by the standards of their profession. If a doctor acts in accordance with the practice of a responsible body of practitioners, then the doctor is not negligent, even if others would have taken a different and more efficacious approach.

cardiotoxicity Damage to the heart muscle, sometimes due to medications a patient is taking.

circumstantial speech A speech pattern characterised by rambling, unnecessary comments and irrelevant details (also known as circumstantiality). Individuals exhibiting circumstantial speech have difficulty 'getting to the point' – their focus wanders to other unnecessary topics or ideas. They are only talking about circumstances instead of answering the question.

clonus A set of involuntary and rhythmic muscular contractions and relaxations. It is a sign of certain neurological conditions, particularly associated with upper motor neuron lesions involving descending motor pathways, and in many cases is accompanied by spasticity.

cognitive dysfunction An unusually poor mental function, associated with confusion, forgetfulness and difficulty concentrating.

collaborative process Achieving a desired outcome in the most efficient and effective way possible by paying attention to how people work together in an equitable partnership.

co-morbid substance misuse See dual diagnosis.

concordance The extent to which a patient correctly follows medical advice. It often refers to medication adherence but may also involve non-adherence to self-directed physiotherapy exercises or other courses of therapy. Both the patient and the healthcare provider affect adherence, and a positive nurse–patient relationship is the most important factor.

creatine phosphokinase (CPK) An enzyme whose elevated levels in the blood are a marker for myocardial infarction (heart attack).

Cushing's syndrome A disease caused by increased production of cortisol or by excessive use of cortisol or other steroid hormones.

decimal   Relating to a system of numbers and arithmetic based on the number 10.

decompensation   The deterioration of a previously working structure or system. It can occur due to tiredness, stress, illness or old age. Decompensation also describes an inability to compensate for these.

deoxyribonucleic acid (DNA)   A substance present in nearly all living organisms that carries genetic information.

diaphoresis   Excessive, abnormal sweating in relation to the environment and activity level. It tends to affect the entire body rather than a part of the body. This condition is also sometimes called secondary hyperhidrosis.

dual diagnosis   Also known as co-morbid substance misuse, a dual condition where a person suffers from a mental illness and a substance abuse problem. The term can be used broadly (e.g. depression, alcoholism), or it can be restricted to specify severe mental illness and substance use disorder.

dyslipidaemia   An abnormal amount of fat, including cholesterol, in the blood. Most dyslipidaemias are hyperlipidaemias, an elevation of lipids in the blood, often due to lifestyle and diet. Prolonged elevation of insulin levels in the blood can lead to dyslipidaemia.

ego-syntonic   A psychological term referring to behaviours, values or feelings that are in harmony with – or acceptable to – the needs and goals of one's ideal self-image.

empirical study   A study relying on – or derived from – observation or experiment.

enterohepatic circulation   The circulation of biliary acids, bilirubin, drugs or other substances from the liver to the bile, followed by entry into the small intestine, absorption by the enterocyte and transport back to the liver.

eosinophilia   A condition in which the eosinophil count in the peripheral blood exceeds 0.5×10 /1 ($500/\mu L$). A marked increase in non-blood tissue eosinophil count upon histopathologic examination is diagnostic for tissue eosinophilia. Several causes are known, with the most common being some form of allergic reaction or parasitic infection.

excitatory amino acid transporter (EAAT)   Part of a family of glutamate transporter proteins that remove glutamate from the synaptic cleft and extra synaptic sites into the glial cells and neurons.

exfoliative dermatitis   Scaly eruption of most of the skin.

expressed emotion   A qualitative measure of the amount of emotion displayed, typically in the family setting, usually by a family or caretakers. Theoretically, a high level of expressed emotion in the home can worsen the prognosis in patients with mental illness, or act as a potential risk factor for the development of psychiatric disease.

extrapyramidal side effects A group of symptoms that can occur when taking antipsychotic medications. These symptoms include akathisia, slurred speech, dystonia, slowness of movements and muscular rigidity.

follicle-stimulating hormone (FSH) A hormone found in humans that regulates growth, pubertal development and reproductive processes of the body.

fraction A numerical quantity that is not a whole number (e.g. three-quarters or one-fifth).

genome The genetic material of an organism. It consists of DNA (or RNA in RNA viruses). The genome includes both genes (the coding regions) and non-coding DNA, as well as mitochondrial DNA and chloroplast DNA.

glial cells Supportive cells surrounding neurons in the central nervous system that do not conduct electrical impulses.

globus pallidus Also known as paleo-striatum or dorsal pallidum; a subcortical structure of the brain that consists of two adjacent segments, one external (known as globus pallidus externa) and one internal (known as globus pallidus interna). It is part of the telencephalon but retains close functional ties with the subthalamus in the diencephalon, both of which are part of the extrapyramidal motor system.

glucuronic acid A carboxylic acid derived from glucose, the basic form of sugar in the human body. It is formed when glucose interacts with oxygen and creates a slightly different structure, through oxidation. This acid's main function is to combine with toxins and eliminate them from the body.

haemodialysis A method for removing waste products such as creatinine and urea, as well as free water, from the blood when the kidneys have failed.

half-life The period it takes for a medicine being metabolised to decrease by half.

hallucinogens Drugs that cause profound distortions in a person's perceptions of reality. Under the influence of such drugs (e.g. LSD), people can see images, hear sounds and feel sensations that seem real but do not exist.

homeostasis Maintenance of a stable equilibrium in the body, especially by adjusting physiological processes.

hyperchromic anaemia Any type of anaemia in which the red blood cells are paler than normal. This decrease in redness is due to a disproportionate reduction of red cell haemoglobin in proportion to the volume of the cell.

hyperprolactinaemia The presence of abnormally high levels of prolactin in the blood.

hyperreflexia Overactive or exaggerated reflexes, such as twitching.

hypoglycaemia   A condition that occurs when blood sugar (glucose) is too low.

hypokalaemia   A low level of potassium in the blood serum. Symptoms may include feeling tired, leg cramps, weakness, and constipation. Low potassium also increases the risk of an abnormal heart rhythm, which is often too slow and can cause cardiac arrest.

hyponatraemia   An electrolyte disturbance in which the sodium concentration in the blood is lower than normal. It is a serum sodium concentration of less than 135 mmol/L. It is quite often a complication of other physical illness, such as vomiting or diarrhoea, where there is a loss of sodium.

hypophosphataemia   An electrolyte disorder in which there is a low level of phosphate in the blood. Symptoms may include weakness, trouble breathing, and loss of appetite. Complications may include seizures, coma, rhabdomyolysis or softening of the bones.

hypothyroidism   A condition in which the thyroid gland does not make enough thyroid hormone, which can result in symptoms such as increased sensitivity to cold, constipation, depression, fatigue or feeling slowed down, and heavier menstrual flow.

iatrogenic   Induced inadvertently by a doctor or surgeon, or by medical treatment or diagnostic procedures.

idiopathic   Used to describe medical conditions arising spontaneously or from an unknown cause.

idiosyncratic response   A subjective or unusual response to a drug that is peculiar to the individual who manifests the response. The cause of such a response is not readily understood.

insight   From a psychiatric perspective, to see ourselves as others see us.

intubation   The placement of a flexible plastic tube into the trachea to maintain an open airway or to serve as a conduit through which to administer certain medicines. It is frequently performed in critical care conditions.

Leigh syndrome   An inherited neurometabolic disorder that affects the central nervous system. Normal levels of thiamine, thiamine monophosphate and thiamine diphosphate are commonly found, but there is a reduced or absent level of thiamine triphosphate. This is believed to be caused by a blockage in the enzyme thiamine-diphosphate kinase, and therefore treatment in some patients would be to take thiamine triphosphate daily.

leucocytosis   A condition in which the white blood cell count is above the normal range in the blood. It is frequently a sign of an inflammatory response, most commonly the result of infection, but may also occur following certain parasitic infections or bone tumours, as well as leukaemia. It may also occur after strenuous exercise, convulsions such as epilepsy, emotional stress, pregnancy and labour, anaesthesia, as a side effect of medication, and noradrenaline administration.

luteinising hormone (LH)   Also known as lutropin, a hormone produced by the anterior pituitary gland. It triggers the ovulation process in women. It is called the interstitial cell-stimulating hormone (ICSH) in males and is responsible for stimulating the production of testosterone.

lymphadenopathy   A disease affecting the lymph nodes where they enlarge.

lymphocytopenia   The condition of having an abnormally low level of lymphocytes (types of white blood cells) in the blood. It is also called lymphopenia. The opposite is lymphocytosis, which refers to an excessive level of lymphocytes.

metabolite   A substance produced by metabolism or by a metabolic process.

myelin   The fatty substance that covers and protects nerves. It allows efficient conduction of action potentials down the axon. It consists of 70 per cent lipids and phospholipids and 30 per cent proteins.

myoclonus   A term used to describe the jerking or twitching of a muscle. It can be a symptom of an underlying medical condition that requires medical attention. This involuntary muscle movement can take a wide variety of forms, appearing in any muscle in the body at any time, depending on the underlying cause of the myoclonus.

neutropenia   A condition where a person has a low level of neutrophils. Neutrophils are types of white blood cells that help to fight infection by destroying harmful bacteria and fungi (yeast) that invade the body. Neutrophils are made in the bone marrow. Bone marrow is the spongy tissue found in larger bones such as the pelvis, vertebrae and ribs.

orthostatic hypotension   Also known as postural hypotension, this is a form of hypotension in which the blood pressure suddenly falls when the person stands up or stretches. The decrease is most pronounced after resting. Many psychotropic medications, especially antipsychotics, cause orthostatic hypotension.

per cent   One part in every hundred (e.g. 25 per cent is 25 out of 100).

pharmacotherapy   Treatment of disease with medicines.

phosphorylated   The attachment of a phosphoryl molecule group to another molecule to add energy to that molecule. It is critical for many cellular processes in biology. Protein phosphorylation is especially important for their function; for example, this modification activates (or deactivates) enzymes, thereby regulating their function.

plasmapheresis   A method of removing blood plasma from the body by withdrawing blood, separating it into plasma and cells, and transfusing the cells back into the bloodstream. It is usually performed to remove antibodies in treating autoimmune conditions.

probenecid   A medication that increases uric acid excretion in the urine. It is primarily used in treating gout and hyperuricemia.

psychoactive Describes a chemical that crosses the blood–brain barrier and acts primarily upon the central nervous system, where it affects brain function, resulting in changes in perception, mood, consciousness, cognition and behaviour.

psychotropic medication Medication that affects the mind, emotions and behaviour. Psychotropic medications include most medicines used to treat psychiatric symptoms.

reticular activating system (RAS) A diffuse network of nerve pathways in the brainstem connecting the spinal cord, the cerebrum and the cerebellum, as well as mediating the overall level of consciousness.

secondary delusions Delusions influenced by the person's background or current situation (e.g. ethnic or sexual orientation, religious beliefs).

sedation An act of calming by administering certain medicines.

Socratic questioning A form of disciplined questioning that can be used to pursue thoughts in many directions and for many purposes, including to explore complex ideas, to get to the truth of things, to open up issues and problems, to uncover assumptions, to analyse concepts, to distinguish what we know from what we do not know, to follow logical consequences of thought, or to control discussions. It is based on the foundation that thinking has structured logic, and allows underlying thoughts to be questioned. Socratic questioning is systematic, disciplined and deep, and usually focuses on fundamental concepts, principles, theories, issues or problems.

spindle coma An electroclinical entity in which physiological sleep patterns, such as sleep spindles in the 12–14 Hz range, occur synchronously in patients with altered consciousness.

steady state A condition in the body whereby drug blood serum levels do not change over time, or in which any one change is continually balanced by another, such as the stable condition of a system in equilibrium.

subtherapeutic Below the dosage levels used to treat diseases.

sulphuric acid A mineral acid composed of the elements sulphur, oxygen and hydrogen. It is a colourless, odourless and syrupy liquid that is soluble in water, and is synthesised in reactions that generate heat (exothermic).

syncope Temporary loss of consciousness caused by low blood pressure.

tardive dyskinesia A movement disorder caused by long-term use of antipsychotic medications. It is characterised by uncontrolled facial movements such as a protruding tongue, chewing or sucking motions, and making faces.

therapeutic alliance Within the context of psychotherapy, the collaborative relationship between the therapist and the client. The therapeutic alliance can have three components: an agreement between the therapist and the client about the goals of treatment, an agreement about the therapy tasks needed to accomplish those goals, and the emotional bond developed between the therapist and the client that allows the client to make therapeutic progress.

therapeutic drug levels Laboratory tests that look for the presence and the amount of specific drugs in the blood.

thiazide A diuretic medicine that increases the amount of water passed through the kidneys.

titrating Incremental increase or decrease in drug dosage to a level that provides the optimal therapeutic effect.

transaminases Any of a group of enzymes that catalyse the transfer of the amino group ($-NH_2$) of an amino acid to a carbonyl compound such as a -keto acid (also known as aminotransferase).

tricyclics Antidepressant drugs named after their chemical structure, which has three rings of atoms.

trigeminal neuralgia A nerve disorder that causes a stabbing or electric shock-like pain in parts of the face.

validity In research, the degree to which a study accurately reflects or assesses the specific concept that the researcher is attempting to measure.

variance Measures how far a set of numbers are spread out from their average value.

veracity Conformity to facts; accuracy.

vesicular glutamate transporter (VGLUT) A family of excitatory neurotransmitter transporter proteins that move glutamate mainly across a membrane. They are encoded by the SLC17A7 gene.

References

Adelufosi, A.O., Abayomi, O. and Ojo, T.M. (2015) Pyridoxal 5 phosphate for neuroleptic-induced tardive dyskinesia. *Cochrane Database of Systematic Reviews*, 4, CD010501. Available at: http://dx.doi.org/10.1002/14651858.CD010501.pub2

Aitken, M. and Gorokhovich, L. (2013) Advancing the responsible use of medicines: applying levers for change. Available at: http://dx.doi.org/10.2139/ssrn.2222541

Al Khalili, Y. and Jain, S. (2019) Carbamazepine toxicity. In *StatPearls*, Treasure Island (FL): StatPearls Publishing StatPearls Publishing LLC.

Alloy, L.B. and Abramson, L.Y. (1988) Depressive realism: four theoretical perspectives. In L.B. Alloy (ed.), *Cognitive Processes in Depression*. New York: Guilford Press, pp223–65.

Alyahya, B., Friesen, M., Nauche, B. and Laliberte, M. (2018) Acute lamotrigine overdose: a systematic review of published adult and pediatric cases. *Clinical Toxicology*, 56(2): 81–9.

Alzheimer's Society (2018) *Optimising Treatment and Care for People with Behavioural and Psychological Symptoms of Dementia*. Available at: www.alzheimers.org.uk/sites/default/files/2018-08/Optimising%20treatment%20and%20care%20-%20best%20practice%20guide.pdf?downloadID=609

Amador, X.F. and David, A. (2004) *Insight and Psychosis: Awareness of Illness in Schizophrenia and Related Disorders*. Oxford: Oxford University Press.

Amann, B., Born, C., Crespo, J.M., Pomarol-Clotet, E. and McKenna, P. (2011) Lamotrigine: when and where does it act in affective disorders? A systematic review. *Journal of Psychopharmacology*, 25(10): 1289–94.

Amato, D., Kruyer, A., Samaha, A.-N. and Heinz, A. (2019) Hypofunctional dopamine uptake and antipsychotic treatment-resistant schizophrenia. *Frontiers in Psychiatry*, 10: 314. Available at: http://dx.doi.org/10.3389/fpsyt.2019.00314

Amato, D., Vernon, A.C. and Papaleo, F. (2018) Dopamine, the antipsychotic molecule: a perspective on mechanisms underlying antipsychotic response variability. *Neuroscience & Biobehavioral Reviews*, 85: 146–59.

Anacker, C., O'Donnell, K.J. and Meaney, M.J. (2014) Early life adversity and the epigenetic programming of hypothalamic-pituitary-adrenal function. *Dialogues in Clinical Neuroscience*, 16(3): 321–33.

Anand, K.S., Dhikav, V., Sachdeva, A. and Mishra, P. (2016) Perceived caregiver stress in Alzheimer's disease and mild cognitive impairment: a case control study. *Annals of Indian Academy of Neurology*, 19(1): 58–62.

Anderson, P. and Baumberg, B. (2006) Alcohol in Europe – public health perspective: report summary. *Drugs: Education, Prevention and Policy*, 13(6): 483–8.

Andrisano, C., Chiesa, A. and Serretti, A. (2013) Newer antidepressants and panic disorder: a meta-analysis. *International Clinical Psychopharmacology*, 28(1): 33–45.

Aquino, C.C. and Lang, A.E. (2014) Tardive dyskinesia syndromes: current concepts. *Parkinsonism & Related Disorders*, 20(S1): 113–17.

Asmal, L., Flegar, S.J., Wang, J., Rummel-Kluge, C., Komossa, K. and Leucht, S. (2013) Quetiapine versus other atypical antipsychotics for schizophrenia. *Cochrane Database of Systematic Reviews*, 11, CD006625. Available at: http://dx.doi.org/10.1002/14651858. CD006625.pub3

Baird-Gunning, J., Lea-Henry, T., Hoegberg, L.C.G., Gosselin, S. and Roberts, D.M. (2017) Lithium poisoning. *Journal of Intensive Care Medicine*, 32(4): 249–63.

Bala, A., Nguyen, H.M.T. and Hellstrom, W.J.G. (2018) Post-SSRI sexual dysfunction: a literature review. *Sexual Medicine Reviews*, 6(1): 29–34.

Baldwin, D., Woods, R., Lawson, R. and Taylor, D. (2011) Efficacy of drug treatments for generalised anxiety disorder: systematic review and meta-analysis. *BMJ*, 342: d1199. Available at: http://dx.doi.org/10.1136/bmj.d1199

Baldwin, D.S., Asakura, S., Koyama, T., Hayano, T., Hagino, A., Reines, E. and Larsen, K. (2016) Efficacy of escitalopram in the treatment of social anxiety disorder: a meta-analysis versus placebo. *European Neuropsychopharmacology*, 26(6): 1062–9.

Baldwin, D.S., den Boer, J.A., Lyndon, G., Emir, B., Schweizer, E. and Haswell, H. (2015) Efficacy and safety of pregabalin in generalised anxiety disorder: a critical review of the literature. *Journal of Psychopharmacology*, 29(10): 1047–60.

Balon, R. (2007) *Practical Management of the Side Effects of Psychotropic Drugs*. New York: Marcel Dekker.

Bandura, A. (1977) *Social Learning Theory*. Englewood Cliffs, NJ: Prentice Hall.

Bao, Y.P., Liu, Z.M., Epstein, D.H., Du, C., Shi, J. and Lu, L. (2009) A meta-analysis of retention in methadone maintenance by dose and dosing strategy. *American Journal of Drug and Alcohol Abuse*, 35(1): 28–33.

Barber, P., Brown, R. and Martin, D. (2016) *Mental Health Law in England and Wales: A Guide for Mental Health Professionals*. Exeter: Learning Matters.

Barnes, T.R. (1989) A rating scale for drug-induced akathisia. *British Journal of Psychiatry*, 154: 672–6.

Barrons, R. and Roberts, N. (2010) The role of carbamazepine and oxcarbazepine in alcohol withdrawal syndrome. *Journal of Clinical Pharmacy and Therapeutics*, 35(2): 153–67.

Baxter, A.J., Scott, K.M., Vos, T. and Whiteford, H.A. (2013) Global prevalence of anxiety disorders: a systematic review and meta-regression. *Psychological Medicine*, 43(5): 897–910.

Baxter, A.J., Vos, T., Scott, K.M., Ferrari, A.J. and Whiteford, H.A. (2014) The global burden of anxiety disorders in 2010. *Psychological Medicine*, 44(11): 2363–74.

Baxter, K. (ed.) (2011) *Stockley's Drug Interactions Pocket Companion*. London: Pharmaceutical Press.

Beauchamp, T.L. and Childress, J.F. (2001) *Principles of Biomedical Ethics*. Oxford: Oxford University Press.

Beauchamp, T.L. and Walters, L. (1999) Ethical theory and bioethics. *Contemporary Issues in Bioethics*, pp1–32.

Beck, A. (1976) *Cognitive Therapy and the Emotional Disorders*. New York: International Universities Press.

Berghmans, R., Dickenson, D. and Meulen, R.T. (2004) Mental capacity: in search of alternative perspectives. *Health Care Analysis*, 12(4): 251–63.

Bester, J., Cole, C.M. and Kodish, E. (2016) The limits of informed consent for an overwhelmed patient: clinicians' role in protecting patients and preventing overwhelm. *AMA Journal of Ethics*, 18(9): 869–86.

Bhat, S., Dao, D.T., Terrillion, C.E., Arad, M., Smith, R.J., Soldatov, N.M. and Gould, T.D. (2012) CACNA1C (Cav1.2) in the pathophysiology of psychiatric disease. *Progress in Neurobiology*, 99(1): 1–14.

Blackwell, B. (1998) From compliance to alliance: a quarter century of research. In B. Blackwell (ed.), *Treatment Compliance and the Therapeutic Alliance*. Amsterdam: Harwood Academic, pp1–15.

Blomstrom, A., Gardner, R.M., Dalman, C., Yolken, R.H. and Karlsson, H. (2015) Influence of maternal infections on neonatal acute phase proteins and their interaction in the development of non-affective psychosis. *Translational Psychiatry*, 5(2): e502. Available at: http://dx.doi.org/10.1038/tp.2014.142

Bond, D.J., Kauer-Sant'Anna, M., Lam, R.W. and Yatham, L.N. (2010) Weight gain, obesity, and metabolic indices following a first manic episode: prospective 12-month data from the Systematic Treatment Optimization Program for Early Mania (STOP-EM)', *Journal of Affective Disorders*, 124(1–2): 108–17.

Bond, K. and Anderson, I.M. (2015) Psychoeducation for relapse prevention in bipolar disorder: a systematic review of efficacy in randomized controlled trials. *Bipolar Disorders*, 17(4): 349–62.

Bonnet, U. and Scherbaum, N. (2017) How addictive are gabapentin and pregabalin? A systematic review. *European Neuropsychopharmacology*, 27(12): 1185–215.

Borrelli, B., Riekert, K.A., Weinstein, A. and Rathier, L. (2007) Brief motivational interviewing as a clinical strategy to promote asthma medication adherence. *Journal of Allergy and Clinical Immunology*, 120(5): 1023–30.

Bostoen, S., Seeman, P., Vanderheyden, P. and Vauquelin, G. (2012) Clozapine, atypical antipsychotics, and the benefits of fast-off D2 dopamine receptor antagonism. *Naunyn-Schmiedeberg's Archives of Pharmacology*, 385(4): 337–72.

Bouhanick, B., Meliani, S., Doucet, J., Bauduceau, B., Verny, C., Chamontin, B. and Le Floch, J.P. (2014) Orthostatic hypotension is associated with more severe hypertension in elderly autonomous diabetic patients from the French Gerodiab study at inclusion. *Annales de Cardiologie et d'Angéiologie*, 63(3): 176–82.

Bretler, T., Weisberg, H., Koren, O. and Neuman, H. (2019) The effects of antipsychotic medications on microbiome and weight gain in children and adolescents. *BMC Medicine*, 17(1): 112. Available at: http://dx.doi.org/10.1186/s12916-019-1346-1

Brissos, S., Veguilla, M.R., Taylor, D. and Balanza-Martinez, V. (2014) The role of long-acting injectable antipsychotics in schizophrenia: a critical appraisal. *Therapeutic Advances in Psychopharmacology*, 4(5): 198–219.

British Medical Association (BMA) (2018) *Consent Toolkit.* Available at: https://cse.google.com/cse?cx=partner-pub-2698861478625135:7463904445&ie=UTF-8&q=guidande%20on%20consnet%2C%20the%20general%20pharmaceutical%20council%20%23

Brołsen, K. and Naranjo, C.A. (2001) Review of pharmacokinetic and pharmacodynamic interaction studies with citalopram. *European Neuropsychopharmacology*, 11(4): 275–83.

Calhoun, A., King, C., Khoury, R. and Grossberg, G.T. (2018) An evaluation of memantine ER + donepezil for the treatment of Alzheimer's disease. *Expert Opinion on Pharmacotherapy*, 19(15): 1711–17.

Carlson, G.A. and Goodwin, F.K. (1973) The stages of mania: a longitudinal analylsis of the manic episode. *JAMA*, 28(2): 221–8.

Carlsson, A. and Lindqvist, M. (1963) Effect of chlorpromazine or haloperidol on formation of 3methoxytyramine and normetanephrine in mouse brain. *Acta Pharmacologica et Toxicologica*, 20: 140–4.

Carmona, S., Hardy, J. and Guerreiro, R. (2018) The genetic landscape of Alzheimer disease. *Handbook of Clinical Neurology*, 148: 395–408.

Castano-Ramirez, O.M., Sepulveda-Arias, J.C., Duica, K., Diaz Zuluaga, A.M., Vargas, C. and Lopez-Jaramillo, C. (2018) Inflammatory markers in the staging of bipolar disorder: a systematic review of the literature. *Revista Colombiana de Psiquiatría*, 47(2): 119–28.

Caton, C.L., Goldstein, J.M., Serrano, O. and Bender, R. (1984) The impact of discharge planning on chronic schizophrenic patients. *Hospital and Community Psychiatry*, 35(3): 255–62.

Chakrabarti, S. (2018) Treatment alliance and adherence in bipolar disorder. *World Journal of Psychiatry*, 8(5): 114–24.

Chaudhry, I., Neelam, K., Duddu, V. and Husain, N. (2008) Ethnicity and psychopharmacology. *Journal of Psychopharmacology*, 22(6): 673–80.

Chen, C.-H., Chen, C.-Y. and Lin, K.-M. (2008) Ethnopsychopharmacology. *International Review of Psychiatry*, 20(5): 452–9.

Chen, R., Zhu, X., Capitao, L.P., Zhang, H., Luo, J., Wang, X., Xi, Y., Song, X., Feng, Y., Cao, L. and Malhi, G.S. (2019) Psychoeducation for psychiatric inpatients following remission of a manic episode in bipolar I disorder: a randomized controlled trial. *Bipolar Disorders*, 21(1): 76–85.

Chen, Y.D., Zhang, J., Wang, Y., Yuan, J.L. and Hu, W.L. (2016) Efficacy of cholinesterase inhibitors in vascular dementia: an updated meta-analysis. *European Neurology*, 75(3–4): 132–41.

Chesney, E., Goodwin, G.M. and Fazel, S. (2014) Risks of all-cause and suicide mortality in mental disorders: a meta-review. *World Psychiatry*, 13(2): 153–60.

Chessick, C.A., Allen, M.H., Thase, M., Batista Miralha da Cunha, A.B., Kapczinski, F.F., de Lima, M.S. and dos Santos Souza, J.J. (2006) Azapirones for generalized anxiety disorder. *Cochrane Database of Systematic Reviews*, 3, CD006115. Available at: http://dx.doi.org/10.1002/14651858.cd006115

Cipriani, A., Reid, K., Young, A.H., Macritchie, K. and Geddes, J. (2013) Valproic acid, valproate and divalproex in the maintenance treatment of bipolar disorder. *Cochrane Database of Systematic Reviews*, 10, CD003196. Available at: http://dx.doi.org/10.1002/14651858.CD003196.pub2

Clark, D.A. and Beck, A. (2011) *Cognitive Therapy for Anxiety Disorders: Science and Practice.* London: Guilford Press.

Cohn, K. (2007) Developing effective communication skills. *Journal of Oncology Practice*, 3(6): 314–17.

Coleman, J.J. and Pontefract, S.K. (2016) Adverse drug reactions. *Clinical Medicine*, 16(5): 481–5.

Connolly, A., Taylor, D., Sparshatt, A. and Cornelius, V. (2011) Antipsychotic prescribing in Black and White hospitalised patients. *Journal of Psychopharmacology*, 25(5): 704–9.

Cornwall, J. (2011) Are nursing students safe when choosing gluteal intramuscular injection locations? *Australasian Medical Journal*, 4(6): 315–21.

Cosgrove, K.P. (2010) Imaging receptor changes in human drug abusers. *Current Topics in Behavioral Neurosciences*, 3: 199–217.

Cousins, D.H., Gerrett, D. and Warner, B. (2012) A review of medication incidents reported to the National Reporting and Learning System in England and Wales over 6 years (2005–2010). *British Journal of Clinical Pharmacology*, 74(4): 597–604.

Cox, L.E. (2002) Social support, medication compliance and HIV/AIDS. *Social Work in Health Care*, 35(1–2): 425–60.

Cunningham Owens, D.G. (2014) *A Guide to the Extrapyramidal Side-Effects of Antipsychotic Drugs.* Cambridge: Cambridge University Press.

Cutler, R.L., Fernandez-Llimos, F., Frommer, M., Benrimoj, C. and Garcia-Cardenas, V. (2018) Economic impact of medication non-adherence by disease groups: a systematic review. *BMJ Open*, 8(1): e016982. Available at: http://dx.doi.org/10.1136/bmjopen-2017-016982

Cvjetkovic-Bosnjak, M., Soldatovic-Stajic, B., Babovic, S.S., Boskovic, K. and Jovicevic, M. (2015) Pregabalin versus sertraline in generalized anxiety disorder: an open label study. *European Review for Medical and Pharmacological Sciences*, 19(11): 2120–4.

Czobor, P., Van Dorn, R.A., Citrome, L., Kahn, R.S., Fleischhacker, W.W. and Volavka, J. (2015) Treatment adherence in schizophrenia: a patient-level meta-analysis of combined CATIE and EUFEST studies. *European Neuropsychopharmacology*, 25(8): 1158–66.

Dal Molin, A., McMillan, S.C., Zenerino, F., Rattone, V., Grubich, S., Guazzini, A. and Rasero, L. (2012) Validity and reliability of the Italian Constipation Assessment Scale. *International Journal of Palliative Nursing*, 18(7): 321–5.

Davis, K.L., Kahn, R.S., Ko, G. and Davidson, M. (1991) Dopamine in schizophrenia: a review and reconceptualization. *American Journal of Psychiatry*, 148(11): 1474–86.

Degenhardt, L., Baxter, A.J., Lee, Y.Y., Hall, W., Sara, G.E., Johns, N., Flaxman, A., Whiteford, H.A. and Vos, T. (2014) The global epidemiology and burden of psychostimulant dependence: findings from the Global Burden of Disease Study 2010. *Drug and Alcohol Dependence*, 137: 36–47.

Dembler-Stamm, T., Fiebig, J., Heinz, A. and Gallinat, J. (2018) Sexual dysfunction in unmedicated patients with schizophrenia and in healthy controls. *Pharmacopsychiatry*, 51(6): 251–6.

Demjaha, A., Lappin, J.M., Stahl, D., Patel, M.X., MacCabe, J.H., Howes, O.D., Heslin, M., Reininghaus, U.A., Donoghue, K., Lomas, B., Charalambides, M., Onyejiaka, A., Fearon, P., Jones, P., Doody, G., Morgan, C., Dazzan, P. and Murray, R.M. (2017) Antipsychotic treatment resistance in first-episode psychosis: prevalence, subtypes and predictors. *Psychological Medicine*, 47(11): 1981–9.

Department of Health (DoH) (1999) *Saving Lives: Our Healthier Nation*. London: DoH.

Department of Health (DoH) (2006) *Immunisation Against Infectious Disease*. London: DoH.

Dimond, B. (2014) *Legal Aspects of Consent*, 2nd edition. Luton: Andrews UK.

Dorevitch, A., Aronzon, R. and Zilberman, L. (1993) Medication maintenance of chronic schizophrenic out-patients by a psychiatric clinical pharmacist: 10-year follow-up study. *Journal of Clinical Pharmacy and Therapeutics*, 18(3): 183–6.

Dries, D.L., Exner, D.V., Gersh, B.J., Cooper, H.A., Carson, P.E. and Domanski, M.J. (1999) Racial differences in the outcome of left ventricular dysfunction. *New England Journal of Medicine*, 340(8): 609–16.

Drummond, D.C. (2004) An alcohol strategy for England: the good, the bad and the ugly. *Alcohol and Alcoholism*, 39(5): 377–9.

Dubicka, B., Hadley, S. and Roberts, C. (2006) Suicidal behaviour in youths with depression treated with new-generation antidepressants: meta-analysis. *British Journal of Psychiatry*, 189(5): 393–8.

Dunkley, E.J., Isbister, G.K., Sibbritt, D., Dawson, A.H. and Whyte, I.M. (2003) The Hunter Serotonin Toxicity Criteria: simple and accurate diagnostic decision rules for serotonin toxicity. *QJM*, 96(9): 635–42.

Edwards, I.R. and Aronson, J.K. (2000) Adverse drug reactions: definitions, diagnosis, and management. *The Lancet*, 356(9237): 1255–9.

Edwards, S.J., Hamilton, V., Nherera, L. and Trevor, N. (2013) Lithium or an atypical antipsychotic drug in the management of treatment-resistant depression: a systematic review and economic evaluation. *Health Technology Assessment*, 17(54): 1–190.

Egerton, A., Chaddock, C.A., Winton-Brown, T.T., Bloomfield, M.A.P., Bhattacharyya, S., Allen, P., McGuire, P.K. and Howes, O.D. (2013) Presynaptic striatal dopamine dysfunction in people at ultra-high risk for psychosis: findings in a second cohort. *Biological Psychiatry*, 74(2): 106–12.

Elwyn, G., Edwards, A. and Kinnersley, P. (1999) Shared decision-making in primary care: the neglected second half of the consultation. *British Journal of General Practice*, 49(443): 477–82.

Epstein, O., Perkin, G.D., de Bono, D.P. and Cookson, J. (2008) The abdomen. *Clinical Examination*, 4th edition. Edinburgh: Mosby Elsevier.

European Medicinces Agency (EMA) (2018) *Pharmacovigilance: Overview.* Available at: www.ema.europa.eu/en/human-regulatory/overview/pharmacovigilance-overview

Fallowfield, L., Ford, S. and Lewis, S. (1994) Information preferences of patients with cancer. *The Lancet*, 344(8936): 1576. Available at: https://doi.org/10.1016/S0140-6736(94)90386-7

Ferner, R.E. and Aronson, J.K. (2010) Preventability of drug-related harms: part I – a systematic review. *Drug Safety*, 33(11): 985–94.

Fleeman, N., Dundar, Y., Dickson, R., Jorgensen, A., Pushpakom, S., McLeod, C., Pirmohamed, M. and Walley, T. (2011) Cytochrome P450 testing for prescribing antipsychotics in adults with schizophrenia: systematic review and meta-analyses. *Pharmacogenomics Journal*, 11(1): 1–14.

Foebel, A.D., Onder, G., Finne-Soveri, H., Lukas, A., Denkinger, M.D., Carfi, A., Vetrano, D.L., Brandi, V., Bernabei, R. and Liperoti, R. (2016) Physical restraint and antipsychotic medication use among nursing home residents with dementia. *Journal of the American Medical Directors Association*, 17(2): 184–e9–14.

Ford, M.J., Hennessey, I. and Japp, A. (2005) *Introduction to Clinical Examination.* Elsevier Health Sciences.

Forsman, J., Taipale, H., Masterman, T., Tiihonen, J. and Tanskanen, A. (2019) Adherence to psychotropic medication in completed suicide in Sweden 2006–2013: a forensic-toxicological matched case-control study. *European Journal of Clinical Pharmacology*, 75(10): 1421–30.

Frank, A.F. and Gunderson, J.G. (1990) The role of the therapeutic alliance in the treatment of schizophrenia: relationship to course and outcome. *Archives of General Psychiatry*, 47(3): 228–36.

Freud, S. (1957) Mourning and melancholia. In *The Standard Edition of the Complete Psychological Works of Sigmund Freud, Volume XIV (1914–1916): On the History of the Psycho-Analytic Movement, Papers on Metapsychology and Other Works*, pp237–58.

Fricke-Galindo, I., Jung-Cook, H., Llerena, A. and Lopez-Lopez, M. (2016) Interethnic variability of pharmacogenetic biomarkers in Mexican healthy volunteers: a report from the RIBEF (Ibero-American Network of Pharmacogenetics and Pharmacogenomics). *Drug Metabolism and Personalized Therapy*, 31(2): 61–81.

Frogley, C., Taylor, D., Dickens, G. and Picchioni, M. (2012) A systematic review of the evidence of clozapine's anti-aggressive effects. *International Journal of Neuropsychopharmacology*, 15(9): 1351–71.

Frontier Economics (2014) *Exploring the Costs of Unsafe Care in the NHS: A Report Prepared for the Department of Health*. London: Frontier Economics.

Furukawa, T.A., McGuire, H. and Barbui, C. (2003) Low dosage tricyclic antidepressants for depression. *Cochrane Database of Systematic Reviews*, 3, CD003197. Available at: http://dx.doi.org/10.1002/14651858.CD003197

Furukawa, T.A., Watanabe, N. and Churchill, R. (2007) Combined psychotherapy plus antidepressants for panic disorder with or without agoraphobia. *Cochrane Database of Systematic Reviews*, 1, CD004364. Available at: https://doi.org/10.1002/14651858.CD004364

Gabbard, G.O. (2005) Does psychoanalysis have a future? Yes. *Canadian Journal of Psychiatry*, 50(12): 741–2.

Garcia, S., Martinez-Cengotitabengoa, M., Lopez-Zurbano, S., Zorrilla, I., Lopez, P., Vieta, E. and Gonzalez-Pinto, A. (2016) Adherence to antipsychotic medication in bipolar disorder and schizophrenic patients: a systematic review. *Journal of Clinical Psychopharmacology*, 36(4): 355–71.

Garcia-Doval, I., LeCleach, L., Bocquet, H., Otero, X.L. and Roujeau, J.C. (2000) Toxic epidermal necrolysis and Stevens-Johnson syndrome: does early withdrawal of causative drugs decrease the risk of death? *Archives of Dermatology*, 136(3): 323–7.

Garg, S.K., Kumar, N., Bhargava, V.K. and Prabhakar, S.K. (1998) Effect of grapefruit juice on carbamazepine bioavailability in patients with epilepsy. *Clinical Pharmacology & Therapeutics*, 64(3): 286–8.

Gauthier, S., Vellas, B., Farlow, M. and Burn, D. (2006) Aggressive course of disease in dementia. *Alzheimer's & Dementia*, 2(3): 210–17.

Geddes, J.R., Goodwin, G.M., Rendell, J., Azorin, J.M., Cipriani, A., Ostacher, M.J., Morriss, R., Alder, N. and Juszczak, E. (2010) Lithium plus valproate combination therapy versus monotherapy for relapse prevention in bipolar I disorder (BALANCE): a randomised open-label trial. *The Lancet*, 375(9712): 385–95.

Geerts, P., Martinez, G. and Schreiner, A. (2013) Attitudes towards the administration of long-acting antipsychotics: a survey of physicians and nurses. *BMC Psychiatry*, 13: 58. Available at: http://dx.doi.org/10.1186/1471-244x-13-58

General Medical Council (GMC) (1998) *Seeking Patients' Consent: The Ethical Considerations*. London: GMC.

Generoso, M.B., Trevizol, A.P., Kasper, S., Cho, H.J., Cordeiro, Q. and Shiozawa, P. (2017) Pregabalin for generalized anxiety disorder: an updated systematic review and meta-analysis. *International Clinical Psychopharmacology*, 32(1): 49–55.

Gibb, B. (2012) *The Rough Guide to the Brain*. New York: Rough Guides.

Girardi, P., Brugnoli, R., Manfredi, G. and Sani, G. (2016) Lithium in bipolar disorder: optimizing therapy using prolonged-release formulations. *Drugs in R&D*, 16(4): 293–302.

Goldberg, H.L. (1979) Buspirone: a new antianxiety agent not chemically related to any presently marketed drugs [proceedings]. *Psychopharmacology Bulletin*, 15(2): 90–2.

Goldberg, J.F. and Ernst, C.L. (2018) *Managing the Side Effects of Psychotropic Medications*. Arlington, VA: APA Publishing.

Gomez, A.F., Barthel, A.L. and Hofmann, S.G. (2018) Comparing the efficacy of benzodiazepines and serotonergic anti-depressants for adults with generalized anxiety disorder: a meta-analytic review. *Expert Opinion on Pharmacotherapy*, 19(8): 883–94.

Gossop, M. (1990) The development of a short opiate withdrawal scale (SOWS). *Addictive Behaviors*, 15(5): 487–90.

Gray, R., Rofail, D., Allen, J. and Newey, T. (2005) A survey of patient satisfaction with and subjective experiences of treatment with antipsychotic medication. *Journal of Advanced Nursing*, 52(1): 31–7.

Griffith, R. and Tengnah, C. (2017) *Law and Professional Issues in Nursing*, 4th edition. Exeter: Learning Matters.

Guina, J., Rossetter, S.R., DeRhodes, B.J., Nahhas, R.W. and Welton, R.S. (2015) Benzodiazepines for PTSD: a systematic review and meta-analysis. *Journal of Psychiatric Practice*, 21(4): 281–303.

Guy, W. (1976) Assessment manual for psychopathology: revised edn 502. In, Washington DC: Department of Education, Health and Welfare, pp534–7.

Hammad, T.A., Laughren, T. and Racoosin, J. (2006) Suicidality in pediatric patients treated with antidepressant drugs. *Archives of General Psychiatry*, 63(3): 332–9.

Hammond, C.J., Niciu, M.J., Drew, S. and Arias, A.J. (2015) Anticonvulsants for the treatment of alcohol withdrawal syndrome and alcohol use disorders. *CNS Drugs*, 29(4): 293–311.

Hashemi, J. and Movahedian, A. (2006) Lithium ratio in bipolar patients in Isfahan, Iran. *Journal of Research in Medical Sciences*, 11: 257–62.

Haynes, R.B., Ackloo, E., Sahota, N., McDonald, H.P. and Yao, X. (2008) Interventions for enhancing medication adherence. *Cochrane Database of Systematic Reviews*, 2, CD000011. Available at: https://doi.org/10.1002/14651858.CD000011.pub3

Hazari, N., Kate, N. and Grover, S. (2013) Clozapine and tardive movement disorders: a review. *Asian Journal of Psychiatry*, 6(6): 439–51.

He, M., Deng, C. and Huang, X.F. (2013) The role of hypothalamic H1 receptor antagonism in antipsychotic-induced weight gain. *CNS Drugs*, 27(6): 423–34.

Hendrick, J. (2000) *Law and Ethics in Nursing and Health Care*. Cheltenham: Nelson Thornes.

Hepler, C.D. and Strand, L.M. (1990) Opportunities and responsibilities in pharmaceutical care. *American Journal of Health-System Pharmacy*, 47(3): 533–43.

Herbeck, D.M., West, J.C., Ruditis, I., Duffy, F.F., Fitek, D.J., Bell, C.C. and Snowden, L.R. (2004) Variations in use of second-generation antipsychotic medication by race among adult psychiatric patients. *Psychiatric Services*, 55(6): 677–84.

Holt, R.I.G. (2019) Association between antipsychotic medication use and diabetes. *Current Diabetes Reports*, 19(10): 96. Available at: https://doi.org/10.1007/s11892-019-1220-8

Horne, R., Weinman, J., Barber, N., Elliott, R., Morgan, M., Cribb, A. and Kellar, I. (2005) *Concordance, Adherence and Compliance in Medicine Taking: Report for the National Co-ordinating Centre for NHS Service Delivery and Organisation R&D (NCCSDO)*. London: NCCSDO.

Hort, J., O'Brien, J.T., Gainotti, G., Pirttila, T., Popescu, B.O., Rektorova, I., Sorbi, S. and Scheltens, P. (2010) EFNS guidelines for the diagnosis and management of Alzheimer's disease. *European Journal of Neurology*, 17(10): 1236–48.

Hoskins, M., Pearce, J., Bethell, A., Dankova, L., Barbui, C., Tol, W.A., van Ommeren, M., de Jong, J., Seedat, S., Chen, H. and Bisson, J.I. (2015) Pharmacotherapy for post-traumatic stress disorder: systematic review and meta-analysis. *British Journal of Psychiatry*, 206(2): 93–100.

Hovington, C.L. and Lepage, M. (2012) Neurocognition and neuroimaging of persistent negative symptoms of schizophrenia. *Expert Review of Neurotherapeutics*, 12(1): 53–69.

Huhn, M., Tardy, M., Spineli, L., Kissling, W., Förstl, H., Pitschel-Walz, G., Leucht, C., Samara, M., Dold, M. and Leucht, S. (2014) Efficacy of pharmacotherapy and psychotherapy for adult psychiatric disorders: a systematic overview of meta-analyses. *JAMA Psychiatry*, 71(6): 706–15.

Hung, C.I. (2014) Factors predicting adherence to antidepressant treatment. *Current Opinion in Psychiatry*, 27(5): 344–9.

Husain, Z., Reddy, B.Y. and Schwartz, R.A. (2013) DRESS syndrome: part I – clinical perspectives. *Journal of the American Academy of Dermatology*, 68(5): 693.e1–693.e14. Available at: http://dx.doi.org/https://doi.org/10.1016/j.jaad.2013.01.033

Iacobucci, G. (2018) MHRA bans valproate prescribing for women not in pregnancy prevention programme. *BMJ*, 361: k1823. Available at: http://dx.doi.org/10.1136/bmj.k1823

Inder, M., Lacey, C. and Crowe, M. (2019) Participation in decision-making about medication: a qualitative analysis of medication adherence. *International Journal of Mental Health Nursing*, 28(1): 181–9.

International Conference on Harmonisation Good Clinical Practice (ICH GCP) (2014) *Glossary*. Available at: https://ichgcp.net/1-glossary

Issari, Y., Jakubovski, E., Bartley, C.A., Pittenger, C. and Bloch, M.H. (2016) Early onset of response with selective serotonin reuptake inhibitors in obsessive-compulsive disorder: a meta-analysis. *Journal of Clinical Psychiatry*, 77(5): e605–11. Available at: http://dx.doi.org/10.4088/JCP.14r09758

Jakubovski, E., Johnson, J.A., Nasir, M., Muller-Vahl, K. and Bloch, M.H. (2019) Systematic review and meta-analysis: dose-response curve of SSRIs and SNRIs in anxiety disorders. *Depression and Anxiety*, 36(3): 198–212.

Jankel, C.A. and Fitterman, L.K. (1993) Epidemiology of drug-drug interactions as a cause of hospital admissions. *Drug Safety*, 9(1): 51–9.

Jevon, P. (2016) *Clinical Examination Skills*. Oxford: John Wiley & Sons.

Joachim, H. (1890) *Papyros Ebers: The First Complete Translation from Egyptian*. Berlin: G. Reimer.

John, A. and Stevenson, T. (1995) A basic guide to the principles of drug therapy. *British Journal of Nursing*, 4(20): 1194–8.

Jones, P.B., Barnes, T.R., Davies, L., Dunn, G., Lloyd, H., Hayhurst, K.P., Murray, R.M., Markwick, A. and Lewis, S.W. (2006) Randomized controlled trial of the effect on quality of life of second- vs first-generation antipsychotic drugs in schizophrenia: Cost Utility of the Latest Antipsychotic Drugs in Schizophrenia Study (CUtLASS 1). *Archives of General Psychiatry*, 63(10): 1079–87.

Jonsdottir, H., Opjordsmoen, S., Birkenaes, A.B., Simonsen, C., Engh, J.A., Ringen, P.A., Vaskinn, A., Friis, S., Sundet, K. and Andreassen, O.A. (2013) Predictors of medication adherence in patients with schizophrenia and bipolar disorder. *Acta Psychiatrica Scandinavica*, 127(1): 23–33.

Julius, R.J., Novitsky, M.A., Jr. and Dubin, W.R. (2009) Medication adherence: a review of the literature and implications for clinical practice. *Journal of Psychiatric Practice*, 15(1): 34–44.

Kandiah, N., Pai, M.C., Senanarong, V., Looi, I., Ampil, E., Park, K.W., Karanam, A.K. and Christopher, S. (2017) Rivastigmine: the advantages of dual inhibition of acetylcholinesterase and butyrylcholinesterase and its role in subcortical vascular dementia and Parkinson's disease dementia. *Clinical Interventions in Aging*, 12: 697–707.

Kane, J. and Garcia-Ribera, C. (2009) Antipsychotic long-acting (depot) injections for the treatment of schizophrenia. *British Journal of Psychiatry*, 195(S52): 63–7.

Kane, J., Honigfeld, G., Singer, J. and Meltzer, H. (1988) Clozapine for the treatment-resistant schizophrenic: a double-blind comparison with chlorpromazine. *Archives of General Psychiatry*, 45(9): 789–96.

Kapur, S. and Seeman, P. (2001) Does fast dissociation from the dopamine d(2) receptor explain the action of atypical antipsychotics? A new hypothesis. *American Journal of Psychiatry*, 158(3): 360–9.

Kapur, S., Agid, O., Mizrahi, R. and Li, M. (2006) How antipsychotics work: from receptors to reality. *NeuroRX*, 3(1): 10–21.

Kapur, S., Mizrahi, R. and Li, M. (2005) From dopamine to salience to psychosis: linking biology, pharmacology and phenomenology of psychosis. *Schizophrenia Research*, 79(1): 59–68.

Kasckow, J., Felmet, K. and Zisook, S. (2011) Managing suicide risk in patients with schizophrenia. *CNS Drugs*, 25(2): 129–43.

Kashner, T.M., Rader, L.E., Rodell, D.E., Beck, C.M., Rodell, L.R. and Muller, K. (1991) Family characteristics, substance abuse, and hospitalization patterns of patients with schizophrenia. *Hospital and Community Psychiatry*, 42(2): 195–6.

Keeler, B.E., Lallemand, P., Patel, M.M., de Castro Bras, L.E. and Clemens, S. (2016) Opposing aging-related shift of excitatory dopamine D1 and inhibitory D3 receptor protein expression in striatum and spinal cord. *Journal of Neurophysiology*, 115(1): 363–9.

Kendler, K.S., Myers, J. and Prescott, C.A. (2007) Specificity of genetic and environmental risk factors for symptoms of cannabis, cocaine, alcohol, caffeine, and nicotine dependence. *Archives of General Psychiatry*, 64(11): 1313–20.

Kessler, R.C., Petukhova, M., Sampson, N.A., Zaslavsky, A.M. and Wittchen, H.U. (2012) Twelve-month and lifetime prevalence and lifetime morbid risk of anxiety and mood disorders in the United States. *International Journal of Methods in Psychiatric Research*, 21(3): 169–84.

Khandaker, G.M., Zimbron, J., Lewis, G. and Jones, P.B. (2013) Prenatal maternal infection, neurodevelopment and adult schizophrenia: a systematic review of population-based studies. *Psychological Medicine*, 43(2): 239–57.

Kinderman, P. and Bentall, R.P. (1997) Causal attributions in paranoia and depression: internal, personal, and situational attributions for negative events. *Journal of Abnormal Psychology*, 106(2): 341–5.

Kinney, C. (1999) *Coping with Schizophrenia: The Significance of Appraisal*. Unpublished thesis, University of Manchester.

Kishi, T., Oya, K. and Iwata, N. (2016) Long-acting injectable antipsychotics for the prevention of relapse in patients with recent-onset psychotic disorders: a systematic review and meta-analysis of randomized controlled trials. *Psychiatry Research*, 246: 750–5.

Knapp, M., King, D., Pugner, K. and Lapuerta, P. (2004) Non-adherence to antipsychotic medication regimens: associations with resource use and costs. *British Journal of Psychiatry*, 184(6): 509–16.

Knegtering, H., Boks, M., Blijd, C., Castelein, S., van den Bosch, R.J. and Wiersma, D. (2006) A randomized open-label comparison of the impact of olanzapine versus risperidone on sexual functioning. *Journal of Sex & Marital Therapy*, 32(4): 315–26.

Kotlinska-Lemieszek, A., Klepstad, P. and Haugen, D.F. (2019) Clinically significant drug-drug interactions involving medications used for symptom control in patients with advanced malignant disease: a systematic review. *Journal of Pain and Symptom Management*, 57(5): 989–98.

Kottow, M. (2004) The battering of informed consent. *Journal of Medical Ethics*, 30(6): 565–9.

Kotyuk, E., Farkas, J., Magi, A., Eisinger, A., Király, O., Vereczkei, A., Barta, C., Griffiths, M.D., Kökönyei, G. and Székely, A. (2019) The psychological and genetic factors of the addictive behaviors (PGA) study. *International Journal of Methods in Psychiatric Research*, 28(1): e1748. Available at: https://doi.org/10.1002/mpr.1748

Krupnick, J.L., Sotsky, S.M., Simmens, S., Moyer, J., Elkin, I., Watkins, J. and Pilkonis, P.A. (1996) The role of the therapeutic alliance in psychotherapy and pharmacotherapy outcome: findings in the National Institute of Mental Health Treatment of Depression Collaborative Research Program. *Journal of Consulting and Clinical Psychology,* 64(3): 532–9.

Kuepper, R., Skinbjerg, M. and Abi-Dargham, A. (2012) The dopamine dysfunction in schizophrenia revisited: new insights into topography and course. *Handbook of Experimental Pharmacology,* 212: 1–26.

Landen, M., Hogberg, P. and Thase, M.E. (2005) Incidence of sexual side effects in refractory depression during treatment with citalopram or paroxetine. *Journal of Clinical Psychiatry,* 66(1): 100–6.

Laoutidis, Z.G. and Luckhaus, C. (2014) 5-HT2A receptor antagonists for the treatment of neuroleptic-induced akathisia: a systematic review and meta-analysis. *International Journal of Neuropsychopharmacology,* 17(5): 823–32.

Lawson, E. and Hennefer, D. (2010) *Medicines Management in Adult Nursing.* Exeter: Learning Matters.

Leahy, R. (2006) *Roadblocks in Cognitive-Behavioral Therapy: Transforming Challenges into Opportunities for Change.* London: Guilford Press.

Leucht, C., Heres, S., Kane, J.M., Kissling, W., Davis, J.M. and Leucht, S. (2011) Oral versus depot antipsychotic drugs for schizophrenia: a critical systematic review and meta-analysis of randomised long-term trials. *Schizophrenia Research,* 127(1–3): 83–92.

Leucht, S., Cipriani, A., Spineli, L., Mavridis, D., Orey, D., Richter, F., Samara, M., Barbui, C., Engel, R.R., Geddes, J.R., Kissling, W., Stapf, M.P., Lassig, B., Salanti, G. and Davis, J.M. (2013) Comparative efficacy and tolerability of 15 antipsychotic drugs in schizophrenia: a multiple-treatments meta-analysis. *The Lancet,* 382(9896): 951–62.

Leventhal, H.O.R. and Ian, B. (2012) The common-sense model of self-regulation of health and illness. In L. Cameron and H.O.R. Leventhal (eds), *The Self-Regulation of Health and Illness Behaviour.* London: Routledge, pp56–79.

Levy, J. (1982) A particular kind of negative therapeutic reaction based on Freud's 'borrowed guilt'. *International Journal of Psychoanalysis,* 63(3): 361–8.

Lewis, S.W., Davies, L., Jones, P.B., Barnes, T.R., Murray, R.M., Kerwin, R., Taylor, D., Hayhurst, K.P., Markwick, A., Lloyd, H. and Dunn, G. (2006) Randomised controlled trials of conventional antipsychotic versus new atypical drugs, and new atypical drugs versus clozapine, in people with schizophrenia responding poorly to, or intolerant of, current drug treatment. *Health Technology Assessment,* 10(17): iii–iv, ix–xi, 1–165.

Li, X., Zhu, L., Zhou, C., Liu, J., Du, H., Wang, C. and Fang, S. (2018) Efficacy and tolerability of short-term duloxetine treatment in adults with generalized anxiety disorder: a meta-analysis. *PLOS One,* 13(3): e0194501. Available at: http://dx.doi.org/10.1371/journal.pone.0194501

Lilford, P. and Hughes, J.C. (2018) Biomarkers and the diagnosis of preclinical dementia. *BJPsych Advances,* 24(6): 422–30.

Lin, K.M., Poland, R.E. and Nagasaki, G. (1993) *Psychopharmacology and Psychobiology of Ethnicity*. Washington: American Psychiatric Press.

Lin, K.M., Poland, R.E., Lau, J.K. and Rubin, R.T. (1988) Haloperidol and prolactin concentrations in Asians and Caucasians. *Journal of Clinical Psychopharmacology*, 8(3): 195–201.

Lindstrom, L., Lindstrom, E., Nilsson, M. and Hoistad, M. (2017) Maintenance therapy with second generation antipsychotics for bipolar disorder: a systematic review and meta-analysis. *Journal of Affective Disorders*, 213: 138–50.

Lohoff, F.W. (2010) Overview of the genetics of major depressive disorder. *Current Psychiatry Reports*, 12(6): 539–46.

Lopez-Munoz, F. and Alamo, C. (2009) Historical evolution of the neurotransmission concept. *Journal of Neural Transmission*, 116(5): 515–33.

Luker, K. and Wolfson, D. (1999) *Medicines Management for Clinical Nurses*. Oxford: Blackwell Science.

Luscher, B., Shen, Q. and Sahir, N. (2011) The GABAergic deficit hypothesis of major depressive disorder. *Molecular Psychiatry*, 16(4): 383–406.

Lyketsos, C.G., Colenda, C.C., Beck, C., Blank, K., Doraiswamy, M.P., Kalunian, D.A. and Yaffe, K. (2006) Position statement of the American Association for Geriatric Psychiatry regarding principles of care for patients with dementia resulting from Alzheimer disease. *American Journal of Geriatric Psychiatry*, 14(7): 561–73.

Macfarlane, A. and Greenhalgh, T. (2018) Sodium valproate in pregnancy: what are the risks and should we use a shared decision-making approach? *BMC Pregnancy and Childbirth*, 18(1): 200. Available at: http://dx.doi.org/10.1186/s12884-018-1842-x

Malhi, G.S., Tanious, M. and Berk, M. (2012a) Mania: diagnosis and treatment recommendations. *Current Psychiatry Reports*, 14(6): 676–86.

Malhi, G.S., Tanious, M., Das, P. and Berk, M. (2012b) The science and practice of lithium therapy. *Australian and New Zealand Journal of Psychiatry*, 46(3): 192–211.

Malkin, B. (2008) Are techniques used for intramuscular injection based on research evidence? *Nursing Times*, 104(50–1): 48–51.

Mallinger, J.B. and Lamberti, J.S. (2006) Clozapine: should race affect prescribing guidelines? *Schizophrenia Research*, 83(1): 107–8.

Manoguerra, A.S., Erdman, A.R., Woolf, A.D., Chyka, P.A., Caravati, E.M., Scharman, E.J., Booze, L.L., Christianson, G., Nelson, L.S., Cobaugh, D.J. and Troutman, W.G. (2008) Valproic acid poisoning: an evidence-based consensus guideline for out-of-hospital management. *Clinical Toxicology*, 46(7): 661–76.

Marcus, S.C., Zummo, J., Pettit, A.R., Stoddard, J. and Doshi, J.A. (2015) Antipsychotic adherence and rehospitalization in schizophrenia patients receiving oral versus long-acting injectable antipsychotics following hospital discharge. *Journal of Managed Care & Specialty Pharmacy*, 21(9): 754–68.

Marder, S.R., Mebane, A., Chien, C.P., Winslade, W.J., Swann, E. and Van Putten, T. (1983) A comparison of patients who refuse and consent to neuroleptic treatment. *American Journal of Psychiatry*, 140(4): 470–2.

Maron, E. and Nutt, D. (2017) Biological markers of generalized anxiety disorder. *Dialogues in Clinical Neuroscience*, 19(2): 147–58.

Marques, T.R., Levine, S.Z., Reichenberg, A., Kahn, R., Derks, E.M., Fleischhacker, W.W., Rabinowitz, J. and Kapur, S. (2014) How antipsychotics impact the different dimensions of schizophrenia: a test of competing hypotheses. *European Neuropsychopharmacology*, 24(8): 1279–88.

Martin, G. and Sabbagh, M. (2010) *Palliative Care for Advanced Alzheimer's and Dementia: Guidelines and Standards for Evidence-Based Care*. New York: Springer.

Masimirembwa, C.M. and Hasler, J.A. (1997) Genetic polymorphism of drug metabolising enzymes in African populations: implications for the use of neuroleptics and antidepressants. *Brain Research Bulletin*, 44(5): 561–71.

Masters, K.P. and Carr, B.M. (2009) Survey of pharmacists and physicians on drug interactions between combined oral contraceptives and broad-spectrum antibiotics. *Pharmacy Practice*, 7(3): 139–44.

Mattick, R.P., Breen, C., Kimber, J. and Davoli, M. (2014) Buprenorphine maintenance versus placebo or methadone maintenance for opioid dependence. *Cochrane Database of Systematic Reviews*, 2, CD002207. Available at: https://doi.org/10.1002/14651858.CD002207.pub4

Mavranezouli, I., Meader, N., Cape, J. and Kendall, T. (2013) The cost effectiveness of pharmacological treatments for generalized anxiety disorder. *Pharmacoeconomics*, 31(4): 317–33.

McCarthy, M., Addington-Hall, J. and Altmann, D. (1997) The experience of dying with dementia: a retrospective study. *International Journal of Geriatric Psychiatry*, 12(3): 404–9.

McCutcheon, R., Beck, K., Jauhar, S. and Howes, O.D. (2017) Defining the locus of dopaminergic dysfunction in schizophrenia: a meta-analysis and test of the mesolimbic hypothesis. *Schizophrenia Bulletin*, 44(6): 1301–11.

McShane, R., Westby, M.J., Roberts, E., Minakaran, N., Schneider, L., Farrimond, L.E., Maayan, N., Ware, J. and Debarros, J. (2019) Memantine for dementia. *Cochrane Database of Systematic Reviews*, 3, CD003154. Available at: http://dx.doi.org/10.1002/14651858.CD003154.pub6

Mechanic, D., McAlpine, D., Rosenfield, S. and Davis, D. (1994) Effects of illness attribution and depression on the quality-of-life among persons with serious mental-illness. *Social Science & Medicine*, 39(2): 155–64.

Medicines and Healthcare Products Regulatory Agency (MHRA) (2004) *Annual Reports and Accounts 2004/05*. Available at: https://assets.publishing.service.gov.uk/government/uploads/system/uploads/attachment_data/file/228822/0719.pdf

Meltzer, H.Y. (2013) Update on typical and atypical antipsychotic drugs. *Annual Review of Medicine*, 64: 393–406.

Menard, C., Hodes, G.E. and Russo, S.J. (2016) Pathogenesis of depression: insights from human and rodent studies. *Neuroscience*, 321: 138–62.

Meyer, J.M. (2011) Pharmacotherapy of psychosis and mania. In L.L. Brunton, B.A. Chabner and B.C. Knollmann (eds), *Goodman and Gilman's the Pharmacological Basis of Therapeutics*. New York: McGraw-Hill, pp417–56.

Miller, D.D., Caroff, S.N., Davis, S.M., Rosenheck, R.A., McEvoy, J.P., Saltz, B.L., Riggio, S., Chakos, M.H., Swartz, M.S., Keefe, R.S., Stroup, T.S. and Lieberman, J.A. (2008) Extrapyramidal side-effects of antipsychotics in a randomised trial. *British Journal of Psychiatry*, 193(4): 279–88.

Miller, W.R. and Rollick, S. (2012) *Motivational Interviewing: Preparing People to Change*, 3rd edition. London: Guilford Press.

Mineur, Y.S. and Picciotto, M.R. (2010) Nicotine receptors and depression: revisiting and revising the cholinergic hypothesis. *Trends in Pharmacological Sciences*, 31(12): 580–6.

Mitchell, N.D. and Baker, G.B. (2010) An update on the role of glutamate in the pathophysiology of depression. *Acta Psychiatrica Scandinavica*, 122(3): 192–210.

Mittelman, M. (2003) *Counseling the Alzheimer's Care Giver: A Resource for Healthcare Professionals*. Chicago, IL: American Medical Association Press.

Mondaini, N., Gontero, P., Giubilei, G., Lombardi, G., Cai, T., Gavazzi, A. and Bartoletti, R. (2007) Finasteride 5 mg and sexual side effects: how many of these are related to a nocebo phenomenon? *Journal of Sexual Medicine*, 4(6): 1708–12.

Montgomery, S.A., Tobias, K., Zornberg, G.L., Kasper, S. and Pande, A.C. (2006) Efficacy and safety of pregabalin in the treatment of generalized anxiety disorder: a 6-week, multicenter, randomized, double-blind, placebo-controlled comparison of pregabalin and venlafaxine. *Journal of Clinical Psychiatry*, 67(5): 771–82.

Moon, A.L., Haan, N., Wilkinson, L.S., Thomas, K.L. and Hall, J. (2018) CACNA1C: association with psychiatric disorders, behavior, and neurogenesis. *Schizophrenia Bulletin*, 44(5): 958–65.

Morris, G.H. and Chenail, R.J. (2013) *The Talk of the Clinic: Explorations in the Analysis of Medical and Therapeutic Discourse*. London: Routledge.

Munkholm, K., Vinberg, M. and Vedel Kessing, L. (2013) Cytokines in bipolar disorder: a systematic review and meta-analysis. *Journal of Affective Disorders*, 144(1–2): 16–27.

Munro, I. and Edward, K.L. (2008) Mental illness and substance use: an Australian perspective. *International Journal of Mental Health Nursing*, 17(4): 255–60.

Mutsatsa, S. (2015) *Physical Healthcare and Promotion in Mental Health Nursing*. London: SAGE.

Naranjo, C.A., Busto, U., Sellers, E.M., Sandor, P., Ruiz, I., Roberts, E.A., Janecek, E., Domecq, C. and Greenblatt, D.J. (1981) A method for estimating the probability of adverse drug reactions. *Clinical Pharmacology & Therapeutics*, 30(2): 239–45.

National Institute for Health and Care Excellence (NICE) (2007) *Methadone and Buprenorphine for the Management of Opioid Dependence*. Available at: www.nice.org.uk/Guidance/TA114

National Institute for Health and Care Excellence (NICE) (2009a) *Medicines Adherence: Involving Patients in Decisions About Prescribed Medicines and Supporting Adherence.* Available at: www.nice.org.uk/guidance/cg76

National Institute for Health and Care Excellence (NICE) (2009b) *The NICE Guidelines on the Treatment and Management of Depression (Updated Edition).* Available at: www.nice.org.uk/guidance/cg90

National Institute for Health and Care Excellence (NICE) (2010) *Alcohol Use Disorders: Physical Complications.* Available at: www.nice.org.uk/guidance/cg100

National Institute for Health and Care Excellence (NICE) (2011) *Generalised Anxiety Disorder and Panic Disorder in Adults: Management.* Available at: www.nice.org.uk/guidance/cg113

National Institute for Health and Care Excellence (NICE) (2013) *Aripiprazole for Treating Moderate to Severe Manic Episodes in Adolescents with Bipolar Disorder.* Available at: www.nice.org.uk/guidance/TA292

National Institute for Health and Care Excellence (NICE) (2014) *Bipolar Disorder: Assessment and Management.* Available at: www.nice.org.uk/guidance/cg185

National Institute for Health and Care Excellence (NICE) (2015a) *Depression in Children and Young People: Identification and Management.* Available at: www.nice.org.uk/guidance/cg28

National Institute for Health and Care Excellence (NICE) (2015b) *Overview: First-Choice Antidepressant Use in Adults with Depression or Generalised Anxiety Disorder.* Available at: www.nice.org.uk/advice/ktt8

National Institute for Health and Care Excellence (NICE) (2015c) *Quality Statement 4: Treatment with Clozapine.* Available at: www.nice.org.uk/guidance/qs80/chapter/quality-statement-4-treatment-with-clozapine#:~:text=Clozapine%20is%20the%20only%20drug,intolerant%20of%2C%20conventional%20antipsychotic%20drugs

National Institute for Health and Care Excellence (NICE) (2016) *Evidence Context: First-Choice Antidepressant Use in Adults with Depression or Generalised Anxiety Disorder.* Available at: www.nice.org.uk/advice/ktt8/chapter/evidence-context

National Institute for Health and Care Excellence (NICE) (2017) *Alcohol-Use Disorders: Diagnosis and Management of Physical Complications.* Available at: www.nice.org.uk/guidance/cg100/chapter/Context

National Institute for Health and Care Excellence (NICE) (2018a) *Dementia: Assessment, Management and Support for People Living with Dementia and Their Carers.* Available at: www.nice.org.uk/guidance/ng97

National Institute for Health and Care Excellence (NICE) (2018b) *Evidence and Interpretation: Donepezil, Galantamine, Rivastigmine and Memantine for the Treatment of Alzheimer's Disease.* Available at: www.nice.org.uk/guidance/ta217/chapter/4-Evidence-and-interpretation

National Patient Safety Agency (NPSA) (2007) *Safety in Doses: Medication Safety Incidents in the NHS.* Available at: http://data.parliament.uk/DepositedPapers/Files/DEP2008-1788/DEP2008-1788.pdf

National Prescribing Centre (NPC) (1999) Signposts for prescribing nurses: general principles of good prescribing. *Prescribing Nurse Bulletin*, 1(1): 1–4.

Nemade, R., Reiss, N., Dombeck (2017) *Historical Understandings of Depression.* Available at: www.mentalhelp.net/articles/historical-understandings-of-depression/

Nieuwlaat, R., Wilczynski, N., Navarro, T., Hobson, N., Jeffery, R., Keepanasseril, A., Agoritsas, T., Mistry, N., Iorio, A., Jack, S., Sivaramalingam, B., Iserman, E., Mustafa, R.A., Jedraszewski, D., Cotoi, C. and Haynes, R.B. (2014) Interventions for enhancing medication adherence. *Cochrane Database of Systematic Reviews*, 11, CD000011. Available at: http://dx.doi.org/10.1002/14651858.CD000011.pub4

Nursing and Midwifery Council (NMC) (2010) *Standards for Pre-Registration Nursing Education.* Available at: www.nmc.org.uk/globalassets/sitedocuments/standards/nmc-standards-for-pre-registration-nursing-education.pdf

Nursing and Midwifery Council (NMC) (2018a) *Standards of Proficiency for Registered Nurses.* Available at: www.nmc.org.uk/standards/standards-for-nurses/standards-of-proficiency-for-registered-nurses/

Nursing and Midwifery Council (NMC) (2018b) *The Code.* Available at: www.nmc.org.uk/standards/code/

Nuttall, D. and Rutt-Howard, J. (2015) *The Textbook of Non-Medical Prescribing.* Oxford: John Wiley & Sons.

O'Brien, A. (2016) Comparing the risk of tardive dyskinesia in older adults with first-generation and second-generation antipsychotics: a systematic review and meta-analysis. *International Journal of Geriatric Psychiatry*, 31(7): 683–93.

O'Brien, M., Spires, A. and Andrews, K. (2011) *Introduction to Medicines Management in Nursing.* Exeter: Learning Matters.

Offidani, E., Guidi, J., Tomba, E. and Fava, G.A. (2013) Efficacy and tolerability of benzodiazepines versus antidepressants in anxiety disorders: a systematic review and meta-analysis. *Psychotherapy and Psychosomatics*, 82(6): 355–62.

Okazaki, M., Adachi, N., Akanuma, N., Hara, K., Ito, M., Kato, M. and Onuma, T. (2014) Do antipsychotic drugs increase seizure frequency in epilepsy patients? *European Neuropsychopharmacology*, 24(11): 1738–44.

Olfson, M., Mechanic, D., Hansell, S., Boyer, C.A., Walkup, J. and Weiden, P.J. (2000) Predicting medication noncompliance after hospital discharge among patients with schizophrenia. *Psychiatric Services*, 51(2): 216–22.

Orr, C., Deshpande, S., Sawh, S., Jones, P.M. and Vasudev, K. (2017) Asenapine for the treatment of psychotic disorders. *Canadian Journal of Psychiatry*, 62(2): 123–37.

Otowa, T., Maher, B.S., Aggen, S.H., McClay, J.L., van den Oord, E.J. and Hettema, J.M. (2014) Genome-wide and gene-based association studies of anxiety disorders in European and African American samples. *PLOS One*, 9(11): e112559. Available at: http://dx.doi.org/10.1371/journal.pone.0112559

Patel, L. and Grossberg, G.T. (2011) Combination therapy for Alzheimer's disease. *Drugs & Aging*, 28(7): 539–46.

Peuskens, J., Pani, L., Detraux, J. and De Hert, M. (2014) The effects of novel and newly approved antipsychotics on serum prolactin levels: a comprehensive review. *CNS Drugs*, 28(5): 421–53.

Pharoah, F., Mari, J., Rathbone, J. and Wong, W. (2010) Family intervention for schizophrenia. *Cochrane Database of Systematic Reviews*, 12, CD000088. Available at: http://dx.doi.org/10.1002/14651858.CD000088.pub2

Phillips, M.L. and Swartz, H.A. (2014) A critical appraisal of neuroimaging studies of bipolar disorder: toward a new conceptualization of underlying neural circuitry and a road map for future research. *American Journal of Psychiatry*, 171(8): 829–43.

Pilowsky, L.S., Costa, D.C., Ell, P.J., Murray, R.M., Verhoeff, N. and Kerwin, R.W. (1993) Antipsychotic medication, D2 dopamine receptor blockade and clinical response: a 123I IBZM SPET (single photon emission tomography) study. *Psychological Medicine*, 23(3): 791–7.

Pirmohamed, M., James, S., Meakin, S., Green, C., Scott, A.K., Walley, T.J., Farrar, K., Park, B.K. and Breckenridge, A.M. (2004) Adverse drug reactions as cause of admission to hospital: prospective analysis of 18,820 patients. *BMJ*, 329(7456): 15–19.

Plotkin, L.L., Bordunovskii, V.N., Bazarova, E.N. and Smirnov, D.M. (2008) Hepatic protection in patients with generalized purulent peritonitis complicated by sepsis. *Anesteziol Reanimatol*, 4: 39–40.

Polanczyk, G.V., Salum, G.A., Sugaya, L.S., Caye, A. and Rohde, L.A. (2015) Annual research review: a meta-analysis of the worldwide prevalence of mental disorders in children and adolescents. *Journal of Child Psychology and Psychiatry*, 56(3): 345–65.

Posternak, M.A. and Zimmerman, M. (2005) Is there a delay in the antidepressant effect? A meta-analysis. *Journal of Clinical Psychiatry*, 66(2): 148–58.

Potkin, S., Raoufinia, A., Mallikaarjun, S., Bricmont, P., Peters-Strickland, T., Kasper, W., Baker, R.A., Eramo, A., Sanchez, R. and McQuade, R. (2013) Safety and tolerability of once monthly aripiprazole treatment initiation in adults with schizophrenia stabilized on selected atypical oral antipsychotics other than aripiprazole. *Current Medical Research and Opinion*, 29(10): 1241–51.

Pound P., Britten N., Morgan M., Yardley L., Pope C., Daker-White G., et al. (2005) Resisting medicines: a synthesis of qualitative studies of medicine taking. *Soc Sci Med.*, 61(1): 133–55.

Pratt, N., Roughead, E.E., Salter, A. and Ryan, P. (2012) Choice of observational study design impacts on measurement of antipsychotic risks in the elderly: a systematic review. *BMC Medical Research Methodology*, 12(72). Available at: https://doi.org/10.1186/1471-2288-12-72

Preston, J.D., O'Neal, J.H. and Talaga, M.C. (2017) *A Handbook of Clinical Psychopharmacology*, 8th edition. Oakland, CA: New Harbinger.

Prochaska, J.O. and Diclemente, C.C. (1984) Self change processes, self efficacy and decisional balance across five stages of smoking cessation. *Progress in Clinical and Biological Research*, 156: 131–40.

Puyat, J.H., Daw, J.R., Cunningham, C.M., Law, M.R., Wong, S.T., Greyson, D.L. and Morgan, S.G. (2013) Racial and ethnic disparities in the use of antipsychotic medication: a systematic review and meta-analysis. *Social Psychiatry and Psychiatric Epidemiology*, 48(12): 1861–72.

Qurashi, I., Kapur, N. and Appleby, L. (2006) A prospective study of noncompliance with medication, suicidal ideation, and suicidal behavior in recently discharged psychiatric inpatients. *Archives of Suicide Research*, 10(1): 61–7.

Rabins, P.V., Slavney, P.R., Lyketsos, C.G. and Lipsey, J.R. (2008) Overview of psychiatric symptoms and syndromes. In P.V. Rabins, P.R. Slavney, C.G. Lyketsos and J.R. Lipsey (eds), *Psychiatric Aspects of Neurologic Diseases: Practical Approaches to Patient Care*, New York: Oxford University Press, p41.

Radua, J., Borgwardt, S., Crescini, A., Mataix-Cols, D., Meyer-Lindenberg, A., McGuire, P.K. and Fusar-Poli, P. (2012) Multimodal meta-analysis of structural and functional brain changes in first episode psychosis and the effects of antipsychotic medication. *Neuroscience & Biobehavioral Reviews*, 36(10): 2325–33.

Rahe, C., Unrath, M. and Berger, K. (2014) Dietary patterns and the risk of depression in adults: a systematic review of observational studies. *European Journal of Nutrition*, 53(4): 997–1013.

Rahmani, F., Ebrahimi, H., Ranjbar, F., Razavi, S.S. and Asghari, E. (2016) The effect of group psychoeducation program on medication adherence in patients with bipolar mood disorders: a randomized controlled trial. *Journal of Caring Sciences*, 5(4): 287–97.

Rao, S., Paulson, J., Donahue, R., Soubra, M., Brown, K. and Attaluri, A. (2009) Investigation of dried plums in constipation: a randomized controlled trial. *American Journal of Gastroenterology*, 104: S496.

Ravichandran, D., Gopalakrishnan, R., Kuruvilla, A. and Jacob, K.S. (2019) Sexual dysfunction in drug-naive or drug-free male patients with psychosis: prevalence and risk factors. *Indian Journal of Psychological Medicine*, 41(5): 434–9.

Ravindran, L.N. and Stein, M.B. (2010) The pharmacologic treatment of anxiety disorders: a review of progress. *Journal of Clinical Psychiatry*, 71(7): 839–54.

Reimers, A. (2019) Lamotrigine, bipolar disorder, and the pill-free week. *Bipolar Disorders*, 21(4): 372–3.

Reisberg, B., Doody, R., Stoffler, A., Schmitt, F., Ferris, S. and Mobius, H.J. (2003) Memantine in moderate-to-severe Alzheimer's disease. *New England Journal of Medicine*, 348(14): 1333–41.

Ribeiro, E.L.A., de Mendonca Lima, T., Vieira, M.E.B., Storpirtis, S. and Aguiar, P.M. (2018) Efficacy and safety of aripiprazole for the treatment of schizophrenia: an overview of systematic reviews. *European Journal of Clinical Pharmacology*, 74(10): 1215–33.

Richardson, M., McCabe, R. and Priebe, S. (2013) Are attitudes towards medication adherence associated with medication adherence behaviours among patients with psychosis? A systematic review and meta analysis. *Social Psychiatry and Psychiatric Epidemiology*, 48(4): 649–57.

Ritchie, R. and Roser, M. (2019) *Drug Use*. Available at: https://ourworldindata.org/drug-use

Rosner, S., Hackl-Herrwerth, A., Leucht, S., Vecchi, S., Srisurapanont, M. and Soyka, M. (2010) Opioid antagonists for alcohol dependence. *Cochrane Database of Systematic Reviews*, 12, CD001867. Available at: https://doi.org/10.1002/14651858.CD001867.pub3

Royal College of Nursing (RCN) (2011) *Informed Consent in Health and Social Care Research: RCN Guidance for Nurses*. London: RCN.

Royal Pharmaceutical Society (RPS) (2015) *Prescribing Competency Framework*. Available at: www.rpharms.com/resources/frameworks/prescribers-competency-framework

Royal Pharmaceutical Society (RPS) (2019) *Professional Guidance on the Administration of Medicines in Healthcare Settings*. Available at: www.rpharms.com/Portals/0/RPS%20 document%20library/Open%20access/Professional%20standards/SSHM%20and%20 Admin/Admin%20of%20Meds%20prof%20guidance.pdf?ver=2019-01-23-145026-567

Rudorfer, M.V., Lane, E.A., Chang, W.H., Zhang, M.D. and Potter, W.Z. (1984) Desipramine pharmacokinetics in Chinese and Caucasian volunteers. *British Journal of Clinical Pharmacology*, 17(4): 433–40.

Rybakowski, J.K. (2018) Challenging the negative perception of lithium and optimizing its long-term administration. *Frontiers in Molecular Neuroscience*, 11: 349. Available at: http://dx.doi.org/10.3389/fnmol.2018.00349

Safran, J.D., Muran, J.C. and Eubanks-Carter, C. (2011) Repairing alliance ruptures. *Psychotherapy*, 48(1): 80–7.

Saini, P., Chantler, K. and Kapur, N. (2018) GPs' views and perspectives on patient non-adherence to treatment in primary care prior to suicide. *Journal of Mental Health*, 27(2): 112–19.

Sajatovic, M., Davies, M., Bauer, M.S., McBride, L., Hays, R.W., Safavi, R. and Jenkins, J. (2005) Attitudes regarding the collaborative practice model and treatment adherence among individuals with bipolar disorder. *Comprehensive Psychiatry*, 46(4): 272–7.

Say, R.E. and Thomson, R. (2003) The importance of patient preferences in treatment decisions: challenges for doctors. *BMJ*, 327(7414): 542–5.

Schatzberg, A.F., Haddad, P., Kaplan, E.M., Lejoyeux, M., Rosenbaum, J.F., Young, A.H. and Zajecka, J. (1997) Serotonin reuptake inhibitor discontinuation syndrome: a hypothetical definition. *Journal of Clinical Psychiatry*, 58(S7): 5–10.

Schooler, N.R., Levine, J., Severe, J.B., Brauzer, B., DiMascio, A., Klerman, G.L. and Tuason, V.B. (1980) Prevention of relapse in schizophrenia: an evaluation of fluphenazine decanoate. *Archives of General Psychiatry*, 37(1): 16–24.

Scott, J., Colom, F., Pope, M., Reinares, M. and Vieta, E. (2012) The prognostic role of perceived criticism, medication adherence and family knowledge in bipolar disorders. *Journal of Affective Disorders*, 142(1–3): 72–6.

Sellwood, W., Tarrier, N., Quinn, J. and Barrowclough, C. (2003) The family and compliance in schizophrenia: the influence of clinical variables, relatives' knowledge and expressed emotion. *Psychological Medicine*, 33(1): 91–6.

Sendt, K.V., Tracy, D.K. and Bhattacharyya, S. (2015) A systematic review of factors influencing adherence to antipsychotic medication in schizophrenia-spectrum disorders. *Psychiatry Research*, 225(1–2): 14–30.

Serretti, A. and Chiesa, A. (2011) A meta-analysis of sexual dysfunction in psychiatric patients taking antipsychotics. *International Clinical Psychopharmacology*, 26(3): 130–40.

Severus, E., Taylor, M.J., Sauer, C., Pfennig, A., Ritter, P., Bauer, M. and Geddes, J.R. (2014) Lithium for prevention of mood episodes in bipolar disorders: systematic review and meta-analysis. *International Journal of Bipolar Disorders*, 2: 15. Available at: http://dx.doi.org/10.1186/s40345-014-0015-8

Shah, N. (2005a) Taking a history: conclusion and closure. *Student BMJ*, 13: 358–9.

Shah, N. (2005b) Taking a history: introduction and the presenting complaint. *Student BMJ*, 13: 314–15.

Shirzadi, A.A. and Ghaemi, S.N. (2006) Side effects of atypical antipsychotics: extrapyramidal symptoms and the metabolic syndrome. *Harvard Review of Psychiatry*, 14(3): 152–64.

Silver, J.M., Shin, C. and McNamara, J.O. (1991) Antiepileptogenic effects of conventional anticonvulsants in the kindling model of epilepsy. *Annals of Neurology*, 29(4): 356–63.

Slifstein, M., van de Giessen, E., Van Snellenberg, J., Thompson, J.L., Narendran, R., Gil, R., Hackett, E., Girgis, R., Ojeil, N., Moore, H., D'Souza, D., Malison, R.T., Huang, Y., Lim, K., Nabulsi, N., Carson, R.E., Lieberman, J.A. and Abi-Dargham, A. (2015) Deficits in prefrontal cortical and extrastriatal dopamine release in schizophrenia: a positron emission tomographic functional magnetic resonance imaging study. *JAMA Psychiatry*, 72(4): 316–24.

Sloboda, Z., Glantz, M.D. and Tarter, R.E. (2012) Revisiting the concepts of risk and protective factors for understanding the etiology and development of substance use and substance use disorders: implications for prevention. *Substance Use & Misuse*, 47(8–9): 944–62.

Smialowska, M., Szewczyk, B., Wozniak, M., Wawrzak-Wlecial, A. and Domin, H. (2013) Glial degeneration as a model of depression. *Pharmacological Reports*, 65(6): 1572–9.

Smink, B.E., Egberts, A.C., Lusthof, K.J., Uges, D.R. and de Gier, J.J. (2010) The relationship between benzodiazepine use and traffic accidents: a systematic literature review. *CNS Drugs*, 24(8): 639–53.

Soares-Weiser, K., Maayan, N. and Bergman, H. (2018) Vitamin E for antipsychotic-induced tardive dyskinesia. *Cochrane Database of Systematic Reviews*, 1, CD000209. Available at: http://dx.doi.org/10.1002/14651858.CD000209.pub3

Soomro, G.M., Altman, D., Rajagopal, S. and Oakley-Browne, M. (2008) Selective serotonin re-uptake inhibitors (SSRIs) versus placebo for obsessive compulsive disorder (OCD). *Cochrane Database of Systematic Reviews*, 1, CD001765. Available at: http://dx.doi.org/10.1002/14651858.CD001765.pub3

Sparks, J.A. and Duncan, B.L. (2013) Outside the black box: re-assessing pediatric antidepressant prescription. *Journal of the Canadian Academy of Child and Adolescent Psychiatry*, 22(3): 240–6.

Spiller, H.A. (2001) Management of carbamazepine overdose. *Pediatric Emergency Care*, 17(6).

Sramek, J.J. and Pi, E.H. (1996) Ethnicity and antidepressant response. *Mount Sinai Journal of Medicine*, 63(5–6): 320–5.

Stahl, E.A., Breen, G., Forstner, A.J., McQuillin, A., Ripke, S., Trubetskoy, V., Mattheisen, M., Wang, Y., Coleman, J.R.I., Gaspar, H.A., de Leeuw, C.A., Steinberg, S., Pavlides, J.M.W., Trzaskowski, M., Byrne, E.M., Pers, T.H., Holmans, P.A., Richards, A.L., Abbott, L., Agerbo, E., Akil, H., Albani, D., Alliey-Rodriguez, N., Als, T.D., Anjorin, A., Antilla, V., Awasthi, S., Badner, J.A., Bækvad-Hansen, M., Barchas, J.D., Bass, N., Bauer, M., Belliveau, R., Bergen, S.E., Pedersen, C.B., Bøen, E., Boks, M.P., Boocock, J., Budde, M., Bunney, W., Burmeister, M., Bybjerg-Grauholm, J., Byerley, W., Casas, M., Cerrato, F., Cervantes, P., Chambert, K., Charney, A.W., Chen, D., Churchhouse, C., Clarke, T.-K., Coryell, W., Craig, D.W., Cruceanu, C., Curtis, D., Czerski, P.M., Dale, A.M., de Jong, S., Degenhardt, F., Del-Favero, J., DePaulo, J.R., Djurovic, S., Dobbyn, A.L., Dumont, A., Elvsåshagen, T., Escott-Price, V., Fan, C.C., Fischer, S.B., Flickinger, M., Foroud, T.M., Forty, L., Frank, J., Fraser, C., Freimer, N.B., Frisén, L., Gade, K., Gage, D., Garnham, J., Giambartolomei, C., Pedersen, M.G., Goldstein, J., Gordon, S.D., Gordon-Smith, K., Green, E.K., Green, M.J., Greenwood, T.A., Grove, J., Guan, W., Guzman-Parra, J., Hamshere, M.L., Hautzinger, M., Heilbronner, U., Herms, S., Hipolito, M., Hoffmann, P., Holland, D., Huckins, L., Jamain, S., Johnson, J.S., Juréus, A., et al. (2019) Genome-wide association study identifies 30 loci associated with bipolar disorder. *Nature Genetics*, 51(5): 793–803.

Stahl, S.M. (2013) *Stahl's Essential Psychopharmacology: The Prescriber's Guide*, 4th edition. Cambridge: Cambridge University Press.

Starcevic, V. (2014) The reappraisal of benzodiazepines in the treatment of anxiety and related disorders. *Expert Review of Neurotherapeutics*, 14(11): 1275–86.

Stargrove, B.M., Treasure, J. and McKee, D.L. (2008) *Herb, Nutrient, and Drug Interactions: Clinical Implications and Therapeutic Strategies*. St Louis, MO: Mosby.

Stip, E. and Tourjman, V. (2010) Aripiprazole in schizophrenia and schizoaffective disorder: a review. *Clinical Therapeutics*, 32(S1): 3–20.

Strickland, T.L., Lin, K.M., Fu, P., Anderson, D. and Zheng, Y. (1995) Comparison of lithium ratio between African-American and Caucasian bipolar patients. *Biological Psychiatry*, 37(5): 325–30.

Stroup, T.S., Lieberman, J.A., McEvoy, J.P., Davis, S.M., Swartz, M.S., Keefe, R.S., Miller, A.L., Rosenheck, R.A. and Hsiao, J.K. (2009) Results of phase 3 of the CATIE schizophrenia trial. *Schizophrenia Research*, 107(1): 1–12.

Subotnik, K.L., Ventura, J., Gretchen-Doorly, D., Hellemann, G.S., Agee, E.R., Casaus, L.R., Luo, J.S., Villa, K.F. and Nuechterlein, K.H. (2014) The impact of second-generation antipsychotic adherence on positive and negative symptoms in recent-onset schizophrenia. *Schizophrenia Research*, 159(1): 95–100.

Swansburg, R.C. and Swansburg, R.J. (2002) *Introduction to Management and Leadership for Nurse Managers*, 3rd edition. Burlington, MA: Jones & Bartlett Learning.

Szasz, T. (2009) *Coercion as Cure: A Critical History of Psychiatry*. Piscataway, NJ: Transaction Publishers.

Tangamornsuksan, W., Chaiyakunapruk, N., Somkrua, R., Lohitnavy, M. and Tassaneeyakul, W. (2013) Relationship between the HLA-B*1502 allele and carbamazepine-induced Stevens-Johnson syndrome and toxic epidermal necrolysis: a systematic review and meta-analysis. *JAMA Dermatology*, 149(9): 1025–32.

Tarazi, F.I., Moran-Gates, T., Wong, E.H., Henry, B. and Shahid, M. (2008) Differential regional and dose-related effects of asenapine on dopamine receptor subtypes. *Psychopharmacology*, 198(1): 103–11.

Taylor, D.M., Barnes, T.R.E. and Young, A.H. (2018) *The Maudsley Prescribing Guidelines in Psychiatry*, 13th edition. London: Informa Healthcare.

Taylor, D., Paton, C. and Kerwin, R. (2007) *The Maudsley Prescribing Guidelines*. London: Informa Healthcare.

Taylor, D., Young, C., Esop, R., Paton, C. and Walwyn, R. (2004) Testing for diabetes in hospitalised patients prescribed antipsychotic drugs. *British Journal of Psychiatry*, 185(2): 152–6.

Tenback, D.E. and van Harten, P.N. (2011) Epidemiology and risk factors for (tardive) dyskinesia. In Jonathan Brotchie, E. B. a. P. J., (ed.), *International Review of Neurobiology*. Academic Press, pp211–30.

Tessier, A., Boyer, L., Husky, M., Bayle, F., Llorca, P.M. and Misdrahi, D. (2017) Medication adherence in schizophrenia: the role of insight, therapeutic alliance and perceived trauma associated with psychiatric care. *Psychiatry Research*, 257: 315–21.

Thamby, A. and Jaisoorya, T.S. (2019) Antipsychotic augmentation in the treatment of obsessive-compulsive disorder. *Indian Journal of Psychiatry*, 61(S1): 51–7.

Thompson, L. and McCabe, R. (2012) The effect of clinician-patient alliance and communication on treatment adherence in mental health care: a systematic review. *BMC Psychiatry*, 12(1): 87.

Thomson, R., Edwards, A. and Grey, J. (2005) Risk communication in the clinical consultation. *Clinical Medicine*, 5(5): 465–9.

Tiihonen, J., Haukka, J., Taylor, M., Haddad, P.M., Patel, M.X. and Korhonen, P. (2011) A nationwide cohort study of oral and depot antipsychotics after first hospitalization for schizophrenia. *American Journal of Psychiatry*, 168(6): 603–9.

Tolson, D., Rolland, Y., Andrieu, S., Aquino, J.P., Beard, J., Benetos, A., Berrut, G., Coll-Planas, L., Dong, B., Forette, F., Franco, A., Franzoni, S., Salva, A., Swagerty, D., Trabucchi, M., Vellas, B., Volicer, L. and Morley, J.E. (2011) International Association of Gerontology and Geriatrics: a global agenda for clinical research and quality of care in nursing homes. *Journal of the American Medical Directors Association*, 12(3): 184–9.

Torrey, E.F. (1994) Violent behavior by individuals with serious mental illness. *Hospital and Community Psychiatry*, 45(7): 653–62.

Tortora, G.J. and Derrickson, B.H. (2018) *Principles of Anatomy and Physiology*. Oxford: John Wiley & Sons.

Trivedi, M.H., Rush, A.J., Wisniewski, S.R., Nierenberg, A.A., Warden, D., Ritz, L., Norquist, G., Howland, R.H., Lebowitz, B., McGrath, P.J., Shores-Wilson, K., Biggs, M.M., Balasubramani, G.K. and Fava, M. (2006) Evaluation of outcomes with citalopram for depression using measurement-based care in STAR*D: implications for clinical practice. *American Journal of Psychiatry*, 163(1): 28–40.

Tsai, D.F.-C. (2008) Personhood and autonomy in multicultural health care settings. *Virtual Mentor*, 10(3): 171–6.

Tursi, M.F., Baes, C., Camacho, F.R., Tofoli, S.M. and Juruena, M.F. (2013) Effectiveness of psychoeducation for depression: a systematic review. *Australian and New Zealand Journal of Psychiatry*, 47(11): 1019–31.

Tyrer, P. (2012) Why benzodiazepines are not going away: commentary on benzodiazepines for anxiety disorders. *Advances in Psychiatric Treatment*, 18(4): 259–62.

Tyrer, P., Casey, P.R., Seivewright, H. and Seivewright, N. (1988) A survey of the treatment of anxiety disorders in general practice. *Postgraduate Medical Journal*, 64(S2): 27–31.

Uguz, F. and Sharma, V. (2016) Mood stabilizers during breastfeeding: a systematic review of the recent literature. *Bipolar Disorders*, 18(4): 325–33.

van der Molen, H.F., Zwinderman, K.A.H., Sluiter, J.K. and Frings-Dresen, M.H.W. (2011) Better effect of the use of a needle safety device in combination with an interactive workshop to prevent needle stick injuries. *Safety Science*, 49(8–9): 1180–6.

Van Putten, T., Crumpton, E. and Yale, C. (1976) Drug refusal in schizophrenia and the wish to be crazy. *Archives of General Psychiatry*, 33(12): 1443–6.

Varner, R.V., Ruiz, P. and Small, D.R. (1998) Black and white patients response to antidepressant treatment for major depression. *Psychiatric Quarterly*, 69(2): 117–25.

Volman, S.F., Lammel, S., Margolis, E.B., Kim, Y., Richard, J.M., Roitman, M.F. and Lobo, M.K. (2013) New insights into the specificity and plasticity of reward and aversion encoding in the mesolimbic system. *Journal of Neuroscience*, 33(45): 17569–76.

Waddell, L. and Taylor, M. (2009) Attitudes of patients and mental health staff to antipsychotic long-acting injections: systematic review. *British Journal of Psychiatry*, 195(S52): 43–50.

Wang, Q., Jie, W., Liu, J.H., Yang, J.M. and Gao, T.M. (2017a) An astroglial basis of major depressive disorder? An overview. *Glia*, 65(8): 1227–50.

Wang, X., Chen, Q. and Yang, M. (2017b) Effect of caregivers' expressed emotion on the care burden and rehospitalization rate of schizophrenia. *Patient Prefer Adherence*, 11: 1505–11.

Weiden, P.J., Aquila, R., Dalheim, L. and Standard, J.M. (1997) Switching antipsychotic medications. *Journal of Clinical Psychiatry*, 58(S10): 63–72.

Wells, A. (1997) *Cognitive Therapy of Anxiety Disorders: A Practice Manual and Conceptual Guide.* Chichester: Wiley.

Wester, K., Jonsson, A.K., Spigset, O., Druid, H. and Hagg, S. (2008) Incidence of fatal adverse drug reactions: a population based study. *British Journal of Clinical Pharmacology*, 65(4): 573–9.

Wheeler, H. (2013) *Law, Ethics and Professional Issues for Nursing: A Reflective and Portfolio-Building Approach.* London: Routledge.

Whiskey, E. and Taylor, D. (2007) Restarting clozapine after neutropenia: evaluating the possibilities and practicalities. *CNS Drugs*, 21(1): 25–35.

Wieck, A. and Jones, S. (2018) Dangers of valproate in pregnancy. *BMJ*, 361: k1609. Available at: http://dx.doi.org/10.1136/bmj.k1609

Wiehl, W.O., Hayner, G. and Galloway, G. (1994) Haight Ashbury free clinics' drug detoxification protocols – part 4: alcohol. *Journal of Psychoactive Drugs*, 26(1): 57–9.

Wijayendran, S.B., O'Neill, A. and Bhattacharyya, S. (2018) The effects of cannabis use on salience attribution: a systematic review. *Acta Neuropsychiatrica*, 30(1): 43–57.

Williams, D.J. (2007) Medication errors. *Journal of the Royal College of Physicians*, 37(4): 343–6.

Winograd-Gurvich, C., Fitzgerald, P.B., Georgiou-Karistianis, N., Bradshaw, J.L. and White, O.B. (2006) Negative symptoms: a review of schizophrenia, melancholic depression and Parkinson's disease. *Brain Research Bulletin*, 70(4–6): 312–21.

Woelbert, E., Kirtley, A., Balmer, N. and Dix, S. (2019) How much is spent on mental health research: developing a system for categorising grant funding in the UK. *Lancet Psychiatry*, 6(5): 445–52.

Wong, F.K. and Pi, E.H. (2012) Ethnopsychopharmacology considerations for Asians and Asian Americans. *Asian Journal of Psychiatry*, 5(1): 18–23.

Workman, B. (1999) Safe injection techniques. *Nursing Standard*, 13(39): 47–53.

World Health Organization (WHO) (1972) *International Drug Monitoring: The Role of National Centres*. Geneva: WHO.

World Health Organization (WHO) (2003) *Evidence for Action*. Available at: www.who.int/chp/knowledge/publications/adherence_full_report.pdf

World Health Organization (WHO) (2018) *Alcohol*. Available at: www.who.int/news-room/fact-sheets/detail/alcohol

World Health Organization (WHO) (2019) *Medication Safety in Polypharmacy*. Available at: www.who.int/publications/i/item/medication-safety-in-polypharmacy-technical-report

Your Genome (2016) *How Are Drugs Designed and Developed?* Available at: www.yourgenome.org/facts/how-are-drugs-designed-and-developed

Zai, C.C., Tiwari, A.K., Mazzoco, M., de Luca, V., Müller, D.J., Shaikh, S.A., Lohoff, F.W., Freeman, N., Voineskos, A.N. and Potkin, S.G. (2013) Association study of the vesicular monoamine transporter gene SLC18A2 with tardive dyskinesia. *Journal of Psychiatric Research*, 47(11): 1760–5.

Zeber, J.E., Copeland, L.A., Good, C.B., Fine, M.J., Bauer, M.S. and Kilbourne, A.M. (2008) Therapeutic alliance perceptions and medication adherence in patients with bipolar disorder. *Journal of Affective Disorders*, 107(1–3): 53–62.

Zhao, S., Sampson, S., Xia, J. and Jayaram, M.B. (2015) Psychoeducation (brief) for people with serious mental illness. *Cochrane Database of Systematic Reviews*, 4, CD010823. Available at: http://dx.doi.org/10.1002/14651858.CD010823.pub2

Zheng, W., Xiang, Y.Q., Ng, C.H., Ungvari, G.S., Chiu, H.F. and Xiang, Y.T. (2016) Extract of ginkgo biloba for tardive dyskinesia: meta-analysis of randomized controlled trials. *Pharmacopsychiatry*, 49(3): 107–11.

Zhu, F., Liu, Y., Liu, F., Yang, R., Li, H., Chen, J., Kennedy, D.N., Zhao, J. and Guo, W. (2019) Functional asymmetry of thalamocortical networks in subjects at ultra-high risk for psychosis and first-episode schizophrenia. *European Neuropsychopharmacology*, 29(4): 519–28.

Zimmermann, P.G. (2010) Revisiting IM injections. *American Journal of Nursing*, 110(2): 60–1.

Zorrilla, E.P., Logrip, M.L. and Koob, G.F. (2014) Corticotropin releasing factor: a key role in the neurobiology of addiction. *Frontiers in Neuroendocrinology*, 35(2): 234–44.

Zubin, J. and Spring, B. (1977) Vulnerability: a new view of schizophrenia. *Journal of Abnormal Psychology*, 86(2): 103–26.

Zunszain, P.A., Anacker, C., Cattaneo, A., Carvalho, L.A. and Pariante, C.M. (2011) Glucocorticoids, cytokines and brain abnormalities in depression. *Progress in Neuro-Psychopharmacology & Biological Psychiatry*, 35(3): 722–9.

Index

Note: References in *italics* are to figures, those in **bold** to tables; 'g' refers to the glossary.:

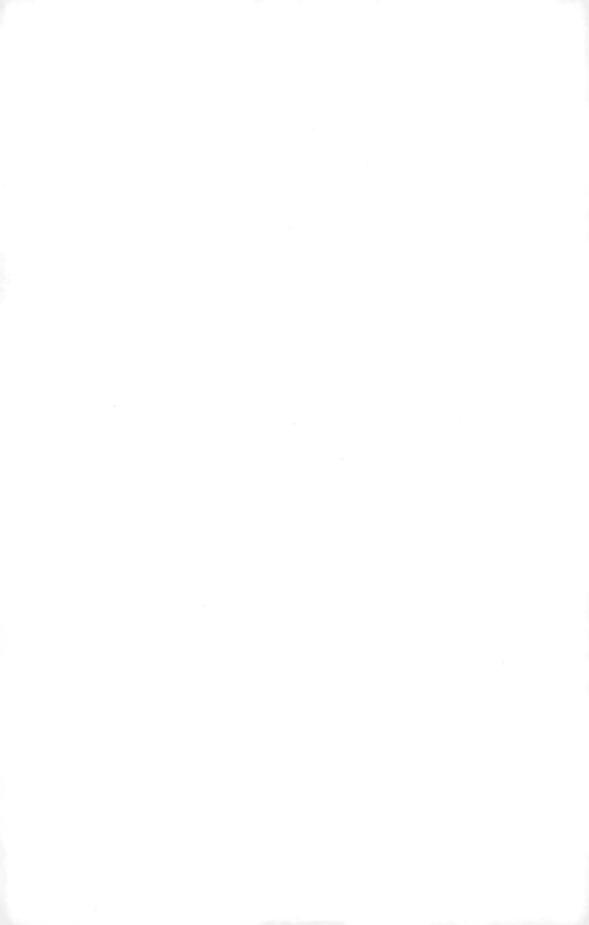